LIPPINCOTT WILLIAMS & WILKINS'

Medical Assisting Exam Review

FOURTH EDITION

for CMA, RMA & CMAS Certification

Helen J. Houser, RN, MSHA, BS, RMA (AMT)

Faculty Medical Assisting
Phoenix College
Phoenix, Arizona

Janet R. Sesser, MS, BS, RMA (AMT)

Academic Regulatory Affairs and Faculty
 Medical Assisting
Phoenix, Arizona

Wolters Kluwer

Philadelphia • Baltimore • New York • London
Buenos Aires • Hong Kong • Sydney • Tokyo

Acquisitions Editor: Jay Campbell
Product Development Editor: Amy Millholen
Editorial Assistant: Tish Rodgers
Marketing Manager: Shauna Kelley
Production Product Manager: Joan Sinclair
Design Coordinator: Stephen Druding
Manufacturing Coordinator: Margie Orzech
Prepress Vendor: S4Carlisle Publishing Services

4th Edition Copyright © 2016 Wolters Kluwer.

9 8 7 6 5

Printed in China

Library of Congress Cataloging-in-Publication Data
Houser, Helen J., author.
  Lippincott Williams & Wilkins' medical assisting exam review for CMA, RMA, and CMAS certification/
Helen J. Houser, Janet R. Sesser. — 4 edition.
      p. ; cm.
  Lippincott Williams and Wilkins' medical assisting exam review for CMA, RMA, and CMAS certification
  Medical assisting exam review for CMA, RMA, and CMAS certification
  Includes index.
  ISBN 978-1-4511-9256-8
  1. Medical assistants—Examinations, questions, etc.   I. Sesser, Janet R., author.   II. Title.   III. Title:
Lippincott Williams and Wilkins' medical assisting exam review for CMA, RMA, and CMAS certification. IV. Title: Medical assisting exam review for CMA, RMA, and CMAS certification.
  [DNLM: 1. Clinical Medicine—methods—Examination Questions. 2. Practice Management, Medical—Examination Questions.   W 18.2]
  R728.8
  610.73'7076—dc23
                                                                                                2015021077

LWW.com

To the commitment of the health-care workers around the world who go beyond borders to respond to people in need during global health challenges such as the Ebola outbreak of 2014, and to the health-care office staff in this country who stand between us and the diseases that can cross the threshold of our communities. You protect us by educating, immunizing, practicing sound aseptic technique throughout the medical office, keeping up with standards, supporting certification and other indicators of competency, and by remaining always vigilant to the health risks of our populations.

About the Authors

Helen J. Houser is a Registered Medical Assistant and a Registered Nurse holding a master of science in healthcare administration. She served as the Director of the Medical Assisting Program at Phoenix College, and her extensive experience involving medical assisting includes serving as Vice President of Phoenix General Hospital, Deer Valley, where she opened and administered medical practices in rural areas. She is a national speaker on such topics as "Immunization Education for Medical Assisting Students," and has received several awards, including the National Institute of Staff and Organizational Development Excellence Award for teaching and two Arizona Governor's Awards for Excellence. Houser lived on the Navajo reservation for 4 years and has extensive experience working with diverse populations. She also serves on the Board of Adelante Healthcare, a community health center system.

Janet R. Sesser, a Registered Medical Assistant, holds a Master of Science in Health Education and a Bachelor of Science in Health Care Management. She is currently the Director of Academic Regulatory Affairs for a private postsecondary school with campuses in Phoenix, Arizona; and Brooklyn and Jamaica, New York. Her background includes working for many years as a practicing medical assistant for various types of practices and as a cardiopulmonary technician. For the past 25 years, she has worked in postsecondary education, teaching and writing allied health curricula. Sesser is actively involved with American Medical Technologists, serving as an appointed member on the AMT Examinations, Qualifications, and Standards Committee. She is a recipient of the Medallion of Merit Award, the highest honor bestowed by AMT to a medical assistant, and a frequent presenter at national and state medical conferences.

Gerry A. Brasin, AS, CMA (AAMA), CPC
Coordinator
Corporate Education
Premier Education Group
Springfield, Massachusetts

Christine Cusano, CMA (AAMA), CPhT, CHI
Senior Regional Director of Education
Lincoln Technical Institute
Brockton, Massachusetts

Donna Domanke-Nuytten, BSN, MSIMC
Professor/Practicum Coordinator
Health Science Technology
Macomb Community College
Warren, Michigan

Anne Gailey, CMA (AAMA)
Instructor
Medical Assisting
Ogeechee Technical College
Statesboro, Georgia

Carolyn Greenwood, BA
Medical Program Director
Medical Assisting and Medical Billing and Coding
Vatterott College
Tulsa, Oklahoma

Sharyn Ketcham, BS, MBA, MHSA
Medical Assisting Program Director
Health Professions, Fitness and Wellness
Phoenix College
Phoenix, Arizona

Carey Mortensen, NCMA
Student Success Manager
Education Department
Southern Careers Institute
Austin, Texas

Kathleen Schreiner, RN/MS
Director of Medical Office Professions
Health Sciences
Montgomery County Community College
Pottstown, Pennsylvania

Dr. Leslie Watkins, DC
Department Chair
Medical Department
Wright Career College
Overland Park, Kansas

Kari Williams, BS, AA
Faculty
Health Professions
Front Range Community College
Longmont, Colorado

Preface

LWW's Medical Assisting Exam Review for CMA, RMA, and CMAS Certifications provides a capstone review for recent graduates from medical assisting and medical administrative specialist programs, and working medical assistants and medical administrative specialists who are preparing to take a national certification exam. Medical assisting faculty find the text an invaluable tool to both validate learning and integrate topics. The decision to write it grew out of our frustrated attempts to find a review book that provided a focused straightforward yet effective approach to preparing for the national medical assisting and medical administrative specialist exams; not a duplication of a primary text.

The *LWW's Medical Assisting Exam Review for CMA, RMA, and CMAS Certification* is more than a review: You can use the first three chapters to develop a unique study plan that is tailored to your individual strengths and weaknesses. Next, you can implement the plan, study the material included in the remainder of the book, and, finally, test your knowledge and retention with the simulated exams.

The book's user-friendly design follows a simple outline format to make the information easy to digest, and we have sequenced topics so they build on each other. For example, medical terminology is one of the early chapters because it is necessary to understand terms in order to understand anatomy, physiology, and additional content areas in subsequent chapters.

Other unique features of *LWW's Medical Assisting Exam Review for CMA, RMA, and CMAS Certification* include the following:

- Material that is succinct, focused, pertinent, and truly up to date, incorporating the national exams' topics
- New and expanded information on emergencies, compliance, Meaningful Use and *ICD-10*, and more
- What exam takers should know about immunizations, VAERS, VISs, and vaccine storage
- New Critical Thinking Case Review at the end of each chapter with critical thinking questions related to the case
- A pretest with an analysis to help you determine your strong and weak study areas
- A method for creating your own study plan and a calendar to help you track it
- A design that incorporates *Bloom's Taxonomy* for teaching with questions and answers and rationale on the same page to avoid flipping back and forth; also,

a sturdy bookmark that includes pertinent abbreviations to cover answers

- Over 2,000 questions; research shows that probably the best way to prepare for a specific exam is to practice answering lots of questions with the content worded differently.
- Practice exams specific to the CMA (AAMA), RMA (AMT), and CMAS (AMT)
- Important review terms with definitions included in each chapter
- Review and study tips pertinent to each chapter
- Test preparation tips for students for whom English is their second language
- Important information for study groups
- Explanation of the major national exams
- Exam-taking strategies and exam-day preparation
- Six timed simulated exams: one for each of the three national exams appear in the back of the book and one for each of the three national exams is on the companion website.

The following are reviewer comments that attest to the effectiveness and practicality of the book's approach:

- "I think that this is one of the best review texts that I have ever seen—very inclusive."
- "This text is excellent and will be recommended to our students to study for the certification exam."
- "The short chapter reviews are very well done and effectively organized."
- "The students need a little levity once in a while. The cartoons are good. Made me smile."
- "Excellent."
- "Invaluable."
- "I use a different book in my review class at this time, but after seeing your text, I will switch."

Our goal is to help you succeed by providing you with the tools and information you need to pass the national medical assisting exams—and to retain that information to ensure a successful career. We have incorporated our expertise, creativity, interest in student success, and even a little humor into this book, and believe we will achieve our goal while helping you achieve yours.

Helen J. Houser, RN, MSHA, BS, RMA (AMT)
Janet R. Sesser, MS, BS, RMA (AMT)

ADDITIONAL RESOURCES

Lippincott Williams & Wilkins' Medical Assisting Exam Review for CMA, RMA, and CMAS Certification includes additional resources for students and instructors that are available on the book's companion website at http://thePoint.lww.com/Houser4e.

INSTRUCTOR RESOURCES

Approved adopting instructors will be given access to the following additional resources:

- PowerPoints
- LMS cartridges

STUDENT RESOURCES

- Interactive Exam Simulator with over 2,000 questions simulating the CMA, RMA, and CMAS national exams
- Electronic flash cards with audio pronunciation
- Audio Glossary

See the inside front cover of this text for more details, including the passcode you will need to gain access to the website.

Acknowledgments

We are extremely grateful for the efforts of the exceptional, dedicated reviewers whose thoughts positively influenced the content of the book. They provided insight and advice to the authors based on their experience and knowledge as seasoned educators and health professionals.

Contents

UNIT 1: The Starting Point

UNIT 2: General Knowledge

UNIT 3: Administrative Practice

UNIT 4: Clinical Practice

UNIT 5: Exam Preparation

The Starting Point

CHAPTER

The Certification Process

Y ou opened this book, so you are probably preparing to take one of the national medical assisting exams or the medical administrative specialist exam. Good idea! If you are a recent graduate of a program, the best time to take the exam is now, while the knowledge is fresh in your mind and your information is up to date. If you are a practicing medical assistant, the best time is still now, and here's why:

- Holding a recognized national certification demonstrates to employers, potential employers (especially if you are moving to another state or changing jobs), patients, and others that you have a standardized body of knowledge. This is an important credential that is recognized and respected by the public.

- Medical assisting was traditionally guided by local informal standards. An increasing number of states now regulate the medical assistant role and credentials through legislation. The different training options and criteria required to be considered a valid medical assistant vary among states, but they all recognize medical assistants who have passed one of the two major national exams, the American Association of Medical Assistants (AAMA) and the American Medical Technologists (AMT) exams.

- Expanding administrative responsibilities now warrants specialization and validation of knowledge through a certification process such as the AMT Certified Medical Administrative Specialist (CMAS).

- Increasing numbers of medical offices are affiliated with health-care organizations accredited by The Joint Commission (TJC) (formerly the Joint Commission on Accreditation of Healthcare Organizations [JCAHO]), the National Committee on Quality Assurance (NCQA), or other agencies. Staff credentials are always inspected, and national certifications are looked on favorably.

- Health care is ever-changing. Preparing for a national exam is a method to keep up with practice, to review the latest standards, and to demonstrate your knowledge of entry-level competencies.

- The Centers for Medicare and Medicare and Medicaid Services (CMS) issued a final rule establishing "meaningful use" requirements that providers must meet to receive funding under the second phase of the federal electronic health record (EHR) incentive program. The final Stage 2 rule allows "credentialed medical assistants" (including certain national certifications) to enter orders into the Computerized Physician Order Entry (CPOE) system for medication, laboratory, and radiology services.

NATIONAL MEDICAL ASSISTING EXAMS

The two major organizations offering nationally recognized medical assisting examinations are the AAMA and the AMT, both of which are respected associations. The question content of both exams is similar, and both use a multiple-choice format. The medical assisting certifications issued by the AAMA or AMT are equally accepted by employers. The eligibility criteria for each exam differ. Your choice of which exam to take may be contingent on these criteria.

THE CERTIFIED MEDICAL ASSISTANT (AAMA)

The certification received after passing the AAMA exam is called Certified Medical Assistant (CMA [AAMA]). Those eligible to take the CMA (AAMA) exam are as follows:

- Graduating students or recent graduates of a medical assisting program accredited by the Commission on Accreditation of Allied Health Education Programs (CAAHEP) or the Accrediting Bureau of Health Education Programs (ABHES); completing students may take the exam 30 days prior to completing their formal program

- Nonrecent graduates (more than 12 months after graduation) of a CAAHEP or ABHES accredited medical

assisting program; candidates will have 60 months from the date of graduation to pass the exam; if a candidate does not pass within this time frame, the candidate will not be eligible for the CMA (AAMA) credential

- CMAs (AAMA) recertifying their credential by way of examination

The examination is computerized and available throughout the year at testing sites. Information on the application, testing locations, dates, and fees can be found at www.aama-ntl.org or by emailing certification@aama-ntl.org or calling or writing to

AAMA Certification Department
20 North Wacker Drive, #1575
Chicago, IL 60606
1-800-228-2262

The CMA (AAMA) exam contains approximately 200 multiple-choice questions with five answer options. Some of the questions are used for trial only and do not count toward your score. There is no indication which questions are the trial questions. The questions are in no particular order. Refer to the tables at the end of this chapter for the content outline and corresponding study chapters. Exam review questions for anatomy and physiology and medical terminology are available on the AAMA Website.

THE REGISTERED MEDICAL ASSISTANT (AMT)

The certification received after passing the AMT medical assisting exam is called Registered Medical Assistant (RMA, AMT). Those eligible to take the RMA exam are as follows:

- Graduates of or students scheduled to graduate from a medical assistant program that holds programmatic accreditation by the ABHES or CAAHEP or students in a postsecondary school or college that holds institutional accreditation by the ABHES or CAAHEP

- Graduates of or students scheduled to graduate from a medical assisting program in a postsecondary school or college that has institutional accreditation by a regional accrediting commission or a national accrediting organization approved by the US Department of Education; the program must include a minimum of

FIGURE 1-1 Insignia of the American Association of Medical Assistants (AAMA).

FIGURE 1-2 Insignia of the American Medical Technologists (AMT).

720 clock hours (or equivalent) of training in medical assisting, including a clinical externship

■ Graduates of or students scheduled to graduate from a formal medical services training program of the US Armed Forces

■ Medical assistants employed in the profession for a minimum of 5 years, no more than 2 years of which may have been as an instructor in the postsecondary medical assistant program

The computerized exam is offered throughout the year at specified testing sites. Information on the application, testing locations, dates, and fees can be found at www.amt1.com or by emailing rma@amt1.com or calling or writing to

AMT
10700 W. Higgins Road, Suite 150
Rosemont, IL 60018
1-847-823-5169

The RMA exam consists of 200 to 210 multiple-choice questions with four answer options. If there are 210 questions, 10 will be trial questions and, as with the AAMA, they do not count toward your score. You have 2 hours to take the exam. The questions are in no particular order. Refer to the tables at the end of this chapter for the content areas and corresponding study chapters. Exam review questions are located on the AMT Website, and for a nominal fee, you may send for a practice exam.

NATIONAL MEDICAL ADMINISTRATIVE SPECIALIST EXAM

At the time of this writing, the AMT is the only nationally recognized organization offering the Medical Administrative Specialist examination. The credential received upon successful completion is the CMAS. Those eligible to take the CMAS exam are as follows:

■ Graduating students or graduates of a medical office administrative program that holds programmatic accreditation or is part of a postsecondary school or college that holds institutional accreditation by the ABHES

■ Graduating students or graduates of a medical office administrative program in a postsecondary school or college that holds institutional accreditation by a regional accrediting commission or a national accrediting organization approved by the US Department of Education; the program must include a minimum of 720 clock hours (or equivalent) of training in medical office administration skills, including a practical externship. The training must include at least the following:

  • Medical records management
  • Health-care insurance processing, billing, and coding

  • Office financial responsibilities
  • Information processing

■ RMAs or equivalent who possess a minimum of 2 years working as a medical office administrative specialists

■ Medical office administrative specialists employed in the profession for a minimum of 5 years

The computerized exam is offered throughout the year at specified testing sites. Information on the application, testing locations, dates, and fees can be found at www.amt1.com or by emailing cmas@amt1.com or calling or writing to

AMT
10700 W. Higgins Road, Suite 150
Rosemont, IL 60018
1-847-823-5169

The CMAS exam consists of 200 to 210 multiple-choice questions with four answer options. If there are 210 questions, 10 will be trial questions, and as with the CMA (AAMA) and RMA, they do not count toward your score. You have 2 hours to complete the exam. The questions are in no particular order. Refer to the tables at the end of this chapter for the content areas and corresponding study chapters. Exam review questions are located on the AMT Website.

MAINTAINING CERTIFICATION

Once you have received your certification, in order to maintain it, you must earn a specific number of continuing education units (CEUs) each year or in a designated number of years. The purpose is to stay current in your field by keeping up to date with changing or new standards and practices. Generally, one CEU is equivalent to 1 clock hour. CEUs may be earned in various ways. The most common are given below:

■ Attending seminars and conferences approved for CEUs by your certifying organization

■ Completing online modules of appropriate topics approved for CEUs by your certifying organization

■ Reading material in journals approved for CEUs by your certifying organization and answering related questions

■ Listening to audio modules approved for CEUs by your certifying organization and completing required exercises or answering related questions

Not only is staying up to date important to maintain your certification, but you are also responsible for staying current in your field as a legal obligation. You will be held accountable for the standards in place at any given time.

ADVICE FROM REAL TEST TAKERS

A graduate, who recently took the certification examination, gives this advice: "Study this book, study the practice exam at the end, and then study this book again." The simulated computerized exam and the simulated written exam with an answer sheet are located in the back of the book. Other real test takers provided the following feedback:

- Do not think that you can pass the exam without studying. You are wasting your time and money.

- There are lots of questions related to anatomy and physiology and medical terminology; the answers are not always straight forward. This book helps you to think critically to answer.

- Know the EKG leads and body cavities.

- Do not feel overwhelmed; study this book chapter by chapter for success; the layout is perfect.

STUDYING

The book is designed for simple, efficient study. The combination of narrative and an outline structure keeps the information succinct, emphasizes what is most likely to be on the exams, and decreases reading time. Material is presented in three areas: the body of the text with illustrations, boxes, and tables; the review terms; and the questions with associated rationale. This method reinforces previous information and provides additional information. Be sure to study all content areas that are applicable to your exam. Refer to the tables at the end of this chapter. The material may be phrased differently throughout the text to ensure understanding because it is unlikely that the wording will appear exactly as it does on the actual exam. Some questions require critical thinking, but the necessary knowledge to formulate the correct answer is contained in the book. Use study techniques that have been successful for you in the past, and incorporate new strategies, as appropriate. Suggestions include the following:

- Inform your family, friends, employer, and fellow employees that you are preparing for the exam. Ask them to support you. Include them in the review process. Ask your family to allow you uninterrupted study time; determine when that time will be and stick to it.

- Read each chapter, and underline or highlight information that needs reinforcement. Reread those areas at different times until you believe you know them. Write down information you cannot remember; writing helps memorization.

- Write difficult information in your own words to assure understanding; ask your employer, a teacher, or a peer if you need assistance.

- Read the important review terms at the end of each chapter.

- Develop flash cards by writing the review term on the front of an index card and the definition on the back. Again, writing enhances the memorization process.

- Look for learning moments. These are times outside of your planned study regimen when you can sneak in some studying, such as during breaks; at lunch; while riding as a passenger in a car or bus, using exercise equipment, or walking the dog; or even during television commercials. Be creative!

- Have friends and family test you using your flash cards.

- Develop rhymes to assist memory (such as, for diabetic coma, "hot and dry, sugar high").

- Use alphabetical connections, for example, arteries ("arteries" begins with an "a") carry blood away ("away" also begins with an "a").

- Incorporate as much repetition as you can.

- Read the review tip boxes at the beginning of each chapter.

- Take lots of practice tests, using the tests in this book and the practice questions from the AAMA and AMT.

- Contact local programs—some offer national exam reviews.

- Cram only if you are confident of your overall knowledge and need only cursory last-minute review.

- Consider joining a study group as additional preparation, but not as your only preparation.

MULTIPLE-CHOICE EXAMS

The national exams consist of multiple-choice questions. The AMT exam has four answer choices for each question; the AAMA exam has five answer choices. The questions have various levels of difficulty. Do not think you will be able to recognize the correct answer without studying if you do not know the topic. The questions purposefully contain what are called decoys. These are words that look similar to the correct answer and can easily confuse you such as "melatonin" and "melanin." Studying and preparedness are the only way to pass any exam. Use these strategies for solving multiple-choice questions:

- Read the question and answer it in your head, and then look for the answer you think is correct in the choices, but do not mark it yet.

- **Read the whole question with each of the choices. Some questions have more than one correct answer,** but one answer is better than the others. Do not mark your answer before considering all of the alternatives. That last choice may be better than the first. A word that is similar but not correct may appear first and act as a decoy.

- Watch your time. Do not spend more than 45 seconds on one question. Come back to it after completing the questions you know.

- Eliminate choices you know are wrong. The more choices you eliminate, the better your chance of selecting the correct one.

- Watch for "all of the above" answers. If you eliminate one answer, "all of the above" cannot be correct.

- Watch for "none of the above." If one answer is correct, "none of the above" is not the answer.

- Use caution with questions that contain the word "except." The answer you are looking for is the opposite of the question. If the question says, "You would use sterile technique in all of the following situations, except," look for the opposite of when "you would use sterile technique," such as when taking a blood pressure. Read "except" questions extra carefully and be sure of what they are asking.

- Watch for words such as "always," "never," "all," and "none." If you can think of one exception to a choice, then that answer is not correct.

- Handle decoys. Some questions lead you to think another answer is correct when you are relatively sure it is not. Read the whole question with each alternative separately. Think about what each question with each answer means. Frequently, this helps confirm your original answer choice.

What about guessing? The scoring on some multiple-choice examinations penalizes test takers for guessing by subtracting additional points for incorrect answers but not for blank answers. Neither the AAMA nor the AMT subtracts additional points for incorrect answers as opposed to blank answers, so use the strategies outlined previously, and if you are still not certain, give it your best guess. The most effective strategy for multiple-choice tests is practice, practice, practice! Practice by trying *all* of the questions in this book.

ENGLISH LANGUAGE LEARNERS

ELL refers to English Language Learners. If English is not your primary language, the following are additional suggestions to assist you in preparing for a national certification exam.

- Do not rush into taking the exam; be prepared.

- Read and follow the previous strategies.

- Buy or borrow the textbook *Test of English as a Foreign Language* (TOEFL). It offers an effective method to evaluate your English. If you have difficulty with this text, consider first taking an English or ELL course at a community college or other school. Taking a course may also increase your employment opportunities.

- English tests called Combined English Language Skills Assessments (CELSA) are available at community colleges for non-English speakers to determine their level of English. A national exam will be difficult to pass if you score below the high school equivalent on the CELSA.

- Obtain an ELL medical terminology book and review it.

- Study with a native English speaker who is motivated and organized (see the next section on study groups).

- If a question on the exam does not seem to make sense to you, look closely at the verb. It may have another meaning different from the one you thought. An example is the word "pose," commonly meaning to assume a posture for a picture or artistic purposes (for example, "She posed for the picture"). Another meaning, more common in tests, is to present an idea for consideration, such as "The doctor posed that the patient may not be taking his medication according to instructions." Consider other verb meanings before answering.

- Select only one answer—the best answer—for multiple-choice questions. In some countries, you may select several correct answers. In the United States, if you select more than one answer, it is marked incorrect.

STUDY GROUPS

Study groups generally consist of three to six people meeting to study or to prepare for a course, test or exam, or project. A group may be more informal, such as a group of friends getting together to study on a Saturday afternoon, or more formal, such as staff members who work in the same medical complex and who have agreed to meet at designated times and places using an agreed-on structure. Study groups have advantages (pros) and disadvantages (cons).

Pros

- Study times and places are designated; people are more motivated to be prepared if others are relying on them.

- The work, such as researching or organizing a topic, is shared.

- One person's weak area may be another's strength, which sometimes makes studying easier.

- You can discuss issues related to the exam, relieve stress, and gain a fresh perspective.

Cons

- Participants must agree on study times and places that are sometimes challenging.

- All members may not participate equally, resulting in more work for some.

- Everyone does not study at the same pace, leaving some behind and others frustrated with the slowness.
- Conversation and other distracters may interfere with study.

Should you organize or join a study group to prepare for a national exam? This is a personal decision. If you are a recent graduate and have a good study group from school, stick with it. If you study best alone, perhaps a group is not for you. If several colleagues that you know or work with are planning to take the exam, a study group could benefit all. The following are tips for working with study groups.

Study Group Advice

- Know the members and look at their performance in school or at work to determine whether they are committed and motivated before inviting them to join the group.
- Select a site and time conducive to study—for example, not the home of a friend who has active, small children.
- Allow only full-time members—coming to just some sessions should not be permitted because a part-time member requires time to catch up. An exception

would be if a person only wants to participate for one or two subjects and the dates and times for those subjects are preestablished.

- Organize an overall study plan with topics, assignments, and a leader for each session. Do this at the first session. It is sometimes difficult but worth the time. There are many options for putting together a plan. One method is to plan an overall review of each topic or to concentrate on specific topics that most members of the group find difficult. Anatomy and physiology is the most challenging area. The group may decide to concentrate on this and study other topics individually.
- Deal with disrupting or distracting members right away; sometimes humor works, for example, "Okay, time out for you until you stop gossiping and get down to work."
- Leave a study group if it is not working for you; simply say, "This is not working for me."
- Remember, the study group is only one tool; use the learning moments, flash cards, and other strategies previously mentioned. After you develop your study plan as described in Chapter 3, you will probably need more hours than the group provides, especially to cover difficult topics.

CONTENT OUTLINES FOR NATIONAL EXAMS AND CORRESPONDING CHAPTERS

Registered Medical Assistant —RMA (AMT)

Work Area	Chapter Locations
I. *General medical assisting knowledge*	
A. **Anatomy and physiology**	Chapters 5, 6, 18, 19, 20, 22, 24
B. **Medical terminology**	Chapters 5, 6, 14, 17, 18, 19, 21, 22
C. **Medical law**	Chapters 4, 9, 11, 21, 24, 25
D. **Medical ethics**	Chapters 4
E. **Human relations**	Chapters 7, 8, 9
F. **Patient education**	Chapters 8, 18, 20, 22, 23, 24
II. *Administrative medical assisting*	
A. **Insurance**	Chapters 4, 13, 14
B. **Financial bookkeeping**	Chapters 4, 15, 16
C. **Medical receptionist/Secretarial/Clerical**	Chapters 7, 9, 10, 11, 12, 16, 24, 25

Certified Medical Assistant —CMA (AAMA)

Content Outline	Chapter Locations
I. *General*	
A. Psychology	Chapters 7, 8, 18
B. Communication	Chapters 7, 8, 9, 16, 18, 20, 22, 23, 24, 25
C. Professionalism	Chapters 1, 3, 7, 16, 25
D. Medical law/Regulatory guidelines	Chapters 4, 8, 9, 11, 12, 13, 14, 15, 16, 17, 21, 24, 25
E. Medical ethics	Chapters 4, 7, 8
F. Risk management, quality assurance, and safety	Chapters 4, 7, 9, 10, 13, 16, 22, 25
G. Medical terminology	Chapters 5, 6, 14, 17, 18, 19, 20, 21, 22, 24
II. *Administrative*	
H. Medical reception	Chapters 4, 7, 9, 10, 13
I. Patient navigator/Advocate	Chapter 8
J. Medical business practices	Chapters 7, 9, 10, 11, 12, 15, 16
K. Establish patient medical record	Chapter 11
L. Scheduling appointments	Chapters 9, 10
M. Practice finances	Chapters 13, 14, 15, 16
III. *Clinical*	
N. Anatomy and physiology	Chapters 5, 6, 18, 19, 20, 22, 24
O. Infection control	Chapters 10, 17, 19, 24, 25
P. Patient intake and documentation of care	Chapters 8, 11, 18, 25
Q. Patient preparation and assisting the provider	Chapters 8, 10, 18, 19, 20, 23, 24, 25
R. Nutrition	Chapter 23
S. Collecting and processing specimens	Chapters 8, 23
T. Diagnostic testing	Chapters 18, 19, 20, 21
U. Pharmacology	Chapters 6, 8, 21, 24
V. Emergency management/Basic first aid	Chapter 25

Certified Medical Administrative Specialist—CMAS (AMT)

Work Area	Chapter Locations
I. *Medical assisting foundations*	
A. Medical terminology	Chapters 5, 6, 17, 18, 20, 21, 22, 23, 24
B. Anatomy and physiology	Chapters 5, 6, 18, 19, 20, 22, 24
C. Legal and ethical considerations	Chapters 4, 7, 11, 13, 14, 15, 16, 24, 25
D. Professionalism	Chapters 1, 4, 7, 8, 9, 18, 19, 22, 24, 25
II. *Basic clinical medical assisting*	
A. Basic health history interview	Chapters 7, 18, 19, 24
B. Basic charting	Chapters 8, 11, 18, 19, 24
C. Vital signs and measurements	Chapters 5, 6, 18
D. Asepsis in the medical office	Chapter 17
E. Examination preparation	Chapters 5, 6, 18, 19, 20
F. Medical office emergencies	Chapters 7, 20, 25
G. Pharmacology	Chapters 5, 24

III. *Medical office clerical assisting*	
A. Appointment management and scheduling	Chapters 7, 10
B. Reception	Chapters 7, 10
C. Communication	Chapters 7, 8, 9, 10, 12, 15, 18, 19, 29, 22, 23, 24, 25
D. Patient information and community resources	Chapters 7, 8, 9, 18, 19, 20, 23, 24, 25
IV. *Medical records management*	
A. Systems	Chapter 11
B. Procedures	Chapter 11
C. Confidentiality	Chapters 4, 7, 8, 9, 11, 18, 24
V. *Health-care insurance processing, coding, and billing*	
A. A. Insurance processing	Chapter 13
B. Coding	Chapter 14
C. Insurance billing and finances	Chapters 4, 14, 15, 16
VI. *Medical office financial management*	
A. Fundamentals of financial management	Chapter 15
B. Patient accounts	Chapters 14, 15
C. Banking	Chapter 15
D. Payroll	Chapter 16
VII. *Medical office information processing*	
A. Fundamentals of computing	Chapter 9
B. Medical office computing applications	Chapters 8, 9, 10, 11, 24
VIII. *Medical office management*	
A. Office communications	Chapters 7, 9, 12
B. Business organization management	Chapters 11, 14, 15, 16
C. Human resources	Chapter 16
D. Safety	Chapters 4, 16, 17, 20, 21, 23, 24, 25
E. Supplies and equipment	Chapters 16, 20, 24, 25
F. Physical office plant	Chapter 16
G. Risk management and quality assurance	Chapters 4, 16

2

Pretest and Analysis

Relax and do not rush when taking the pretest. The purpose is to determine your strengths and weaknesses in the study subjects, not to produce a score. *Do not* time yourself. This test is designed to determine basic knowledge without intimidation. This also allows you to take the pretest in more than one sitting.

All questions are relevant for the CMA (AAMA) and RMA (AMT) exams. Questions 1 through 79 are relevant for the CMAS (AMT) exam. Answer the pretest questions by circling your answer or writing your answers on a separate sheet of paper. Use the special bookmark to cover the answers and work through *all* the questions without stopping to see if you are correct.

PRETEST

1. Which of the following positions is used for the examination of the abdomen?
    A. Prone
    B. Supine
    C. Sims
    D. Fowler
    E. Semi-Fowler

    Answer: **B**
    Subject: Patient Exams and Procedures
    Refer to Chapter 18

2. The two functions of the ear are hearing and:
    A. movement.
    B. equilibrium.
    C. sound production.
    D. maintaining upright position.

    Answer: **B**
    Subject: Anatomy and Physiology
    Refer to Chapter 6

3. The two main divisions of the central nervous system are the:
    A. cerebrum and cerebellum.
    B. hypothalamus and medulla.
    C. spinal cord and brain.
    D. sympathetic and parasympathetic.
    E. endocrine and exocrine.

    Answer: **C**
    Subject: Anatomy and Physiology
    Refer to Chapter 6

4. The portion of the eye that contains rods and cones is the:
    A. lens.
    B. sclera.
    C. conjunctiva.
    D. retina.

    Answer: **D**
    Subject: Anatomy and Physiology
    Refer to Chapter 6

5. The term meaning *muscular pain* is:
    A. myosin.
    B. myoglobin.
    C. myalgia.
    D. myocardium.
    E. myomalacia.

    Answer: **C**
    Subject: Medical Terminology
    Refer to Chapter 5

6. An organizational chart shows the connection of individuals and the reporting structure called the:
    A. chain of infection.
    B. chain of authoritycommand.
    C. team administration.
    D. administrative management.

    Answer: **B**
    Subject: Administration and Compliance
    Refer to Chapter 16

7. Pathogens that thrive in oxygen are called:
    A. antitoxins.
    B. anaerobes.
    C. spores.
    D. aerobes.
    E. oxides.

    Answer: **D**
    Subject: Microorganisms and Asepsis
    Refer to Chapter 17

8. The amount of money the medical office owes
    for supplies and equipment is considered:
    A. accounts payable.
    B. assets.
    C. accounts receivable.
    D. distributions.

    Answer: **A**
    Subject: Financial Practices
    Refer to Chapter 15

9. Balancing a checkbook with the bank statement is called:
    A. tracking.
    B. reconciliation.
    C. disbursement.
    D. justification.
    E. endorsement.

    Answer: **B**
    Subject: Financial Practices
    Refer to Chapter 15

10. The hiring process involves all of the following *except*:
    A. recruiting
    B. interviewing
    C. verifying
    D. training

    Answer: **D**
    Subject: Administration and Compliance
    Refer to Chapter 16

11. The first aid procedure for a suspected fracture includes:
    A. immobilizing the part.
    B. applying an elastic bandage.
    C. straightening the bones involved.
    D. applying heat for pain control.
    E. preparing the patient for physical
        therapy

    Answer: **A**
    Subject: Emergency Preparedness
    Refer to Chapter 25

12. Which condition is commonly characterized
    by a deficiency in insulin production?
    A. Gouty arthritis
    B. Pancreatic cancer
    C. Diabetes mellitus
    D. Anemia
    E. Gastric reflux disease

    Answer: **C**
    Subject: Anatomy and Physiology
    Refer to Chapter 6

13. When deciding whether to purchase or lease
    a piece of equipment, the manager would
    most likely decide to lease:
    A. an expensive piece of equipment.
    B. equipment with high utilization.
    C. equipment with a short guarantee.
    D. equipment that outdates rapidly.

    Answer: **D**
    Subject: Administration and Compliance
    Refer to Chapter 16

14. The heart is divided into right and left sides
    by the:
    A. aorta.
    B. atria.
    C. septum.
    D. valves.
    E. ventricles.

    Answer: **C**
    Subject: Anatomy and Physiology
    Refer to Chapter 6

15. The cardiovascular system includes:
    A. heart and blood vessels.
    B. heart and lungs.
    C. lungs and capillaries.
    D. heart and kidneys.

Answer: **A**
Subject: Anatomy and Physiology
    Refer to Chapter 6

16. A localized dilation of an artery is a(n):
    A. aneurysm.
    B. embolism.
    C. infarction.
    D. stenosis.
    E. thrombus.

Answer: **A**
Subject: Anatomy and Physiology
    Refer to Chapter 6

17. One type of genetic bleeding disorder is:
    A. anemia.
    B. aneurysm.
    C. hemophilia.
    D. leukemia.

Answer: **C**
Subject: Anatomy and Physiology
    Refer to Chapter 6

18. The measurement of height or length and weight is:
    A. auscultation.
    B. manipulation.
    C. palpation.
    D. mensuration.
    E. menstruation.

Answer: **D**
Subject: Patient Exams and Procedures
    Refer to Chapter 18

19. **Gastrectasia** means:
    A. inflammation of the stomach.
    B. ulceration of the stomach.
    C. stretching of the stomach.
    D. surgical repair of the stomach.

Answer: **C**
Subject: Medical Terminology
    Refer to Chapter 5

20. The muscle that expands and contracts during respiration, allowing the lungs to fill and empty air, is the:
    A. pectoralis.
    B. deltoid.
    C. gastrocnemius.
    D. diaphragm.
    E. rectus abdominus.

Answer: **D**
Subject: Anatomy and Physiology
    Refer to Chapter 6

21. The employee's performance appraisal should occur at least:
    A. quarterly.
    B. annually.
    C. semiannually.
    D. biannually.

Answer: **B**
Subject: Administration and Compliance
    Refer to Chapter 16

22. The vocal cords are located in the:
   A. bronchi.
   B. epiglottis.
   C. larynx.
   D. pharynx.
   E. trachea.

Answer: **C**
Subject: Anatomy and Physiology
Refer to Chapter 6

---

23. The most effective method of destroying spores is:
   A. boiling.
   B. disinfecting.
   C. sanitizing.
   D. autoclaving.

Answer: **D**
Subject: Microorganisms and Asepsis
Refer to Chapter 17

---

24. A sphygmomanometer is used to:
   A. measure visual acuity.
   B. listen to heart sounds.
   C. record electrical activity of the heart.
   D. measure blood pressure.
   E. auscultate breath sounds.

Answer: **D**
Subject: Patient Exams and Procedures
Refer to Chapter 18

---

25. When multiple patients are evaluated and prioritized for treatment, it is called:
   A. screening.
   B. triage.
   C. referral.
   D. scheduling.

Answer: **B**
Subject: Emergency Preparedness
Refer to Chapter 25

---

26. During a job interview, the prospective employer may ask questions about all of the following *except*:
   A. certification.
   B. citizenship.
   C. job-related weaknesses.
   D. reason for leaving previous employment.
   E. marital status.

Answer: **E**
Subject: Administration and Compliance
Refer to Chapter 16

---

27. The term **auscultation** means:
   A. tapping.
   B. feeling.
   C. measuring.
   D. listening.

Answer: **D**
Subject: Patient Exams and Procedures
Refer to Chapter 18

---

28. The recommended temperature for effective sterilization in an autoclave is:
   A. 200°F.
   B. 212°F.
   C. 220°F.
   D. 250°F.

Answer: **D**
Subject: Microorganisms and Asepsis
Refer to Chapter 17

29. The organization that established guidelines for occupational exposure to blood is the:
   A. CDC.
   B. FDA.
   C. HCFA.
   D. CMS.
   E. OSHA.

Answer: **E**
Subject: Microorganisms and Asepsis
Refer to Chapter 17

30. Which manual identifies procedural codes for submitting insurance claims?
   A. PPO
   B. ICD
   C. CPT
   D. HMO

Answer: **C**
Subject: Medical Coding and Claims
Refer to Chapter 14

31. The "S" in SOAP charting means:
   A. symptoms.
   B. signs.
   C. source.
   D. subjective.
   E. signature.

Answer: **D**
Subject: Medical Records Management
Refer to Chapter 11

32. The pegboard system of accounting generates which of the following documents?
   A. Cashier's check
   B. Bank statement
   C. Collection letter
   D. Receipt

Answer: **D**
Subject: Financial Practices
Refer to Chapter 15

33. A business letter in which all lines start flush with the left margin is:
   A. simplified style.
   B. modified block style.
   C. modified indented style.
   D. formal.
   E. block style.

Answer: **E**
Subject: Correspondence
Refer to Chapter 12

34. Which of the following acts constitutes negligence?
   A. A patient and physician establishing a professional relationship
   B. Breach of the physician's duty of skill or care
   C. A patient who has a positive outcome as a result of treatment
   D. Revocation of the physician's license

Answer: **B**
Subject: Law and Ethics
Refer to Chapter 4

35. The Employee's Withholding Allowance Certificate is the:
   A. W-2.
   B. W-4.
   C. I-9.
   D. FICA.
   E. Social Security.

Answer: **B**
Subject: Financial Practices
Refer to Chapter 15

36. A file used as a reminder that something must be taken care of on a certain date is called a:
    A. matrix.
    B. tickler.
    C. triage.
    D. chronologic.

Answer: **B**
Subject: Appointment Scheduling and Reception
Refer to Chapter 10

---

37. A set of principles or values is called:
    A. ethics.
    B. legal rights.
    C. opinions.
    D. standards.

Answer: **A**
Subject: Law and Ethics
Refer to Chapter 4

---

38. An instrument used to test neurologic reflexes is a(n):
    A. tuning fork.
    B. audiometer.
    C. sphygmomanometer.
    D. goniometer.
    E. percussion hammer.

Answer: **E**
Subject: Patient Exams and Procedures
Refer to Chapter 18

---

39. Slurred speech and one-sided paralysis are symptoms of:
    A. stroke.
    B. heart attack.
    C. syncope.
    D. epistaxis.

Answer: **A**
Subject: Emergency Preparedness
Refer to Chapter 25

---

40. The abbreviation "mL" means:
    A. microliter.
    B. megaliter.
    C. milliliter.
    D. macroliter.
    E. miniliter.

Answer: **C**
Subject: Pharmacology and Medication Administration
Refer to Chapter 24

---

41. Confirming that the message the listener received is the message you intended to send is called:
    A. observation.
    B. feedback.
    C. empathy.
    D. listening.

Answer: **B**
Subject: Human Behavior and Professional Communication
Refer to Chapter 7

---

42. Insurance that provides protection for wage earners and pays for medical care resulting from an occupational accident is:
    A. workers' compensation.
    B. CHAMPUS.
    C. Medicare.
    D. disability.
    E. Medicaid.

Answer: **A**
Subject: Medical Insurance
Refer to Chapter 13

43. The type of appointment scheduling in which several patients are given appointments in the same block of time is called:
A. grouping.
B. advance booking.
C. wave scheduling.
D. batching.

Answer: **C**
Subject: Appointment Scheduling and Reception
Refer to Chapter 10

44. A drug that relieves nausea and vomiting is classified as an:
A. antispasmodic.
B. anticoagulant.
C. antiemetic.
D. analgesic.
E. antidiarrheal.

Answer: **C**
Subject: Pharmacology and Medication Administration
Refer to Chapter 24

45. Use of chemicals to clean infectious materials from items or surfaces is called:
A. sterilization.
B. disinfection.
C. sanitation.
D. cleansing.

Answer: **B**
Subject: Microorganisms and Asepsis
Refer to Chapter 17

46. Myopia is a condition of:
A. blindness.
B. farsightedness.
C. nearsightedness.
D. loss of peripheral vision.
E. crossed eyes.

Answer: **C**
Subject: Anatomy and Physiology
Refer to Chapter 6

47. A fracture that causes the bone to break through the skin is called:
A. greenstick.
B. simple.
C. spiral.
D. compound.

Answer: **D**
Subject: Emergency Preparedness
Refer to Chapter 25

48. A document requiring a person to appear in court is a:
A. subpoena.
B. deposition.
C. litigation.
D. contract.
E. transcript.

Answer: **A**
Subject: Law and Ethics
Refer to Chapter 4

49. The system used for classifying diseases to facilitate collection of health information is:
A. RBRVS.
B. CPT.
C. ICD.
D. HCFA.

Answer: **C**
Subject: Medical Coding and Claims
Refer to Chapter 14

50. An example of objective information in a patient chart is the:
    A. patient's statement of his or her medical history.
    B. patient's statement of the severity of the pain.
    C. medical professional's note of a red, swollen area.
    D. patient's statement of inability to perform tasks.
    E. medical professional's note that the patient complains of pain.

Answer: **C**
Subject: Medical Records Management
Refer to Chapter 11

51. In communication with patients, an example of an open-ended question would be:
    A. How much pain medication have you taken?
    B. During this illness, did you have an elevated temperature?
    C. Are you allergic to any medications?
    D. What brings you to the doctor today?

Answer: **D**
Subject: Human Behavior and Professional Communication
Refer to Chapter 7

52. The predetermined amount of money paid by the insured party before the insurance company pays medical expenses is referred to as:
    A. capitation.
    B. premium.
    C. indemnity.
    D. coinsurance.
    E. deductible.

Answer: **D**
Subject: Medical Insurance
Refer to Chapter 13

53. When handling third-party requests for information over the telephone, you should ask the caller to:
    A. contact the physician's attorney.
    B. ask the patient to submit written permission.
    C. submit the request in writing.
    D. call back to speak with the physician only.

Answer: **B**
Subject: Administrative Technologies
Refer to Chapter 9

54. To ensure mail delivery the next day, you would send correspondence via:
    A. first class.
    B. registered mail.
    C. certified mail.
    D. express mail.
    E. second-class mail.

Answer: **D**
Subject: Correspondence
Refer to Chapter 12

55. The agency that regulates controlled substances is the:
    A. DEA.
    B. FDA.
    C. CDC.
    D. OSHA.

Answer: **A**
Subject: Pharmacology and Medication Administration
Refer to Chapter 24

56. Orientation of a new staff member would include:
  A. interview.
  B. performance appraisal.
  C. review of policies and procedures.
  D. sending a W-2 form.
  E. checking references.

Answer: **C**
Subject: Administration and Compliance
Refer to Chapter 16

57. The pulse point located bilaterally in the groin is the:
  A. apical.
  B. dorsalis pedis.
  C. femoral.
  D. popliteal.

Answer: **C**
Subject: Patient Exams and Procedures
Refer to Chapter 18

58. Following the indexing rules for filing, which name comes first?
  A. McWilliams
  B. McCally
  C. Mahill
  D. MacHall
  E. McAllister

Answer: **D**
Subject: Medical Records
Refer to Chapter 11

59. When a patient authorizes an insurance company to make payment directly to the physician, it is called:
  A. assignment of benefits.
  B. direct billing.
  C. claims submission.
  D. reimbursement.

Answer: **A**
Subject: Medical Insurance
Refer to Chapter 13

60. A debt incurred but not yet paid is called:
  A. account balance.
  B. accounts payable.
  C. accounts receivable.
  D. credit balance.
  E. adjustment.

Answer: **B**
Subject: Financial Practices
Refer to Chapter 15

61. An instrument used to examine the eyes is a(n):
  A. audiometer.
  B. otoscope.
  C. lensometer.
  D. ophthalmoscope.

Answer: **D**
Subject: Patient Exams and Procedures
Refer to Chapter 18

62. The term **hematuria** means:
  A. infection in the blood.
  B. painful urination.
  C. protein in the urine.
  D. difficult urination.
  E. blood in the urine.

Answer: **E**
Subject: Medical Terminology
Refer to Chapter 5

63. The Centers for Disease Control and Prevention recommends universal precautions that include:
    A. recapping needles when finished using them.
    B. placing all soiled trash in the waste can.
    C. cleaning blood spills with soap and water.
    D. wearing personal protective equipment.

Answer: **D**
Subject: Microorganisms and Asepsis
Refer to Chapter 17

64. The signature on the back of a check is that of the:
    A. payer.
    B. endorser.
    C. disburser.
    D. check maker.
    E. bank.

Answer: **B**
Subject: Financial Practices
Refer to Chapter 15

65. Which pulse site is most commonly used?
    A. Radial artery
    B. Brachial artery
    C. Apical region
    D. Temporal artery

Answer: **A**
Subject: Patient Exams and Procedures
Refer to Chapter 18

66. In the usual physical examination sequence, which area of the body does the physician examine first?
    A. Thorax and lungs
    B. Genital area
    C. Abdomen
    D. Head and neck
    E. Breasts

Answer: **D**
Subject: Patient Exams and Procedures
Refer to Chapter 18

67. The attention line of a business letter is located:
    A. four lines below the date.
    B. three lines below the letterhead.
    C. two lines below the inside address.
    D. two lines below the salutation.

Answer: **C**
Subject: Correspondence
Refer to Chapter 12

68. When a physician's license from one state is accepted by another state, it is called:
    A. endorsement.
    B. acceptance.
    C. reciprocity.
    D. allowance.
    E. transfer.

Answer: **C**
Subject: Law and Ethics
Refer to Chapter 4

69. A patient with 20/30 vision in both eyes can see with:
    A. the right eye at 30 feet what the normal eye sees at 20 feet.
    B. both eyes at 20 feet what the normal eye sees at 30 feet.
    C. the left eye at 20 feet what the normal eye sees at 30 feet.
    D. both eyes at 30 feet what the normal eye sees at 20 feet.

Answer: **B**
Subject: Patient Exams and Procedures
Refer to Chapter 18

70. Which structure is located in the RLQ?
    A. Appendix
    B. Liver
    C. Spleen
    D. Pancreas
    E. Gallbladder

Answer: **A**
Subject: Anatomy and Physiology
Refer to Chapter 6

71. CMS, formerly HCFA, regulates:
    A. prescriptions.
    B. Medicare insurance.
    C. banking institutions.
    D. clinical laboratories.

Answer: **B**
Subject: Medical Insurance
Refer to Chapter 13

72. A patient is placed in Sims' position to examine the:
    A. breasts.
    B. abdomen.
    C. rectum.
    D. heart.
    E. back.

Answer: **C**
Subject: Patient Exams and Procedures
Refer to Chapter 18

73. The ICD-10 codes are:
    A. alphanumeric.
    B. alphabetic.
    C. numeric.
    D. three to five digits dependent on modifiers.

Answer: **A**
Subject: Medical Claims and Coding
Refer to Chapter 14

74. Another term for a **living will** is:
    A. patient's release.
    B. implied contract.
    C. emancipation will.
    D. advance directive.
    E. power of attorney.

Answer: **D**
Subject: Law and Ethics
Refer to Chapter 4

75. A common charting abbreviation used during a complete physical examination is:
    A. UTI.
    B. BID.
    C. HEENT.
    D. NPO.

Answer: **C**
Subject: Patient Exams and Procedures
Refer to Chapter 18

76. First aid treatment for someone experiencing syncope includes:
 A. keeping the person sitting with head lowered to the knees.
 B. inducing vomiting.
 C. giving small amounts of water.
 D. maintaining an open airway.
 E. using an external defibrillator.

Answer: **A**
Subject: Emergency Preparedness
 Refer to Chapter 25

77. A drug classified as an antipyretic would be used to:
 A. lower blood pressure.
 B. decrease cholesterol.
 C. improve breathing.
 D. lower fever.

Answer: **D**
Subject: Pharmacology and Medication Administration
 Refer to Chapter 24

78. Which statement is true about normal values for body temperature?
 A. A rectal temperature is 2° higher than an oral temperature.
 B. An axillary temperature is the most accurate method of determining temperature.
 C. An oral temperature is 1° lower than a rectal temperature.
 D. An oral temperature is the most accurate method of determining temperature.
 E. An axillary temperature is 2° lower than an oral temperature.

Answer: **C**
Subject: Patient Exams and Procedures
 Refer to Chapter 18

79. Vaccines are an example of which kind of immunity?
 A. Natural
 B. Active
 C. Genetic
 D. Congenital

Answer: **B**
Subject: Pharmacology and Medication Administration
 Refer to Chapter 24

80. A substance produced in the body in response to the presence of an antigen is:
 A. atelectasis.
 B. antibody.
 C. inflammation.
 D. allergen.
 E. adrenalin.

Answer: **B**
Subject: Anatomy and Physiology
 Refer to Chapter 6

81. Which of the following is a fat-soluble vitamin?
 A. A
 B. B_6
 C. B_{12}
 D. C

Answer: **A**
Subject: Nutrition
 Refer to Chapter 23

82. A 12-lead electrocardiogram records:
    A. four bipolar, four unipolar, and four pre-cordial leads.
    B. six precordial, two unipolar, and four bipolar leads.
    C. three bipolar, three unipolar, and six precordial leads.
    D. two bipolar, four unipolar, and six pre-cordial leads.
    E. six bipolar, three unipolar, and three precordial leads.

Answer: **C**
Subject: Electrocardiography
Refer to Chapter 20

83. An example of a normal male hematocrit reading would be:
    A. 18 g/dL.
    B. 4,500/mm^3.
    C. 49%.
    D. 33%.

Answer: **C**
Subject: Laboratory Procedures
Refer to Chapter 21

84. One grain is equivalent to:
    A. 100 mg.
    B. 75 mg.
    C. 60 mg.
    D. 15 mg.
    E. 10 mg.

Answer: **C**
Subject: Pharmacology and Medication Administration
Refer to Chapter 24

85. Which of the following is a normal specific gravity reading for urine?
    A. 1.000
    B. 1.010
    C. 1.100
    D. 1.115

Answer: **B**
Subject: Laboratory Procedures
Refer to Chapter 21

86. The device used to record cardiac activity of an ambulatory patient over a 24-hour period is a(n):
    A. echocardiograph.
    B. electrocardiograph.
    C. cardiac ultrasound.
    D. Doppler.
    E. Holter monitor.

Answer: **E**
Subject: Electrocardiography
Refer to Chapter 20

87. What is the document that the government requires to be given to patients explaining the benefits and risks of vaccines?
    A. CMS
    B. SDS
    C. VAERS
    D. VIS

Answer: **D**
Subject: Pharmacology and Medication Administration
Refer to Chapter 24

88. When administering a 1 mL amount of medication by injection, all of the following routes may be used *except*:
    A. intradermal.
    B. subcutaneous.
    C. intramuscular.
    D. intrathecal.
    E. intravascular.

Answer: **A**
Subject: Pharmacology and Medication Administration
Refer to Chapter 24

89. The exam technique that utilizes passive movement of body joints to determine the extent of movement is:
    A. auscultation.
    B. manipulation.
    C. mensuration.
    D. percussion.

Answer: **B**
Subject: Patient Exams and Procedures
Refer to Chapter 18

90. When requesting a clean-catch urine specimen from a female patient, you should instruct the patient to:
    A. empty the bladder in the morning and then collect the second specimen of the day.
    B. void most of the urine into the toilet before collecting the specimen.
    C. cleanse each side of the urinary meatus from front to back.
    D. avoid cleansing the urinary meatus to ensure all artifacts are collected in the urine.
    E. increase fluid intake and then collect a late-day specimen.

Answer: **C**
Subject: Laboratory Procedures
Refer to Chapter 21

91. When performing venipuncture, you should always:
    A. enter the vein with the bevel of the needle placed downward.
    B. enter the vein with the needle at a 45° angle.
    C. recap used needles to avoid accidental needle punctures.
    D. remove the tourniquet before removing the needle from the puncture site.

Answer: **D**
Subject: Laboratory Procedures
Refer to Chapter 21

92. In an electrocardiogram, the standardization mark is:
    A. 1 mm high.
    B. 5 mm high.
    C. 10 mm high.
    D. 20 mm high.
    E. 25 mm high.

Answer: **C**
Subject: Electrocardiography
Refer to Chapter 20

93. A surgical instrument found on a suture re-
    moval tray is a:
    A. scalpel handle.
    B. towel forceps.
    C. needle holder.
    D. thumb forceps.

Answer: **D**
Subject: Medical Office Surgery
Refer to Chapter 19

94. Another term for the chest leads on an elec-
    trocardiogram (ECG) is:
    A. bipolar.
    B. unipolar.
    C. augmented.
    D. precordial.
    E. intercostal.

Answer: **D**
Subject: Electrocardiography
Refer to Chapter 20

95. To obtain a capillary blood specimen, you
    should:
    A. squeeze the tip of the patient's finger.
    B. collect the first drop of blood.
    C. use the patient's index finger.
    D. wipe away the first drop of blood.

Answer: **D**
Subject: Laboratory Procedures
Refer to Chapter 21

96. The proper-size needle for administering an
    intradermal injection is:
    A. 23G 1".
    B. 20G 1½".
    C. 27G ¾".
    D. 25G 1".

Answer: C
Subject: Pharmacology and Medication
Administration
Refer to Chapter 24

97. Which of the following statements is true
    regarding syncope and vertigo?
    A. Vertigo, a specific kind of dizziness, is a
       symptom.
    B. Syncope and vertigo are the same.
    C. Syncope refers to dizziness, and vertigo
       is due to fainting.
    D. Syncope and vertigo are referred to as
       conditions.
    E. Syncope is primarily caused by high
       blood pressure.

Answer: **A**
Subject: Emergency Preparedness
Refer to Chapter 25

98. The best method to deliver deep heat to tis-
    sues is to use:
    A. paraffin bath.
    B. infrared radiation lamp.
    C. whirlpool treatment.
    D. ultrasound therapy.

Answer: **D**
Subject: Physical Modalities
Refer to Chapter 22

99. When preparing a sterile tray for a minor surgical procedure, remember to:
    A. consider the 1-inch border around the perimeter of the tray nonsterile.
    B. place the vial of local anesthetic on the sterile field.
    C. prepare the tray in another location and carry it to the patient's location.
    D. have a sharps container on the sterile field.

Answer: **A**
Subject: Medical Office Surgery
Refer to Chapter 19

100. A physician orders 125 mg of a drug; the available medication on hand is 500 mg/mL. How many milliliters of the drug would you give the patient?
    A. 0.5 mL
    B. 0.4 mL
    C. 0.25 mL
    D. 0.05 mL
    E. 0.04 mL

Answer: **C**
Subject: Pharmacology and Medication Administration
Refer to Chapter 24

101. When performing an ECG, you should:
    A. apply electrodes over bony prominences.
    B. disregard artifacts.
    C. ensure patient comfort.
    D. place lead V1 on the left side of the sternum.

Answer: **C**
Subject: Electrocardiography
Refer to Chapter 20

102. When instructing a patient about a low-cholesterol diet, you should tell the patient to decrease intake of which of the following foods?
    A. Citrus fruit
    B. Green vegetables
    C. Cereal grains
    D. Dairy products
    E. Legumes

Answer: **D**
Subject: Patient Education
Refer to Chapter 8

103. Which of the following is a form of exercise therapy?
    A. Range of motion
    B. Hydrotherapy
    C. Ultrasound
    D. Massage

Answer: **A**
Subject: Physical Modalities
Refer to Chapter 22

104. In an ECG, aVR, aVL, and aVF represent:
    A. bipolar limb leads.
    B. augmented limb leads.
    C. precordial leads.
    D. standard limb leads.
    E. chest leads.

Answer: **B**
Subject: Electrocardiography
Refer to Chapter 20

PRETEST ANALYSIS

The pretest analysis helps you to determine which are your stronger topics and which are your weaker ones, requiring more study. The analysis also assists you in determining how much study time may be needed. There are four steps, which take approximately 15 minutes to complete. This is important time to invest.

ANALYSIS STEP 1

Go back to each question in the pretest. Put a check mark by the answer if:

- Your answer was incorrect.
- Your answer was correct but you were unsure or you required more than 45 seconds to decide on an answer.

ANALYSIS STEP 2

Each answer on the pretest has a subject that corresponds to one of the subjects in Table 2-1, for the CMA (AAMA) and RMA (AMT) exams, or Table 2-2, for the CMAS (AMT) exam. Count the total check marks for each subject. Place the total number of check marks for each subject in the corresponding box on the appropriate table for your exam. If you have no check marks for a subject, place a 0 in the square.

You may, for example, have three answers checked for the subject "Law and Ethics." You would place a 3 in that box.

ANALYSIS STEP 3

The higher the number in each box, the more time you need to study that subject. When all the boxes in Table 2-1 or Table 2-2 are completed, estimate your needed study time this way:

- 0 or 1 in the box: suggests reasonable knowledge of the topic, minimum 1 hour per subject; write "1" on the line "suggested study time: __ hr"
- 2 in the box suggests: partial knowledge of the topic, minimum 2 hours per subject; write "2" on the line "suggested study time: __ hr"
- 3 or higher in the box: suggests limited knowledge of the topic, minimum 3 hours per subject; write "3" on the line "suggested study time: __ hr"

ANALYSIS STEP 4

- Now count all the suggested study hours and place the total in Table 2-3.
- Add all hours in Table 2-3.

The pretest analysis is complete. Your results show you your likely areas of strength and weakness, suggested minimum study times for each subject, and a suggested total review time. Additional time is added in Table 2-3 for Anatomy and Physiology, which has the most content, and for the practice exam. Now you are ready to move on to make your plan using this information.

TABLE 2-1 ▶ Study hours by topic for CMA (AAMA) and RMA (AMT)

General Knowledge	Administrative Practice	Clinical Practice
Law and Ethics Suggested study time: _____ hr ❏	Administrative Technologies Suggested study time: _____ hr ❏	Microorganisms and Asepsis Suggested study time: _____ hr ❏
Medical Terminology Suggested study time: _____ hr ❏	Appointment Scheduling and Reception Suggested study time: _____ hr ❏	Patient Exams and Procedures Suggested study time: _____ hr ❏
Anatomy and Physiology Suggested study time: _____ hr ❏	Medical Records Suggested study time: _____ hr ❏	Medical Office Surgery Suggested study time: _____ hr ❏
Human Behavior and Professional Communication Suggested study time: _____ hr ❏	Correspondence Suggested study time: _____ hr ❏	Electrocardiography Suggested study time: _____ hr ❏
Patient Education Suggested study time: _____ hr ❏	Medical Insurance Suggested study time: _____ hr ❏	Laboratory Procedures Suggested study time: _____ hr ❏
	Medical Coding and Claims Suggested study time: _____ hr ❏	Physical Modalities Suggested study time: _____ hr ❏
	Financial Practices Suggested study time: _____ hr ❏	Nutrition Suggested study time: _____ hr ❏
	Administration and Compliance Suggested study time: _____ hr ❏	Pharmacology and Medication Administration Suggested study time: _____ hr ❏
		Emergency Preparedness Suggested study time: _____ hr ❏

TABLE 2-2 ▶ Study hours by topic for CMAS (AMT)

General Knowledge	Administrative Practice	Clinical Practice
Law and Ethics Suggested study time: _____ hr ❑	Administrative Technologies Suggested study time: _____ hr ❑	Microorganisms and Asepsis Suggested study time: _____ hr ❑
Medical Terminology Suggested study time: _____ hr ❑	Appointment Scheduling and Reception Suggested study time: _____ hr ❑	Patient Exams and Procedures Suggested study time: _____ hr ❑
Anatomy and Physiology Suggested study time: _____ hr ❑	Medical Records Management Suggested study time: _____ hr ❑	Pharmacology and Medication Administration Suggested study time: _____ hr ❑
Human Behavior and Professional Communication Suggested study time: _____ hr ❑	Correspondence Suggested study time: _____ hr ❑	Emergency Preparedness Suggested study time: _____ hr ❑
Patient Education Suggested study time: _____ hr ❑	Medical Insurance Suggested study time: _____ hr ❑	
	Medical Coding and Claims Suggested study time: _____ hr ❑	
	Financial Practices Suggested study time: _____ hr ❑	
	Administration and Compliance Suggested study time: _____ hr ❑	

TABLE 2-3 ▶ Study hours summary

Pretest-suggested study hours	
Extra study hours added for Anatomy and Physiology	4
Timed exam and final prep hours	4
Total suggested minimum study hours	

CHAPTER 3

Creating Your Study Plan

One of the common characteristics among those who pass the exam is that they had a study plan. It is a road map of where you are going and how to get there. Dedication and commitment are essential. They are like fuel for your vehicle—necessary to take you where you want to go.

An 8-week calendar is suggested to give you plenty of time to study. If your exam is already scheduled, you may modify the calendar based on that date. Box 3-1 Staying Motivated provides ideas that might help you stay focused on your study plan. The following steps are guidelines only, and you should change them based on your individual learning needs. Planning is worth the time!

Remove the calendar from the back of the book or use a calendar that you have. Work the following steps:

STEP 1

- Determine how many hours a week you can devote to study; be realistic.
- Refer to Table 2-3 in Chapter 2, which gives your total suggested minimum study hours.
- Use the Study Calendar to assign the study hours for each day.
- Refer to Figure 3-1 as an example.

STEP 2

- Refer to Table 2-1 or 2-2, which gives the total number of hours needed per subject.
- Plug these subjects into the assigned hours on the Study Calendar.
- Use Figure 3-2 as an example of a study week showing subjects assigned to the study hours.

Make your flash cards or other study tools as you go and look for "learning moments" throughout your day. As you progress, shuffle your flash cards so you are reviewing more than one chapter at a time. Also, periodically, go back and answer the questions from previously studied chapters to assure retention.

Sunday	Monday	Tuesday	Wednesday	Thursday	Friday	Saturday
4 total		1 total		1 total		2 total

FIGURE 3-1 **Step 1. Fill in the total number of hours per day you will study. Here is an example week.**

Sunday	Monday	Tuesday	Wednesday	Thursday	Friday	Saturday
4 total 1 hr (Correspondence) 2 hr (Law and Ethics) 1 hr (Medical Terminology)		1 total (Medical Terminology)		1 total (Communication)		2 total Study Group (Anatomy & Physiology)

FIGURE 3-2 **Step 2. Assign subjects to each of the days, according to level of difficulty and number of hours available. Here is an example week.**

BOX 3-1

Staying motivated

You have probably heard the slogan "Just do it!" Adopt this attitude for your exam preparation. Put all "nonessentials" on hold for 8 weeks and dedicate the time to study. Eight weeks go by very quickly. If you fall off your schedule, take a deep breath and jump back on. Let everyone know what you are doing and ask for their support. If you are in a study group, help—do not hinder—each other. Keep in mind the reason you chose to take the exam and stay focused.

Generally, keeping energized is related to physical well-being. Commit to eating healthy meals and snacks. Try to study in pleasant places. Outdoors is great if weather permits and distractions are minimal.

Buy or borrow a little book of inspirational sayings and read one daily. The Internet also has great Websites with inspirational and motivational sayings. Give yourself credit for milestones: When you complete each subject, you should feel a sense of accomplishment. When you complete the study hours for the week, reward yourself in small ways—buy a treat, watch a favorite television show, tell others, or plan a festive event to celebrate the completion of the exam. "Plan your work—then work your plan."

General Knowledge

Law and Ethics

Review Tip:

Legal and ethical decisions arise in every aspect of medical assisting. Examples of legal and ethical practices include ensuring a patient has signed a consent form before releasing information and billing only for services actually performed.

Examples of illegal or unethical practices are knowingly using an incorrect insurance code, failing to report a medication error, or discussing patients with friends. Think about legal and ethical implications that occur in a routine day as you review each chapter.

LAW

Law is a set of rules governing conduct and action that are enforced by a recognized authority. The purposes of law are to

- Regulate conduct
- Punish offenders
- Remedy wrongs
- Benefit society

The two main areas of law are given below:

1. Criminal—laws that govern crimes or wrongs committed against society, an individual, or property in violation of an ordinance; charges are brought forth by the government; a fine or imprisonment can occur. An example is Medicare fraud.

2. Civil—laws that govern crimes or wrongs committed against an individual or property; charges are brought forth by the individual or his representative; compensation (usually monetary) is sought.

The practice of medicine is generally regulated by civil law. Three types of civil law are most frequently involved:

1. Tort law—laws dealing with accidental or intentional harm to a person or property resulting from the wrongdoing of others
2. Contract law—laws dealing with the rights and obligations of enforceable promises
3. Administrative law—laws dealing with requirements and standards of governmental agencies

TORT LAW

A **tort** is a wrongful civil act committed against an individual for which compensation is sought. **Negligence** is a common tort and is defined as failure to exercise the standard of care that a reasonable, comparably trained person would exercise in similar circumstances. The four forms of negligence are:

1. Nonfeasance—failure to act when duty is indicated, resulting in or causing harm
2. Misfeasance—improper performance of an act, resulting in or causing harm
3. Malfeasance—performance of an improper act, resulting in or causing harm
4. Malpractice—failure to act or improper performance of an act or performance of an improper act by a professional (professional negligence); Box 4-1 lists the "Four Ds," which help determine whether a situation is malpractice.

A term used in obvious cases of negligence is *res ipsa loquitur,* meaning "the thing speaks for itself." Another concept is *respondeat superior,* which means "let the master answer." The employer is liable for the actions and conduct of employees while the employees are performing within the scope and job description of their position. This is also called **the law of agency.**

Another common term in the medical practice is *locum tenens,* which means temporarily taking the place

of another; common when a doctor, often contracted, is "filling in" for a time.

ASSOCIATED TERMS

- **Arbitration**—the settlement of a dispute by presenting the circumstances to a third party who decides the outcome; may be binding or nonbinding
- **Mediation**—a third independent party attempts to settle a controversy between two contending parties; differs from arbitration, in that no decision is made by the third party
- **Defendant**—the accused individual in a court of law
- **Plaintiff**—the individual bringing a charge against another in a court of law
- **Deposition**—a formal statement by a person who has promised to tell the truth; may be used in a court of law
- **Common law**—law based on societal customs and recognized by the court; *precedent* is sometimes used synonymously but differs, in that a precedent is a court ruling that is usually cited and upheld in similar cases

Good Samaritan Act As Tort Avoidance

The majority of states have a Good Samaritan Act, which is legislation enacted to encourage off-duty health-care providers to render aid at the scenes of accidents. The Good Samaritan Act protects health-care personnel from liability or tort claims. The care given must have been rendered in good faith and meet the standards of a reasonable and prudent person with similar training. You are *not* covered by the Good Samaritan Act if you are there as part of your health-care position, no matter where the incident occurs. For instance, if you volunteer to give immunizations at a school or to provide first aid at a sporting event, you are volunteering as a health-care professional and are not covered under the act. If you are attending a sporting event as a spectator or participant and render first aid, you are covered under the Good Samaritan Act. If money or other forms of compensation or gifts are accepted from the victim or the representative of the victim for administering help, the Good Samaritan Act no longer applies.

CONTRACT LAW

A **contract** is an obligation resulting from an agreement between two or more parties. Five components are required for a contract to be legal and binding:

1. An offer must be made.
2. The offer must be accepted.
3. An exchange of something of value between the parties must occur; this exchange is often referred to as *consideration.*
4. All parties must be legally capable of accepting the terms; this capability is often referred to as *capacity.*
5. The intent must be legal.

BOX 4-1

The "Four Ds"

The "Four Ds" are used to determine whether a situation is malpractice:

1. Duty—the patient/physician relationship was established
2. Dereliction—the provider neglected a professional obligation to act or acted improperly
3. Direct cause—a negative outcome resulted directly from the provider's actions or failure to act
4. Damages—the patient sustained harm from the negligent act

Contracts may be

- Expressed—written or verbal and describing what each contractual party will do
- Implied—deduced by the actions of the contracting parties (for example, a patient coming to the physician's office seeking treatment)

Consents

Consent for medical care is voluntary permission given by a competent adult or legal agent of the patient (e.g., the parent of a minor child). Consents, as with contracts, may be **expressed** or **implied**. Except in life-threatening emergencies, consent must be **informed**, which requires the physician or an appropriately trained caregiver to explain the information necessary for the patient to make an educated decision regarding the procedure. The health-care professional should provide the following information:

- An explanation of the procedure and the reason for the procedure
- The possible risks and side effects
- Alternative therapies and risks
- Prognosis with and without the procedure
- Any other information that may assist the patient in making an educated decision

Consenters

The following may consent for medical treatment:

- **Competent adult** for self or legal charge (e.g., his or her minor child); someone who has been given a pain medication would not be considered competent at that time
- **Emancipated minor** person under 18 years old legally responsible for his or her own actions and care; state-specific and designated by the court
- **Mature minor** an individual under 18 years of age living apart from parents or guardian, demonstrating maturity, intelligence, economic independence, and experience or a minor married to someone 18 years of age or older
  - Most states have a Mature Minor Rule
  - Documentation required of provider name, date of treatment, criteria used to treat as mature minor
- Minors serving in the armed forces
- Minors seeking treatment for sexually transmitted diseases, birth control, or abortion (state-specific), and out-patient treatment for chemical abuse issues

Advance Directives

Advance directives are special documents signed by the patient, witnessed, and usually notarized that state the patient's wishes for medical decisions should the patient become incapable of making the decisions for himself or herself. Some advance directives are:

- **Living will**—document stating acceptable and unacceptable means to sustain the patient's life in case of terminal conditions
- **Medical (durable) power of attorney**—document stating whom the patient designates to make medical decisions regarding accepting and withholding treatment
- **Designated anatomic donor**—documentation or indication on an existing document (the driver's license in some states) expressing the patient's desire to donate all or specific anatomic organs; **mandated by the Uniform Anatomical Donor Act**
- **Patient Self-Determination Act (PSDA)**—the purpose of the act is for individuals to decide before they become incapacitated on the care they would want or refuse; health-care agencies must ask you whether you have an advance directive and provide information about your rights under state law

ADMINISTRATIVE LAW

Administrative law refers to regulations established and enforced by governmental agencies. Examples include the US Drug Enforcement Agency (DEA), Food and Drug Administration (FDA), and various state-controlled licensing boards, such as nursing boards and boards of medical examiners. Some of the more common governmental regulators and regulations that affect the medical office are:

- **Clinical Laboratory Improvement Amendments (CLIA)**—issues laboratory testing standards for facilities performing specified tests
- **Occupational Safety and Health Administration (OSHA)**—regulates safety in the workplace
- **Internal Revenue Service (IRS)**—regulates federal payroll taxes
- **Equal Employment Opportunity Act (EEOA)**—prohibits employment discrimination because of age, color, national origin, race, religion, or sex
- **Red Flags Rule**—effective June 1, 2010 to combat increasing **medical identity theft** when a person seeking health care uses another person's information or insurance. Two categories determine if a business must comply:
  - **Creditors**—an entity that regularly defers payment for services or arranges the extension of credit; examples are billing patients after the service is rendered, including fees that are billed after insurance payments are received.
  - **Covered account**—a consumer (patient) account that allows multiple payments or transactions; most patient records fall in this category.

■ **Patient Protection and Affordable Care Act**—more commonly known as the Affordable Care Act (ACA) enacted March 23, 2010, with the intent of reforming the health-care system and requiring all citizens to carry health-care insurance or pay a fine (more information located in Chapter 13: Medical Insurance)

Employment Law

Generally, employment law comes under administrative law because it involves administrative rulings that address the rights of employees and employers in the workplace. Medical offices must follow these laws:

■ **Equal Employment Opportunity Commission (EEOC)**—prohibits job discrimination based on race, color, religion, sex, or national origin

■ **Equal Pay Act**—prohibits sex-based pay discrimination for men and women performing the same jobs

■ **Age Discrimination in Employment Act**—prohibits job discrimination for people aged 40 years and older

■ **Americans with Disabilities Act (ADA)**—prohibits discrimination against people with disabilities in employment, transportation, public accommodation, communications, and governmental activities (Fig. 4-1 gives an example)

■ **Americans with Disabilities Act Amendment (ADAA)**—this amendment to the ADA broadens the definition of disability

← 32" Clearance →

FIGURE 4-1 Medical offices must comply with ADA requirements.

■ **Family Medical Leave Act (FMLA)**—allows employees up to 12 job-protected weeks of leave without pay for family or medical needs

■ **Title VII of the Civil Rights Act of 1964**—unwelcome sexual advances, requests for sexual favors, and other verbal or physical conduct of a sexual nature constitutes sexual harassment when submission to or rejection of this conduct explicitly or implicitly affects an individual's employment; unreasonably interferes with an individual's work performance; or creates an intimidating, hostile, or offensive work environment (definition from the EEOC).

■ **Genetic Information Nondiscrimination Act (GINA)** prohibits the use of genetic information to make employment decisions

Licensure

Licensure, the strongest form of professional regulation, is a credential required to practice a profession and issued by an official state agency. This section discusses the physician's license to practice medicine, which is regulated by a state's **Medical Practice Act** and issued by the state's medical board. The license confirms that, after acceptable education and training, the doctor has met minimum standards as defined in the Medical Practice Act. Medical licensure may be obtained through the following:

■ Examination—successful completion of a written or oral state examination

■ Endorsement—acceptance by the state board of a passing score on a recognized national examination

■ Reciprocity—acceptance by the state board of a valid medical license from another state

Renewal of medical licenses is mandatory, and failure to do so results in suspension or revocation. Other causes for suspension or revocation are given below:

■ Conviction of a felony

■ Unprofessional conduct

■ Professional or personal incapacity

Certification, Registration, and Accreditation

Health-care occupations that do not require a license may be subject to a credential called *certification or registration*. This process is often voluntary, with standards developed by a national organization that also administers a national exam. Although governmental agencies are usually not involved in the process, some states require certification or registration for many health-care occupations. Examples are medical assisting, emergency medical technicians (EMTs), paramedics, laboratory technicians, and nursing assistants. These are state-specific.

Accreditation is another form of credentialing, usually involving a health-care facility or organization. It is voluntary, with standards developed by a national organization, after a process including site visits and reports that determine whether the organization meets the standards. Accreditation is not issued by a governmental body. The Joint Commission or TJC (formerly the Joint Commission on Accreditation of Healthcare Organizations or JCAHO) is one example of an accreditation organization.

Schools and training programs may also become accredited, which implies that their graduates have met certain standards. Examples of agencies that accredit specific health-care education schools and programs are

■ Commission on Accreditation of Allied Health Education Programs (CAAHEP)

■ Accrediting Bureau of Health Education Schools (ABHES)

Scope of Practice

In addition to obtaining the appropriate and mandated licensing or certification, all health-care staff is required to stay within their **scope of practice**. The scope of practice is the performance of duties and procedures allowed by law, standards, and educational preparation. As mentioned in Chapter 1, health-care personnel are also responsible for staying current in their field as a legal obligation. The health-care professional will be held accountable for the standards in place at any given time. Failure to act within one's scope of practice could result in immediate dismissal and civil or criminal action dependent on the offense.

Public Duty and Mandatory Reporting

States require physicians and other health-care personnel to report certain information to provide for the health, safety, and welfare of the public.

■ Birth certificates must be completed and submitted to the designated local or state agency by the birth attendant.

■ Death certificates must be completed by the physician in attendance.

■ Deaths that must be reported to the medical examiner include the following:

• Death resulting from violent or criminal activity

• Death from an undetermined cause

• Death without prior medical care

• Death within 24 hours of admission to a health-care facility

■ Each occurrence of specified communicable diseases such as vaccine-preventable diseases, tuberculosis, and sexually transmitted diseases must be reported to the state or county health department. Each medical facility should have a list and reporting forms or go to www.cdc.gov/mmwr/PDF/

■ Suspected abuse or criminal acts must be reported to specific governmental agencies. These acts include the following:

• Child abuse

• Elder abuse

• Spousal abuse/domestic violence (most states)

• Patient abuse

• Injuries by weapons or assault

• Injuries sustained in the commission of a crime

• Suicides or attempted suicides

■ Vaccine administration must be reported to the designated local or state agency in most states. The required information includes the following:

• Date

• Vaccine, lot number, and manufacturer

• Name, title of person administering the vaccine, and place administered

• Any adverse reactions (also reportable to VAERS, the national Vaccine Adverse Events Reporting System; refer Chapter 24)

■ Specified medical surveillance, such as phenylketonuria (PKU) in newborns, must be reported to the designated local or state agency.

ETHICS

Ethics are moral principles, values, and duties. Whereas laws are enforceable regulations set forth by the government, ethics are moral guidelines set forth and formally or informally enforced by peers, professional organizations, and the community. Examples of enforcement for breeches in ethics are censorship of a writer, suspension from a hospital staff, or simply being left out by peers.

■ Standard of conduct—behavior that is valued and usually expected

■ Duties—commitment or obligations to act in a certain moral manner

• Non-malfeasance—an action that avoids harm

• Beneficence—an action that creates benefit

• Fidelity—practice of meeting patient's right to receive competent care and respect, adherence to laws and agreements

• Veracity—truth

• Justice—equitable distribution of benefits and burdens

CODE OF ETHICS

A **code of ethics** is a statement, usually from a professional group, listing the expected behaviors of its members. The code may also set standards and disciplinary

BOX 4-2

AMA principles of medical ethics (adopted June 2001)

I. A physician shall be dedicated to providing competent medical care, with compassion and respect for human dignity and rights.

II. A physician shall uphold the standards of professionalism, be honest in all professional interactions, and strive to report physicians deficient in character or competence, or engaging in fraud or deception, to appropriate entities.

III. A physician shall respect the law and also recognize a responsibility to seek changes in those requirements which are contrary to the best interests of the patient.

IV. A physician shall respect the rights of patients, colleagues, and other health professionals, and shall safeguard patient confidences and privacy within the constraints of the law.

V. A physician shall continue to study, apply, and advance scientific knowledge, maintain a commitment to medical education, make relevant information available to patients, colleagues, and the public, obtain consultation, and use the talents of other health professionals when indicated.

VI. A physician shall, in the provision of appropriate patient care, except in emergencies, be free to choose whom to serve, with whom to associate, and the environment in which to provide medical care.

VII. A physician shall recognize a responsibility to participate in activities contributing to the improvement of the community and the betterment of public health.

VIII. A physician shall, while caring for a patient, regard responsibility to the patient as paramount.

IX. A physician shall support access to medical care for all people.

BOX 4-3

Medical assisting code of ethics

The Code of Ethics of the AAMA shall set forth principles of ethical and moral conduct as they relate to the medical profession and the particular practice of medical assisting.

Members of the AAMA dedicated to the conscientious pursuit of their profession, and thus desiring to merit the high regard of the entire medical profession and the respect of the general public which they serve, do pledge themselves to strive always to:

A. render service with full respect for the dignity of humanity;

B. respect confidential information obtained through employment unless legally authorized or required by responsible performance of duty to divulge such information;

C. uphold the honor and high principles of the profession and accept its disciplines;

D. seek to continually improve the knowledge and skills of medical assistants for the benefit of patients and professional colleagues;

E. participate in additional service activities aimed toward improving the health and well-being of the community.

Reprinted with permission from the American Association of Medical Assistants.

THE PATIENT CARE PARTNERSHIP

In 1973, the American Hospital Association was the first to publish the **Patient's Bill of Rights**. In 2013, it was changed to a document called The Patient Care Partnership. The focus of the partnership is to provide patients with an understanding of expectations, rights, and responsibilities during a hospital stay. Key elements include:

- High-quality hospital care
- A clean and safe environment
- Involvement in your care
- Protection of your privacy
- Help when leaving the hospital
- Help with your billing claims

BIOETHICS

Bioethics is moral issues dealing with biologic studies, research, procedures, policies, and decisions. Some areas of bioethics are:

- Reproduction—artificial insemination, in vitro fertilization (IVF), surrogate parenthood, abortion, fetuses for research purposes

actions for violations, including censure, suspension, fines, or expulsion. The following are examples of early codes of ethics that relate to health care:

- Code of Hammurabi—written 2500 BCE in Babylonia
- Hippocratic Oath—written 400 BCE in Greece by Hippocrates, a physician
- American Medical Association's (AMA) Code of Ethics—first written in 1847 in Philadelphia and revised several times since then to remain current—refer to Box 4-2
- American Association of Medical Assistants (AAMA) Code of Ethics—refer to Box 4-3
- American Medical Technologists' Standards of Practice—refer to Box 4-4

BOX 4-4

American Medical Technologists standards of practice

The American Medical Technologists (AMT) is dedicated to encouraging, establishing, and maintaining the highest standards, traditions, and principles of the disciplines which constitute the allied health professions of the certification agency and the Registry. Members of the Registry and all individuals certified by AMT recognize their professional and ethical responsibilities, not only to their patients, but also to society, to other health-care professionals, and to themselves.

The AMT Board of Directors has adopted the following Standards of Practice which define the essence of competent, honorable, and ethical behavior for an AMT-certified allied health-care professional. Reported violations of these Standards will be referred to the Judiciary Committee and may result in revocation of the individual's certification or other disciplinary sanctions.

I. While engaged in the arts and sciences that constitute the practice of their profession, AMT professionals shall be dedicated to the provision of competent and compassionate service and shall always meet or exceed the applicable standard of care.

II. The AMT professional shall place the health and welfare of the patient above all else.

III. When performing clinical duties and procedures, the AMT professional shall act within the lawful limits of any applicable scope of practice, and when so required shall act under and in accordance with appropriate supervision by an attending physician, dentist, or other licensed practitioner.

IV. The AMT professional shall always respect the rights of patients and of fellow health-care providers, shall comply with all applicable laws and regulations governing the privacy and confidentiality of protected healthcare information, and shall safeguard patient confidences unless legally authorized or compelled to divulge protected health-care information to an authorized individual, law enforcement officer, or other legal or governmental entity.

V. AMT professionals shall strive to increase their technical knowledge, shall continue to learn, and shall continue to apply and share scientific advances in their fields of professional specialization.

VI. The AMT professional shall respect the law and pledges to avoid dishonest, unethical or illegal practices, breaches of fiduciary duty, or abuses of the position of trust into which the professional has been placed as a certified health-care professional.

VII. AMT professionals understand that they shall not make or offer a diagnosis or dispense medical advice unless they are duly licensed practitioners or unless specifically authorized to do so by an attending licensed practitioner acting in accordance with applicable law.

VIII. The AMT professional shall observe and value the judgment of the attending physician, dentist, or other attending licensed practitioner, provided that so doing does not clearly constitute a violation of law or pose an immediate threat to the welfare of the patient.

IX. AMT professionals recognize that they are responsible for any personal wrongdoing, and that they have an obligation to report to the proper authorities any knowledge of professional abuse or unlawful behavior by any party involved in the patient's diagnosis, care, and treatment.

X. The AMT professional pledges to uphold personal honor and integrity and to cooperate in protecting and advancing, by every lawful means, the interests of the AMT and its members.

(Revised by the AMT Board of Directors July 7, 2013)

- Genetics—screening, engineering, testing, cloning, gene therapy
- Death and dying—euthanasia, do-not-resuscitate (DNR) orders, brain death, physician-assisted suicide, right to die
- Transplants—source of donations, financial compensation for donors, priority of recipients, recipients with diseases caused by unhealthy lifestyles
- Resource allocation—cost of health care; funds for research; rationing dependent on age, individual's value to society, and other socioeconomic factors; prolonging life

CONFIDENTIALITY/HEALTH INSURANCE PORTABILITY AND ACCOUNTABILITY ACT

A cornerstone of medical law and ethics, **confidentiality** has long been a standard and expectation in health care. In 1996, the federal government enacted the Health Insurance Portability and Accountability Act (HIPAA). A portion of the act was concerned with the security of the electronic medical record (EMR) and electronic submission of claims that contain sensitive information. In addition, HIPAA outlines what is considered confidential information:

- Names
- Geographic subdivisions smaller than a state
- Dates of birth, admission, discharge, death
- Telephone and fax numbers
- E-mail addresses
- Social security numbers
- Medical records or account numbers
- Health plan beneficiary numbers
- Certificate/license numbers
- Vehicle or device numbers (for example, a pacemaker number)
- Biometric identifiers
- Full-face photos
- Any other unique identifying number, characteristic, or code
- Age older than 89

Patient information can only be released by written consent of the patient, by **subpoena**, or in cases of mandatory reporting, as listed previously. All medical personnel should be aware of the ordinary daily practices in the medical office that may inadvertently lead to breach of patient confidentiality, including the following examples:

- Computer screens and other electronic devices left in sight of unauthorized persons
- Telephone conversations in earshot of others
- Patient sign-in sheets with exposed names
- Messages left on a patient's phone or answering machine with more information than simply to return the call
- Information given to callers who are not positively identified as authorized to receive information
- Information given to family members other than the legal caretaker
- Unattended fax machines and printers
- Unshredded patient material in open areas or trash baskets
- Patient issues discussed in unsecured areas
- Discussions with patients that can be overheard
- Appointment lists posted on exam room doors or other open areas

VULNERABLE POPULATIONS

Many states have enacted legislation protecting **vulnerable populations**, a group of people who may be physically or mentally at risk for harm or exploitation. Generally, infants and children, the elderly, and the disabled are considered vulnerable populations. The case is being made, in some areas, that all patients should be considered vulnerable. To decrease the risk of harm by convicted predators in certain workplace settings, including health care, the state and health-care employers require employees to be screened and fingerprinted. The fingerprints are sent to a federal clearinghouse, where it is determined whether the person has been convicted of a crime. If a criminal record is determined to exist, the person may not be hired.

RISK MANAGEMENT, SAFETY, AND QUALITY IMPROVEMENT

As discussed earlier in this chapter, malpractice has the likelihood of resulting in lawsuits or torts. Other nonmedical areas of a practice, especially those involving safety, may also put the office at risk for lawsuits. These are called *risk factors* (e.g., patients tripping on an electrical cord or sustaining injury due to malfunctioning equipment). Avoiding malpractice and ensuring safety come under an umbrella called **risk management**, which is a process to routinely assess, identify, correct, and monitor any potential hazards or risks to prevent harm and loss. The office's malpractice/liability insurance company can be of assistance in the process and may offer reduced rates for reduced risk. Some common examples of risk management in the medical office are:

- Maintaining a daily temperature chart for refrigerators containing biopharmaceuticals
- Requiring and ensuring that all employees are current in cardiopulmonary resuscitation (CPR)
- Reviewing drug expiration dates and removing all medications due to expire that month
- Replacing fire extinguishers once a year
- Ensuring a system is in place to review and report results of all diagnostic tests
- Using proper containers and techniques for disposal of biohazardous material

Many other examples are given throughout this book and can be found in the topics related to the chapter titles. TJC and the OSHA have made safety a major emphasis in standards and surveys.

An **incident report**, sometimes called an *occurrence report*, is a form usually required when an event occurs in the health-care facility that has the potential of resulting in harm or loss or torts. The incident report may be one specific to that facility or one provided by the facility's insurance company or attorney. The report contains the following information:

- Names and contact information of persons involved in the event
- Date, time, and location of the event
- Brief but complete explanation of the event
- Names and contact information of witnesses
- Any treatment or other actions
- Name(s) of anyone who was notified

Quality improvement (QI), formerly called *quality assurance*, is measuring, improving, and remeasuring patient outcomes based on established criteria or indicators. The emphasis of QI is improved outcomes for patients, whereas the emphasis of risk management is to avoid harm and loss. In some organizations, QI is part of risk management, and in other organizations, QI is a separate committee. Regardless of the organizational structure, the two are interrelated. For example, an insurance company, while reviewing financial losses, discovers that a large percentage of its asthma patients frequently visit the emergency department (ED), which is expensive. To reduce the loss, the insurance company creates a patient education program for its asthmatic patients and provides the medical practices with this program. The result is that the asthmatic patients use the ED less, reducing the company's financial loss. The outcome for the patient is that his or her asthma is better controlled and the quality of life is improved.

Some common indicators are patient immunization rates, percentage of female patients of recommended ages receiving mammograms, percentage of diabetic patients receiving eye exams, and appropriate rationale in prescribing specific antibiotics. The outcomes may be disease prevention or control, early diagnosis, or more rapid recovery.

TERMS

LAW AND ETHICS REVIEW

The following list reviews the terms discussed in this chapter and **provides other important terms that you may see on the exam.**

abandonment withdrawal by a physician from the care of a patient without reasonable notice or provisions for another equally or better qualified provider to assume care; the physician improperly terminates his or her contract with the patient

abuse wrong or improper use

advance directives documents signed by the patient and by witnesses stating the patient's wishes for medical care should he or she become incapacitated

Age Discrimination in Employment Act prohibits job discrimination for people aged 40 years and older

age of majority age at which a person is considered an adult; this is state-dependent, but usually is 18 or 21 years old

Americans with Disabilities Act (ADA) prohibits discrimination against people with disabilities in employment, transportation, public accommodation, communications, and governmental activities

Americans with Disabilities Act Amendment (ADAA) this amendment to the ADA broadens the definition of disability

arbitration the settlement of a dispute by presenting the circumstances to a third party who decides the outcome; may be binding or nonbinding

battery touching a person without his or her consent

beneficence actions that create benefit or good

bioethics moral issues dealing with biologic studies, research, procedures, and decisions

breach violation of a trust

civil law type of law governing crimes or wrongs committed against an individual or property, with charges brought forth by the individual or a representative; compensation (usually monetary) is sought

code of ethics a statement, usually from a professional group, stating the expected behaviors of its members

common law rule based on societal customs and recognized by the court

competent adult a person who has reached the age of majority and is considered of sound mind and not under the influence of drugs or other mind-altering substances

confidentiality protection of patient information from all but authorized persons

contract an agreement between two or more parties

covered account a patient account that allows multiple payments or transactions

criminal law laws that govern crimes or wrongs committed against society or an individual or property in violation of an ordinance, with charges brought forth by the government; fine or imprisonment can occur

defamation injury to a person's character or reputation by false or malicious statements

defendant the accused individual in a court of law

deposition a formal statement by a person who has promised to tell the truth; may be used in a court of law

emancipated minor a person who has not reached the age of majority but is legally responsible for his or her own actions and care; state-specific and designated by the court

endorsement a method of licensure through acceptance of a national examination score

Equal Employment Opportunity Commission (EEOC) federal authority prohibiting job discrimination based on race, color, religion, sex, or national origin

Equal Pay Act prohibits sex-based pay discrimination for men and women performing the same jobs

ethics moral principles or values or duties

expressed consent verbal or written approval

Family Medical Leave Act (FMLA) allows employees up to 12 job-protected weeks of leave without pay for family or medical needs

fee splitting a fraudulent practice in which a physician receives money from another physician solely for referring patients to him or her

fidelity practice of meeting patients' rights to competent care, to respect, and to adherence to laws and agreements

fraud an act of deceiving or misrepresenting

Genetic Information Nondiscrimination Act (GINA) prohibits the use of genetic information to make employment decisions

implied consent a patient's permission in which his or her actions indirectly indicate approval

incident report a form that is usually required when an event occurs in a health-care facility that has the potential to result in harm or loss or tort; sometimes called an occurrence report

informed consent a patient's permission for a procedure, given after receiving all the information necessary to make an educated decision

invasion of privacy releasing patient information to unauthorized parties without the consent of the patient

justice equitable distribution of benefits and burdens

law a set of rules governing conduct and actions; enforced by a recognized authority

law of agency also known as *respondeat superior*, the employer is liable for the actions and conduct of employees while within their job description

libel false or malicious writing against a person's character or reputation

malfeasance performance of an improper act, resulting in or causing harm

malpractice failure to act, improper performance of an act, or performance of an improper act by a professional resulting in or causing harm

mature minor individual under 18 years of age living apart from parents or guardian, demonstrating maturity, intelligence, economic independence, and experience or a minor married to someone 18 years of age or older

mediation a third independent party attempts to settle a controversy between two contending parties; differs from arbitration, in that no decision is offered by the third party

medical identity theft when a person seeking health care fraudulently uses another person's name or insurance

Medical Practice Act laws established by each state to define medical practice, establish educational requirements for physicians, describe licensing and renewal procedures and requirements, determine conditions for revoking or suspending licenses, and prohibit nonqualified individuals with or without a license from practicing medicine

misfeasance improper performance of an act, resulting in or causing harm

negligence commission or omission of an act that resulted in or caused harm

non compos mentis not of sound mind

nonfeasance failure to act when there was a duty to act, resulting in or causing harm

non-malfeasance actions that avoid harm

Patient Care Partnership a list of expectations, rights, and responsibilities for the patient during a hospital stay; published by the American Hospital Association

Patient Protection and Affordable Care Act more commonly known as the Affordable Care Act (ACA) enacted in 2010 with the intent of reforming the health-care system and requiring all citizens to carry health-care insurance or pay a fine

Patient Self-Determination Act (PSDA) the purpose of the act is for individuals to decide before they become incapacitated on the care they would want or refuse.

plaintiff the individual bringing a charge against another in a court of law

quality improvement (QI) measuring, improving, and remeasuring patient outcomes based on established criteria or indicators; formerly called quality assurance

quid pro quo "something for something"; a term generally used in sexual harassment claims, suggesting that career-advancing favors (promotions, raises) would be exchanged for sexual or other favors

reciprocity the acceptance by one state of a license that is issued by another state

Red Flags Rule enacted August 1, 2009, by the Federal Trade Commission to combat medical identity theft

registration a process similar to certification in which an individual, after meeting the criteria of an organization (such as passing an exam), is listed on a state or national registry

release of medical records a form signed by a patient or his or her legal representative allowing a health-care provider to give medical information to a person or agency

reportable incidents events or conditions that, by law, must be reported to a designated authority

res ipsa loquitur "the thing speaks for itself"; used to describe obvious cases of negligence

respondeat superior "let the master answer"; the employer is responsible for the actions of an employee if the employee followed policy and procedure and stayed within the scope of his or her position; also called law of agency

risk management a process to routinely assess, identify, correct, and monitor any potential hazards or risks to prevent harm and loss

scope of practice performance of duties and procedures allowed by law, standards, and educational preparation

slander false or malicious verbal statement made against another

standard of care uniform criterion established by an authority to determine quality or measure of health care or that is recognized as acceptable by usage

statute of limitations a legal time limit in which a person may file suit or authorities may file charges for a violation

subpoena a court order requiring an individual to appear in court on a given date and at a specific time

subpoena duces tecum a court order requiring medical records to be brought to the court on or by a certain date and time

subpoena testicandum a court order to provide testimony

Title VII of the Civil Rights Act of 1964 unwelcome sexual advances, requests for sexual favors, and other verbal or physical conduct of a sexual nature constitutes sexual harassment when submission to or rejection of this conduct explicitly or implicitly affects an individual's employment, unreasonably interferes with an individual's work performance, or creates an intimidating, hostile, or offensive work environment (definition from US Equal Employment Opportunity Commission)

tort a wrongful civil act committed against an individual for which compensation is sought

unbundling collecting higher reimbursement by billing separately for individual components of a procedure rather than for the procedure as a whole

upcoding an illegal practice of billing more than indicated for a procedure by selecting a higher-than-appropriate code

veracity truth

vulnerable populations a group of people who may be physically or mentally at risk for harm or exploitation

REVIEW QUESTIONS

All questions are relevant for all medical assisting and medical administrative assisting certification exams.

1. Informed consent requires that the:
   A. patient have a family member present when the consent form is signed.
   B. medical assistant inform the patient of all possible side effects of the procedure.
   C. attorney witness the signature.
   D. physician treat the patient if it is an emergency.
   E. information provided is enough for the patient to make an educated decision.

   Answer: **E**
   Why: E is the definition of informed consent. A family member or an attorney is not required to be present. The medical assistant may inform the patient of side effects, but side effects are only a portion of informed consent and not enough to make an educated decision.
   Review: Yes ○   No ○

2. Law refers to the:
   A. recognized rule of conduct enforced by a legal authority.
   B. policy used to charge people fees.
   C. Patient's Bill of Rights.
   D. established standards of care.

   Answer: **A**
   Why: A is the definition of law. Charging a fee, the Patient's Bill of Rights, and standards of care are not law.
   Review: Yes ○   No ○

3. The law requires a physician to report to the appropriate authorities:
   A. a person who has received a narcotic drug.
   B. a physician who participates in genetic research.
   C. a physician who conducts an abortion.
   D. a person suspected of elderly abuse.
   E. a person with cancer.

   Answer: **D**
   Why: Elderly abuse is against the law and must be reported to the proper authority. Under normal circumstances, it is not required to report the activities listed in A, B, C, or E.
   Review: Yes ○   No ○

4. Consent for a person's own medical treatment may be given by a:
   A. 17-year-old university student whose parents are paying for school.
   B. 16-year-old who has a baby but is not married and lives at home.
   C. 21-year-old who has taken a narcotic pain medication.
   D. 17-year-old who is in the Navy.

   Answer: **D**
   Why: A person serving in the armed forces, even if a minor, is legally able to consent to his or her own medical treatment. In most states, a person 16 or 17 years old is considered a nonemancipated minor if still dependent on parents. Someone taking narcotic medication is not considered competent because of the narcotic's effects.
   Review: Yes ○   No ○

5. A patient's implied consent usually covers a(n):
   A. organ donation.
   B. electrocardiogram.
   C. blood transfusion.
   D. appendectomy.
   E. release of medical information.

   Answer: **B**
   Why: An electrocardiogram is considered a common procedure in a medical practice and is generally understood to have little risk. Implied consent is sufficient for such procedures. The other procedures usually require expressed consent.
   Review: Yes ○   No ○

6. A **tort** is:
  A. a type of criminal law.
  B. a type of civil law.
  C. exempt from the Good Samaritan Act.
  D. a standard of care.

Answer: **B**
Why: A tort is a type of civil law that deals with accidental or intentional harm to a person or property resulting from the wrongdoing of another. It is not criminal law or exempt from the Good Samaritan Act if malpractice is committed. A standard of care may be addressed in a tort but is not a tort itself.
Review: Yes ◯   No ◯

7. Malfeasance is one form of:
  A. misfeasance.
  B. nonfeasance.
  C. malpractice.
  D. malnutrition.
  E. malformation.

Answer: **C**
Why: Malfeasance is performance of an improper act that results in or causes harm. Malpractice is failure to act or an improper act that results in or causes harm. Malfeasance is a specific type of malpractice. Misfeasance and nonfeasance are different from malfeasance but are also forms of malpractice. Malnutrition and malformation are medical pathology.
Review: Yes ◯   No ◯

8. A physician may obtain his or her license by any of the following *except*:
  A. endorsement.
  B. examination.
  C. reciprocity.
  D. registration.

Answer: **D**
Why: A physician may obtain a license through endorsement, examination, or reciprocity. Registration is not a process for obtaining a license to practice medicine.
Review: Yes ◯   No ◯

9. Advance directives include a:
  A. living memorial.
  B. medical power of attorney.
  C. notarized will.
  D. driver's license.
  E. medical examination.

Answer: **B**
Why: A medical power of attorney gives a designated person the legal authority to make medical decisions for the patient. This is done by the patient while he or she is still competent to make his or her own decisions.
Review: Yes ◯   No ◯

10. *Respondeat superior* refers to:
  A. a subpoena to come to court.
  B. a physician's responsibility for the actions of his or her staff.
  C. "something for something."
  D. "respond to your superiors."

Answer: **B**
Why: *Respondeat superior* means "let the master answer" and refers to the physician's responsibility for the actions of his or her staff.
Review: Yes ◯   No ◯

11. The Good Samaritan Act does not cover a health-care provider who:
  A. renders first aid at the scene of an accident.
  B. volunteers to provide first aid at a charitable "fun run."
  C. helps a person who has fainted at a sporting event.
  D. provides care to a person having a seizure in a restaurant.
  E. provides first aid to a person who has a heart attack in the health-care provider's home.

Answer: **B**
Why: The Good Samaritan Act only covers acts outside of the health-care profession. If you volunteer as a professional, this is considered to be within the formal practice of your profession, and the Good Samaritan Act does not apply.
Review: Yes ◯   No ◯

12. A physician who accepts payment from another physician for the referral of a patient is guilty of:
    A. fee splitting.
    B. bundling.
    C. battery.
    D. abandonment.

Answer: **A**

Why: A physician who accepts money from another physician for referral of a patient is guilty of fee splitting. The physician paying for the referral is also guilty.

Review: Yes ◯   No ◯

13. Failure to act in a manner that a prudent and reasonable person would under similar circumstances is:
    A. negligence.
    B. implied consent.
    C. breach of contract.
    D. fraud.
    E. abuse.

Answer: **A**

Why: Negligence is an omission or commission of an act that a prudent and reasonable person would or would not do in similar circumstances.

Review: Yes ◯   No ◯

14. The "Four Ds" are used to determine malpractice; the following are the "Ds" *except*:
    A. direct cause.
    B. duty.
    C. derelict.
    D. defendant.

Answer: **D**

Why: A defendant is the person charged with an offense, not an element for determining malpractice. The "Four Ds" are duty, derelict, direct cause, and damage.

Review: Yes ◯   No ◯

15. A minor may consent for all of the following *except*:
    A. treatment of syphilis.
    B. abortion.
    C. birth control.
    D. treatment of gonorrhea.
    E. sterilization.

Answer: **E**

Why: A minor cannot consent for his or her sterilization. A minor 12 years of age and older, in most states, may consent for treatment of sexually transmitted diseases, birth control, and abortion.

Review: Yes ◯   No ◯

16. A communicable disease to be reported to the county health department is:
    A. gastroenteritis.
    B. streptococcus.
    C. rubella.
    D. tinnitus.

Answer: **C**

Why: Rubella, or German measles, is a reportable communicable disease. Gastroenteritis, infection of the stomach and small intestine; streptococcus, a bacterial infection; and tinnitus, ringing in the ears, are not required to be reported.

Review: Yes ◯   No ◯

17. Medical examiner cases involve:
    A. deaths.
    B. births.
    C. communicable diseases.
    D. professional misconduct.
    E. *respondeat superior.*

Answer: **A**

Why: Medical examiner cases involve death caused by a criminal act or by violence, death without prior medical care, and death from an undetermined cause.

Review: Yes ◯   No ◯

18. A situation in which the very nature of the injury implicates malpractice is called:
    A. slander.
    B. assault.
    C. defamation.
    D. *res ipsa loquitur.*

Answer: **D**

Why: Res ipsa loquitur means "the thing speaks for itself" and is used in cases in which the malpractice is obvious.

Review: Yes ◯   No ◯

19. The strongest mandatory credential regulated by a state to practice a profession is a(n):
  A. declaration.
  B. licensure.
  C. matriculation.
  D. acceptance.
  E. warranty.

Answer: **B**
Why: Licensure is the strongest mandatory credential. The remaining items are voluntary and usually not issued by a governmental agency.
Review: Yes ◯   No ◯

20. Medical assistants may be:
  A. licensed.
  B. certified.
  C. accredited.
  D. reciprocated.

Answer: **B**
Why: Medical assistants may be certified. They are not licensed by any state; therefore, reciprocity does not apply. Organizations, not individuals, are accredited.
Review: Yes ◯   No ◯

21. Ethics deal with
  A. morals.
  B. *respondeat superior.*
  C. assault.
  D. customs.
  E. religion.

Answer: **A**
Why: Ethics are morals and values. *Respondeat superior* means the physician is responsible for his or her employees; assault is an attack or threat to a person; customs are traditions; religion is the worship of a deity.
Review: Yes ◯   No ◯

22. The Patient Care Partnership was designed to:
  A. reduce hospital charges.
  B. limit number of days in the hospital.
  C. eliminate all medical errors.
  D. involve the patient in their care.
  E. ensure insurance payment of the hospital bill.

Answer: **D**
Why: The Patient Care Partnership was designed to inform patients of expectations during a hospital stay and how they will be involved in their care. There is no assurance of reducing hospital charges, limiting days in the hospital, eliminating medical errors, or ensuring payment of the hospital bill by the insurance company.
Review: Yes ◯   No ◯

23. The first medical code of ethics was written by:
  A. Hippocrates.
  B. Socrates.
  C. the AMA.
  D. Hammurabi.

Answer: **D**
Why: The Code of Hammurabi was written in 2500 BCE. Hippocrates, Socrates, and the American Medical Association (AMA) wrote medical codes of ethics later.
Review: Yes ◯   No ◯

24. Which of the following is considered an ethical issue?
  A. Allocation of resources
  B. Childbirth
  C. Electrical engineering
  D. Appendectomies
  E. Long waits for patients in physician offices

Answer: **A**
Why: Allocation of resources refers to the distribution of funds (money), organs for transplants, needed medical procedures, or other resources, which are ethical issues. Childbirth is a medical or natural process; appendectomies are surgeries. Electrical engineering is a profession. (Long waits are an inconvenience!)
Review: Yes ◯   No ◯

25. A medical assistant publicly criticizes a physician's diagnostic skills. This is an example of:
  A. slander.
  B. veracity.
  C. breach of confidentiality.
  D. malpractice.

Answer: **A**
Why: The definition of slander is a false or malicious statement against another. Veracity means truth; breach of confidentiality refers to releasing protected information without consent; malpractice has to do with specific damages to a patient. Battery is touching a person without consent.
Review: Yes ○   No ○

26. Which of the following conditions must be reported?
  A. Hypertension
  B. Hepatitis B
  C. Hemiplegia
  D. Hemorrhage
  E. Anemia

Answer: **B**
Why: Hepatitis B is a communicable disease that must be reported to the local or state health departments. The other choices are medical conditions that do not require reporting.
Review: Yes ○   No ○

27. A court order instructing the physician to report to court at a certain time and date is:
  A. *quid pro quo.*
  B. a contract.
  C. a subpoena.
  D. consent.

Answer: **C**
Why: A subpoena is a document that mandates a person to appear in court at a given time and date. *Quid pro quo* means "something for something," a favor. A contract is an agreement between parties; consent is permission to perform or do something.
Review: Yes ○   No ○

28. A living will:
  A. names the beneficiaries of the estate.
  B. is an advance directive stating the patient's decisions for medical care before an incapacitating event.
  C. must be drawn up by an attorney.
  D. is subject to estate taxes.
  E. allows a person to give away his or her belongings while still alive.

Answer: **B**
Why: An advance directive is a set of instructions given while a person is fully capacitated. One type of advance directive is the living will, which states the health-care desires of a patient. Advance directives have nothing to do with the estate or estate taxes and do not have to be drawn up by an attorney. No will is needed for selection E.
Review: Yes ○   No ○

29. Dr. Smith is no longer willing to take care of Mr. Watson. If Dr. Smith does not give Mr. Watson proper notification and appropriate time to find a new physician, Dr. Smith is guilty of:
  A. violation of standard of care.
  B. privacy.
  C. failure to act.
  D. abandonment.

Answer: **D**
Why: When a physician withdraws from the care of a patient without reasonable notice or provision for another equally or better qualified provider to assume care, the patient/physician contract is breached and the physician is guilty of abandonment.
Review: Yes ○   No ○

30. The patient puts out his or her arm to allow the physician to cleanse an abrasion. This type of consent is:
  A. implied.
  B. expressed.
  C. contracted.
  D. emergency.
  E. positive.

Answer: **A**
Why: Consent is implied by the patient holding out his or her arm. Expressed consent is verbal or written. The only emergency consent is one that is "life or limb" threatening. The terms "positive" and "contracted" do not apply to consent.
Review: Yes ○   No ○

31. The physician performs an elective surgical procedure without a written consent. The physician is guilty of:
A. a bioethic offense.
B. breach of confidentiality.
C. battery.
D. endorsement.

Answer: **C**
Why: Battery is touching someone without his or her consent. There is no indication that bioethics are involved or that the patient's confidentiality has been breached. Endorsement is one method for a physician to obtain a license to practice medicine.
Review: Yes ○   No ○

32. The purpose of the Good Samaritan Act is to:
A. reward health-care providers for stopping at the scene of an accident.
B. ensure physicians know first aid.
C. protect health-care workers from liability when rendering first aid at an accident scene.
D. avoid having to pay for first aid.
E. encourage more people to go into health-care professions.

Answer: **C**
Why: The Good Samaritan Act was designed to encourage health-care workers to stop at the scene of emergencies by protecting them from liability for civil damages.
Review: Yes ○   No ○

33. Which of the following actions is governed by criminal law?
A. Giving an incorrect medication
B. Discounting
C. Not reporting suspected measles
D. Telling a family member the patient's diagnosis
E. Purposefully overcharging on a Medicare claim

Answer: **E**
Why: Purposefully overcharging on a Medicare claim is considered fraud and is therefore covered under criminal law; the other choices are usually considered civil offenses if charges are made.
Review: Yes ○   No ○

34. A patient is treated for a minor gunshot wound that he states was sustained during a hunting accident. The physician is obligated to report this as part of:
A. implied consent.
B. public duty.
C. mandatory counseling.
D. standard of care.
E. *respondeat superior.*

Answer: **B**
Why: It is the physician's public duty to report all gunshot wounds.
Review: Yes ○   No ○

35. A patient calls to make an appointment and states the symptoms for the office visit. The scheduler says, "That sounds like the flu." The health-care worker violated the:
A. code of ethics.
B. Patient's Bill of Rights.
C. Health Insurance Portability and Accountability Act.
D. scope of practice.

Answer: **D**
Why: A person scheduling appointments has no training or authority to diagnose. A diagnosis can only be made by a physician or mid-level provider such as a physician's assistant or nurse practitioner.
Review: Yes ○   No ○

36. Mandatory reporting is required in all of the following cases *except*:
A. child abuse.
B. unknown cause of death.
C. alcohol abuse.
D. elder abuse.
E. communicable disease.

Answer: **C**
Why: Alcohol abuse is not considered reportable, whereas child abuse, death from an unknown cause, and elder abuse must be reported.
Review: Yes ○   No ○

37. A form of malpractice is **nonfeasance**, which means:
A. failure to act when duty is indicated, resulting in or causing harm.
B. improper performance of an act, resulting in or causing harm.
C. performance of an improper act, resulting in or causing harm.
D. not charging a fee.

Answer: **A**
Why: The definition of nonfeasance is the failure to act when duty is indicated, resulting in or causing harm. B is misfeasance; C is malfeasance; D and E have nothing to do with malpractice.
Review: Yes ○   No ○

38. A physician casts a fracture of the ulna incorrectly. This results in malformation of the arm. The physician could be charged with:
A. misadventure.
B. malunion.
C. tort.
D. torticollis.
E. battery.

Answer: **C**
Why: A tort is accidental or intentional harm to a person or property resulting from the wrongdoing of another. The other choices do not deal with medical wrongdoings.
Review: Yes ○   No ○

39. The medical office must comply with the regulations and standards of:
A. AFL.
B. AAMA.
C. GOP.
D. AARP.
E. OSHA.

Answer: **E**
Why: The Occupational Safety and Health Administration (OSHA) is a regulatory governmental agency; its mandates must be followed or legal actions may be imposed. The American Federation of Labor (AFL), the American Association of Medical Assistants (AAMA), and the Republican Party (GOP) are voluntary special interest organizations.
Review: Yes ○   No ○

40. All of the following are governmental agencies setting standards and regulations that must be followed by medical offices *except*:
A. The Joint Commission.
B. DEA.
C. IRS.
D. FDA.

Answer: **A**
Why: The Joint Commission is the only nongovernmental voluntary agency in this list. The Drug Enforcement Administration (DEA), Internal Revenue Service (IRS), and Food and Drug Administration (FDA) are all governmental agencies with regulations affecting the medical office.
Review: Yes ○   No ○

41. The physician's office shares a patient's medical information with an insurance company. The physician's office did not have the patient's written consent. The office is guilty of:
    A. breach of confidentiality.
    B. slander.
    C. abuse.
    D. breach of respect.

Answer: **A**
Why: Providing a patient's medical information to an outside party without the patient's written consent is a breach of confidentiality.
Review: Yes ○   No ○

42. A wheelchair patient could not use the medical office restroom because it was too small for the wheelchair. This office is in violation of:
    A. CLIA.
    B. FDA.
    C. OSHA.
    D. CDC.
    E. ADA.

Answer: **E**
Why: The Americans with Disabilities Act (ADA) mandates that certain workplaces, including medical offices, must provide accommodations for persons with special needs. CLIA is the Clinical Laboratory Improvement Amendments, FDA is the Food and Drug Administration, OSHA is the Occupational Safety and Health Administration, and CDC is the Centers for Disease Control and Prevention.
Review: Yes ○   No ○

43. The Patient Care Partnership is designed to provide the following *except*:
    A. high-quality hospital care.
    B. a clean and safe environment.
    C. open disclosure of private information.
    D. help when leaving the hospital.

Answer: **C**
Why: The Patient Care Partnership requires health-care providers and hospital staff to protect the patient's privacy at all times during a hospital stay.
Review: Yes ○   No ○

44. A valid contract must:
    A. be paid in full at the beginning of the period covered.
    B. be entered into by competent parties.
    C. always be in writing.
    D. always cover the patient's family.
    E. always have a witness.

Answer: **B**
Why: One of the five components of a valid contract is that all parties must be legally capable of accepting the terms or be competent. The other four requirements are:

■ an offer must be made,

■ the offer must be accepted,

■ an exchange of value between the parties must occur, and

■ the intent must be legal.
Review: Yes ○   No ○

45. The purpose of law is to:
    A. legalize cardiopulmonary training.
    B. provide jobs.
    C. benefit special interest groups.
    D. remedy wrongs.

Answer: **D**
Why: The purposes of law are to regulate conduct, to punish offenders, to remedy wrongs, and to benefit society.
Review: Yes ○   No ○

46. An expressed contract is:
 A. written.
 B. implied.
 C. reportable.
 D. sent via FedEx.
 E. illegal.

Answer: **A**

Why: The definition of an expressed contract is one that is written or verbal and describes what each contractual party will do. A contract is implied when it is deduced by the parties' actions. Contracts are generally not reportable. How contracts are delivered is the decision of the consenting parties. An expressed contract is not illegal.

Review: Yes ○   No ○

47. Written consent for medical care must be:
 A. voluntary.
 B. uninformed.
 C. given for all procedures.
 D. done on a word processor.

Answer: **A**

Why: Consent for medical care is voluntary permission by the appropriate party. Consent should never be uninformed, and written consent is not given for all procedures; for noninvasive procedures with low risk, implied consent is sufficient. Written consent may be in many forms and can even be handwritten.

Review: Yes ○   No ○

48. Examples of ethical cases affected by the law are cases involving:
 A. the right to die.
 B. the use of synthetic drugs.
 C. endoscopy.
 D. licensure.

Answer: **A**

Why: The right to die is an ethical issue addressed by the law in cases such as assisted suicide or euthanasia. The use of synthetic drugs and endoscopy are common practices. Licensure is required by states and comes under administrative law.

Review: Yes ○   No ○

49. Ethical issues are addressed in:
 A. insurance codes.
 B. professional codes.
 C. billing codes.
 D. safety codes.
 E. tort law

Answer: **B**

Why: Professional codes, dating back to 2500 BCE, address moral behavior and ethics. The other codes listed involve medical office procedures.

Review: Yes ○   No ○

50. In cases of public safety:
 A. the laws protecting the general population usually take precedence over an individual's rights.
 B. the AMA is often consulted.
 C. a person cannot go in public with a communicable disease.
 D. the government must uphold all expectations of The Patient Care Partnership.

Answer: **A**

Why: The laws protecting the public safety take precedence. In instances such as contamination and quarantine, the rights of patients are secondary to the public safety.
The AMA is not generally consulted in these cases, and very few communicable diseases mandate quarantine. The government is not obligated to uphold nongovernmental agencies' Patient Care Partnership.

Review: Yes ○   No ○

51. A medical assistant could be held liable for the actions of:
 A. a patient.
 B. the insurance company.
 C. a coworker.
 D. the court.
 E. the hospital

Answer: **C**

Why: A medical assistant who knowingly withholds information involving illegal and, in some cases, immoral actions of a coworker could be held liable. He or she is not responsible for the actions of the patient, insurance company, or court.

Review: Yes ○   No ○

52. A favorable patient outcome resulting from the quality improvement process may be preventing:
    A. illness.
    B. an increase in insurance rates.
    C. financial loss.
    D. incident reports.

Answer: **A**

Why: Preventing illness is directly related to the patient and quality of care; preventing an increase in insurance rates, preventing financial loss, and preventing incident reports are components of risk management.

Review: Yes ○   No ○

53. All of the following are examples of risk management *except*:
    A. ensuring the coffee pot is turned off at the end of the day.
    B. giving the patient an injection ordered by the physician.
    C. checking the emergency cart.
    D. reporting a frayed lamp wire.
    E. repairing a tear in the carpet to prevent tripping.

Answer: **B**

Why: Ensuring the coffee pot is turned off and reporting a frayed wire are intended to prevent fire (loss); checking the emergency cart is intended to provide an appropriate standard of care if an emergency occurs (prevent harm and loss). However, giving the patient an injection is part of the prescribed patient's treatment. It is not considered risk management.

Review: Yes ○   No ○

54. The AMA Principles of Medical Ethics require a physician to:
    A. belong to the AMA.
    B. treat patients on Medicare.
    C. contribute to political action campaigns (PAC).
    D. report other physicians deficient in character or competence.

Answer: **D**

Why: Article II of the AMA Principles of Medical Ethics states, "A physician shall uphold the standards of professionalism, be honest in all professional interactions, and strive to report physicians deficient in character or competence, or engaging in fraud or deception, to appropriate entities." The other answers may be implied but do not specifically deal with ethics.

Review: Yes ○   No ○

55. What prohibits job discrimination for race, color, religion, sex, or national origin?
    A. EEOC
    B. FMLA
    C. ADA
    D. Equal Pay Act
    E. HIPAA

Answer: **A**

Why: The Equal Employment Opportunity Commission (EEOC) is the agency that prohibits job discrimination for race, color, religion, sex, or national origin. The FMLA involves family leave; the ADA prohibits discrimination against people with disabilities; the Equal Pay Act requires equal pay for equal work; and HIPAA involves confidentiality in health care.

Review: Yes ○   No ○

56. Employment law is generally considered:
    A. criminal law.
    B. tort law.
    C. bioethics.
    D. contract law.
    E. administrative law.

Answer: **E**

Why: Employment law concerns administrative regulations for the workplace. Criminal law and tort law are not limited to a specific venue. Contract law concerns an agreement between two parties, and bioethics are not laws.

Review: Yes ○   No ○

57. The purpose of the Red Flags Rule is to:
    A. have national holidays off.
    B. watch for Medicare fraud.
    C. guard for medical identity theft.
    D. check references before hiring.

Answer: **C**

Why: The Red Flags Rule was enacted by the Federal Trade Commission August 2009 for the purpose of legislating certain businesses to implement a program to prevent, detect, and mitigate medical identity theft.

Review: Yes ○   No ○

CRITICAL THINKING CASE REVIEW

The medical assistant administered an incorrect injectable medication. The patient was retained in the office for an extended amount of time with no adverse outcome. When the error was explained to the patient she was extremely upset and stated she was going to sue the medical office for malpractice.

1. Administering an incorrect medication might be considered:
   A. non-malfeasance
   B. misfeasance
   C. nonfeasance
   D. negligence
   E. *res ipsa loquitur*

   Answer: **B**
   Why: Misfeasance is the improper performance of an act resulting in or causing harm. The improper medication was given and if harm resulted the act would be misfeasance. Non-malfeasance is an action that avoids harm; nonfeasance involves a failure to act; negligence is failure to exercise the standard of care which also applies in this case, but misfeasance is the more specific answer. *Res ipsa loquitur* means "the thing speaks for itself."
   Review: Yes ○   No ○

2. The patient threatened to take legal action known as a(n):
   A. breach of contract
   B. advance directive
   C. violation of OSHA
   D. tort

   Answer: **D**
   Why: A tort is a wrongful civil act committed against an individual.
   Review: Yes ○   No ○

3. The case did not meet which of the following "Ds" to determine malpractice?
   A. Duty
   B. Dereliction
   C. Direct cause
   D. Damage
   E. Drug

   Answer: **D**
   Why: The patient did not suffer any damage or harm from the medication error.
   Review: Yes ○   No ○

4. Although the medical assistant was responsible, the physician would also be held responsible under *respondeat superior* meaning "let the master answer," this is also referred to as:
   A. *res ipsa loquitur*
   B. implied consent
   C. law of agency
   D. Red Flags Rule
   E. scope of practice

   Answer: **C**
   Why: The law of agency and *respondeat superior* mean the employer is liable for the actions and conduct of employees while performing within their job description. Implied consent is the patient's unwritten or nonverbal consent understood through an action. Red Flags Rule involves fraudulent patient identity to seek medical care and scope of practice refers to performance of duties and procedures as allowed by law, standards, and educational preparation.
   Review: Yes ○   No ○

5. The medical assistant violated:
   A. scope of practice
   B. standard of care
   C. bioethics
   D. HIPAA

   Answer: **B**
   Why: The standard of care is uniform criterion established by an authority to determine quality health care or recognized as acceptable by usage. Giving correct medication is both quality health care and recognized acceptable usage.
   Review: Yes ○   No ○

5

Medical Terminology

Medical terminology is a significant portion of the national exams. Questions in other chapters may be answered by knowing the meaning of the term. Medical terminology is comparable to a foreign language. You may pick up pieces and phrases just by being around those who speak it, but you could not expect to pass an exam in that language without some study. If you are a medical assistant or medical administrative specialist who received on-the-job training, this may apply to you, especially if you have been working in a specialty practice (e.g., obstetrics, where the terminology is basically limited to the female reproductive system). Certification exam questions may require you to select not only the meaning but also the *correct spelling of a term.*

WORD PARTS

A medical term may have three parts—the prefix, the root, and the suffix. The meaning is found by deciphering the clues as in Figure 5-1.

1. Root—meaning or central part of the word; it often refers to a body part (nearly all medical terms have a root)

   Example of a root: THERMIA (state of heat)

2. Prefix—beginning of the word; it modifies the root (not all medical terms have a prefix)

   Example of a prefix: HYPER (high or excessive)

3. Suffix—ending of the word; it modifies the root and usually refers to a condition, procedure, or action (not all medical terms have a suffix)

   Example of a suffix: -IC (indicating a condition)

   Example of a term with a prefix, root, and suffix: HYPERTHERMIC (abnormally high temperature)
   Prefix: hyper- = high, above, super

Root: therm/o = related to temperature
Suffix: -ic = condition/state related to the root

Example of a word with a root and suffix but no prefix: TONSILLECTOMY (removal of tonsils) = TONSIL + ECTOMY (removal of); the correct spelling of this word is a frequent question.
Example of a word without a suffix: BI LATERAL (having two sides) = BI (two) + LATERAL (side)

Think of an example of a medical term for each of the prefixes (Box 5-1), suffixes (Box 5-2), and roots (Box 5-3). Medical terminology is difficult and may require more time. Use the Review Tip. Consider adding another week to your study plan if you are not comfortable with the material.

BOX 5-1

Common prefixes and meanings

a/an-: absence of	epi-: on, attached to, over	multi-: many
ab-: away from	ex-: out	neo-: new
ad-: toward	hemi-: half	para-: beside
ante-: before	hemo/hemat-: pertaining to blood	per-: through
anti-: against	hyper-: high, excessive	peri-: around, enclosing
auto-: self	hypo-: below	poly-: many
bi-: both, two	inter-: between	post-: after
bio-: life	intra-: within	pre-: before
circum-: around	iso-: equall	primi-: first
con-: with, together	itho-:stone	retro-: back, behind
contra-: against, opposite	mal-: bad	semi-: half
dis-: apart, separate	mega-: large	sub-: under
dys-: painful, difficult	meso-: middle	super-: excessive
ec-: out	meta-: beyond	supra-: above
ecto-: outside of	micro-: very small	syn-: together, with
en-: in	milli-: one-thousandth	
endo-: within	mono-: one, single	

BOX 5-2

Common suffixes and meanings

-ad: toward	-ism: condition of	-phobia: abnormal fear
-al: relating to	-itis: inflammation	-plasia: formation
-ectomy: removal of	-logist: specialist in	-plasty: surgical repair
-emesis: vomiting	-logy: study of	-ptosis: drooping
-genic: producing	-lysis: destruction of	-rrhage: burst forth
-genetic: origin-related	-megaly: enlargement	-rrhea: discharge
-graph: recording instrument	-meter: measurement instrument	-scope: viewing instrument
-graphy: recording process	-oma: tumor	-scopy: procedure using a scope
-iasis: abnormal	-osis: condition of	-stomy: creating a surgical opening
-iatric: treatment of	-pathy: disease	-tomy: incision into
-iatry: field of medicine	-penia: abnormal decrease	-tripsy: crushing
-ic: relating to	-philia: abnormal attraction	

BOX 5-3

Common roots and meanings

aden/o: gland
arteri/o: artery
arthr/o: joint
audi/o: hearing
blephar/o: eyelid
bucc/o: cheek
burs/o: bursa
calc/i: stone
cardi/o: heart
cervic/o: neck, neck of an organ
cholecyst/o: gallbladder
conjunctiv/o: conjunctiva
cost/o: rib
crani/o: skull
cutane/o: skin
cyan/o: blue
cyst/o: bladder
cyt/o: cell
derm/o: skin
dors/o: back
encephal/o: brain
fasci/o: fibrous tissue
fibr/o: connective tissue
gastr/o: stomach
gingiv/o: gum
glyc/o: sugar, glucose
*gynec/o: pertaining to female

hepat/o: liver
hist/o: tissue
hyst/o: uterus
ir/o: iris
kal/i: potassium
lacrim/o: tear
lamin/o: lamina
lapar/o: abdomen
leuk/o: white
lip/o: fat
metr/o: uterus
myel/o: spinal cord
my/o: muscle
nephr/o: kidney
neur/o: nerve
onc/o: tumoronchy/o: fingernails or toenails
opt/o: vision
oste/o: bone
pector/o: chest
pneumon/o: lung
psych/o: mind
retin/o: retina
rhin/o: nose
synovi/o: lining the joint
tend/o: tendon
ven/o: vein

*Gynecomastia is an exception and refers to enlarged breasts, usually of the male.

FIGURE 5-1 **Winning at medical terminology requires deciphering clues**

MEDICAL TERMINOLOGY REVIEW AIDS

The following words and word parts will help with breaking down and building other medical terms and determining their meaning.

BODY PLANES

- Median or midline plane—a lengthwise plane through the midline running front to back dividing the body into equal right and left halves
- Sagittal plane—a lengthwise plane parallel to the midline running front to back dividing the body or any part of it into unequal right and left sides or parts
- Coronal or frontal plane—a lengthwise plane running side to side dividing the body into front and back parts
- Transverse or horizontal plane—a crosswise plane dividing the body into upper and lower parts

DIRECTIONAL TERMS

Directional terms make it possible to say that something is above, below, to the left or right of, behind or in front of, or nearer or farther from something else.

- Superior—toward the head end or toward the upper part of the body
- Inferior—farther away from the head or toward the lower part of the body
- Anterior or ventral—on the front or abdominal side of the body
- Posterior or dorsal—on the backside of the body
- Proximal—nearer a point of reference, usually the trunk or middle of the body
- Distal—farther away from a point of reference
- Medial—closer to the midline of the body
- Lateral—toward the side of the body or away from the midline
- Internal or deep—on the inside of the body
- External or superficial—on or close to the outside of the body

LOCATING TERMS

- Cephalic or cranial—referring to the head or head end
- Caudal—referring to the tail or tail end
- Palmar—referring to the front (while standing in anatomical position) or palm of the hand
- Plantar—referring to the sole or bottom of the foot

DIAGNOSTIC, SYMPTOMATIC, AND RELATED SUFFIXES

- -algia—pain
- -cele—hernia, swelling
- -genesis (-gen)—forming, producing
- -gram—record, a writing
- -graph—instrument for recording
- -iasis—abnormal condition
- -itis—inflammation
- -malacia—softening
- -oid—resembling
- -oma—tumor
- -osis—abnormal condition or increase (used primarily with blood cells)
- -pathy—disease
- -penia—decrease, deficiency
- -phagia—eating, swallowing
- -plegia—paralysis
- -rrhage—bursting forth
- -rrhea—discharge, flow
- -rrhexis—rupture
- -stasis—standing still
- -stenosis—narrowing, stricture

SPELLING CAUTION

The exams contain questions that require you to select correct spelling. Words with the following are high probability:

- -rrhage (example: hemorrhage)
- -rrhea (example: diarrhea)
- -rrhexis (example: myorrhexis)

SURGICAL PROCEDURES

- -centesis—to puncture in order to aspirate
- -desis—binding or fixation
- -ectomy—excision, surgical removal of
- -lithotomy—incision for removal of stones
- -otomy—incision into
- -pexy—suspension or fixation
- -plasty—repair or surgical reconstruction of
- -scopy—inspection/examination through a lighted scope
- -stomy—creation of a new opening for drainage

TERMS

MEDICAL TERMINOLOGY REVIEW

(*Suggestion:* use these terms to make flash cards.)

ab- away from, absent

abdominocentesis surgical puncture of the abdomen to remove fluid

acrocyanosis blue condition of the extremities

adenoma tumor of a gland

adrenomegaly enlargement of the adrenal gland(s)

-algesia pain, sensitivity to pain

analgesia take away pain, free from pain

anteroposterior passing from front to rear

antipyretic against fever; fever-reducing

aplasia lack of formation or development; usually refers to an organ

arteriosclerosis thickening (hardening) of the arteries

arthritis inflammation of the joints

bradycardia slow heart rate (pulse)

cardiomegaly enlargement of the heart

cervicofacial pertaining to the face and neck

chiroplasty surgical repair of the hands

cholecystitis inflammation of the gallbladder

cyanosis bluish condition of the skin

cystitis bladder inflammation

cytology study of cells

cytoscopy microscopic examination of cells

dacryocystitis inflammation of a tear sac

dactyl/o digit, finger or toe

dermatosis any skin lesion or eruption

dextr/o right

duodenoscopy inspection of the duodenum with a scope

dyskinesia difficult or painful movement

dyspepsia indigestion or painful digestion

-emia pertaining to the blood

encephal/o pertaining to the brain

encephalitis inflammation of the brain

endocarditis inflammation of the inside lining of the heart

enteritis inflammation of the small intestine

gastrectasia stretching of the stomach

gastritis inflammation of the stomach

gingivoglossitis inflammation of the gums and tongue

gynecopathy any disease of the female reproductive system

hemiplegia paralysis of one half of the body

hemostasis to stop or control bleeding

hepatomegaly enlargement of the liver

hyperplasia excessive formation of cells or tissue

hypoglycemia less-than-normal blood glucose level

hypothermia below normal temperature

hysterorrhaphy suturing of the uterus

inter- between, in the midst

intracerebral within the main part of the brain

intravascular within a vessel

laparotomy incision of the abdominal wall

leukopenia decreased white cells

lipectomy excision of fatty tissue

litholysis destruction of a stone

-logy the study of

lymphadenitis inflammation of the lymph glands/nodes

-lysis destruction, destroy, dissolution

-malacia softening of tissue

mammoplasty surgical reconstruction of the breast

meningocele herniation of the meninges

menostasis suppression of menses

metrorrhexis rupture of the uterus

myc/o fungus or mold

nasopharyngeal pertaining to nose and throat

necrosis death of tissue or bone

nephrolysis destruction of kidney tissue

nephropathy disease of the kidney

neuralgia pain in the nerves

neuropathy disease of the nerves

neurotripsy surgical crushing of a nerve

onychocryptosis an ingrown (hidden) nail, finger or toe

onychomycosis condition of fungus of the nails

oophorectomy excision of an ovary

orchidectomy surgical removal of a testicle

osteoarthropathy disease of joints and bones

osteocyte bone cell

otalgia pain in the ear

-pepsis digestion

peri- around, about

phag/o to ingest or eat

phleborrhexis rupture of a vein

-phonia voice

pneum/o air

pneumon/o lung

posteromedial middle of the back, middle of backside

proctorrhagia hemorrhage from the rectum

pyeloplasty surgical repair of the renal pelvis

pyogenesis formation of pus

retinopathy disease of the retina

retroperitoneal behind the peritoneum

rhinorrhea flow or discharge from the nose

-rrhagia burst forth, hemorrhage

-rrhexis rupture of a vessel, organ, or tissue

splenomegaly enlargement of the spleen

-stasis to stop or control

sten/o narrowing

stomatomycosis condition of fungus in the mouth

-stomy forming a new opening

subpulmonary below the lungs

tachycardia increased heart rate (pulse)

tenodynia painful tendon

thrombectomy surgical removal of a blood clot

transthorax across the chest

tympan/o eardrum, drumlike

unilateral on one side

vas/o vessel or duct

REVIEW QUESTIONS

All questions are relevant for all medical assisting and medical administrative certification exams.

1. The word root **vas/o** means:
   A. vein.
   B. artery.
   C. vessel.
   D. capillary.

   Answer: **C**
   Why: vas/o = vessel or duct
   Review: Yes ○   No ○

2. The word root **pneumon/o** means:
   A. air.
   B. breathing.
   C. bronchus.
   D. pleura.
   E. lung.

   Answer: **E**
   Why: pneumon/o = lung
   Review: Yes ○   No ○

3. The suffix **-rrhexis** means:
   A. discharge.
   B. pain.
   C. flow.
   D. rupture.

   Answer: **D**
   Why: -rrhexis = rupture of a vessel, organ, or tissue
   Review: Yes ○   No ○

4. The word root **my/o** means:
   A. muscle.
   B. many.
   C. middle.
   D. mold.
   E. mucus.

   Answer: **A**
   Why: my/o= muscle
   Review: Yes ○   No ○

5. The term **rhinorrhea** means:
   A. inflammation of the nose.
   B. suturing of the nostrils.
   C. discharge from the nose.
   D. enlargement of the nose.

   Answer: **C**
   Why: rhin/o = nose -rrhea = flow or discharge
   Review: Yes ○   No ○

6. The term **hepatomegaly** means:
   A. dysfunction of the kidneys.
   B. underdevelopment of the liver.
   C. increased production of blood cells.
   D. enlargement of the liver.
   E. hemorrhage from the liver.

   Answer: **D**
   Why: hepat/o = liver -megaly = enlargement
   Review: Yes ○   No ○

7. The suffix **-lysis** refers to:
   A. formation.
   B. hardening.
   C. abnormal.
   D. destruction.

   Answer: **D**
   Why: -lysis = dissolution or destruction
   Review: Yes ○   No ○

8. The word root **phag/o** means:
   A. grow.
   B. chew.
   C. repair.
   D. narrow.
   E. ingest.

Answer: **E**
Why: phag/o = to ingest or eat
Review: Yes ◯   No ◯

9. The term for *voice* is:
   A. phobia.
   B. ptosis.
   C. phasia.
   D. phonia.

Answer: **D**
Why: -phonia, phon/o = voice
Review: Yes ◯   No ◯

10. The term **-malacia** means:
   A. accumulation.
   B. drooping.
   C. softening.
   D. constriction.
   E. hardening.

Answer: **C**
Why: -malacia = softening of tissues
Review: Yes ◯   No ◯

11. The term **neuropathy** means:
   A. inflammation of the nerves.
   B. hardening of the nerves.
   C. disease of the nerves.
   D. surgical removal of nerves.

Answer: **C**
Why: neur/o = nerves -pathy = disease, disease process
Review: Yes ◯   No ◯

12. The suffix **-rrhagia** means:
   A. rupture.
   B. inflammation.
   C. painful.
   D. surgical suturing.
   E. burst forth.

Answer: **E**
Why: -rrhagia = bursting forth
Review: Yes ◯   No ◯

13. The term **gastritis** means:
   A. disease of the gallbladder.
   B. flow from the duodenum.
   C. inflammation of the stomach.
   D. rupture of the spleen.

Answer: **C**
Why: gastr/o = stomach -itis = inflammation
Review: Yes ◯   No ◯

14. Inflammation of the joints is known as:
   A. tendonitis.
   B. bursitis.
   C. osteitis.
   D. arthritis.
   E. myositis.

Answer: **D**
Why: arthr/o = joints -itis = inflammation
Review: Yes ◯   No ◯

15. The term **hypoglycemia** means:
   A. elevated blood glucose level.
   B. lower-than-normal blood glucose level.
   C. presence of sugar in the blood.
   D. elevated sodium level.

Answer: **B**
Why: hypo- = low, under normal level glyc/o = sugar, glucose -emia = pertaining to blood
Review: Yes ◯   No ◯

16. The term **otalgia** means:
   A. discharge from the ear.
   B. disease of the ear.
   C. pain in the ear.
   D. inflammation of the ear.
   E. opening in the ear.

Answer: **C**
Why: ot/o = ear -algia = pain
Review: Yes ○   No ○

17. The medical term that means *to control bleeding* is:
   A. hemostasis.
   B. hemophilia.
   C. hematoma.
   D. hemoccult.

Answer: **A**
Why: hem/o = blood -stasis = to stop or control
Review: Yes ○   No ○

18. The term **enteritis** means:
   A. inflammation of the colon.
   B. disease of the large intestine.
   C. inflammation of the small intestine.
   D. disease of the esophagus.
   E. inflammation of the mouth.

Answer: **C**
Why: enter/o = small intestine -itis = inflammation
Review: Yes ○   No ○

19. The term meaning *indigestion* or *painful digestion* is:
   A. dyspnea.
   B. dysphagia.
   C. dysplasia.
   D. dyspepsia.

Answer: **D**
Why: dys- = painful or difficult -pepsis = digestion
Review: Yes ○   No ○

20. The medical term used to describe any skin lesion or eruption is:
   A. dermatomycosis.
   B. dermatoplasty.
   C. dermatoid.
   D. dermatoma.
   E. dermatosis.

Answer: **E**
Why: dermat/o = skin -osis = any condition, process
Review: Yes ○   No ○

21. The term meaning *bladder inflammation* is:
   A. cystorrhexis.
   B. cystocele.
   C. cystalgia.
   D. cystitis.

Answer: **D**
Why: cyst/o = bladder or sac -itis = inflammation
Review: Yes ○   No ○

22. The term **bradycardia** means:
   A. slow blood pressure.
   B. increased blood flow.
   C. slow heart rate.
   D. increased heart rate.
   E. slow blood flow.

Answer: **C**
Why: brady- = slow cardi/o = the heart -a = pertaining to
Review: Yes ○   No ○

23. The word part **-algesia** means:
   A. against.
   B. pertaining to.
   C. pain.
   D. without.

Answer: **C**
Why: -algesia = sensation of pain
Review: Yes ○   No ○

24. The word part **dextr/o** means:
    A. sugar.
    B. glucose.
    C. left.
    D. back.
    E. right.

Answer: **E**
Why: dextr/o = right or on the right side
Review: Yes ○   No ○

25. The word part **encephal/o** means:
    A. brain.
    B. head.
    C. cerebrum.
    D. skull.

Answer: **A**
Why: encephal/o = inside the head (the brain)
Review: Yes ○   No ○

26. The term **osteocyte** means:
    A. compact bone.
    B. spongy bone.
    C. bone cell.
    D. bone cyst.
    E. bone infection.

Answer: **C**
Why: oste/o = pertaining to bone -cyte = cell
Review: Yes ○   No ○

27. The word part meaning *eardrum* is:
    A. cochle/o.
    B. salping/o.
    C. myring/o.
    D. tympan/o.

Answer: **D**
Why: tympan/o = a structure that is drumlike
Review: Yes ○   No ○

28. The term **oophorectomy** means:
    A. formation of an ovum.
    B. repair of an ovary.
    C. rupture of the uterus.
    D. incision into the uterus.
    E. excision of an ovary.

Answer: **E**
Why: oophor/o = pertaining to the ovary -ectomy
= surgical removal, excision
Review: Yes ○   No ○

29. The term **nephropathy** means:
    A. distention of the bladder.
    B. infection in the kidney.
    C. inflammation of a nerve.
    D. disease of the kidney.

Answer: **D**
Why: nephr/o = kidney -pathy = any disease
Review: Yes ○   No ○

30. The term **acrocyanosis** means a blue condition of the:
    A. extremities.
    B. neck.
    C. face.
    D. torso.
    E. head.

Answer: **A**
Why: acr/o = extremity cyan/o = blue -osis = any
condition
Review: Yes ○   No ○

31. The term **splenomegaly** means:
    A. prolapse of the spleen.
    B. dysfunction of the spleen.
    C. pain in the spleen.
    D. enlargement of the spleen.

Answer: **D**
Why: splen/o = pertaining to the spleen -megaly
= great, enlarged
Review: Yes ○   No ○

32. The medical term meaning *within a vessel* is:
   A. intercellular.
   B. interarterial.
   C. intravascular.
   D. intravalvular.
   E. intra-articular.

Answer: **C**
Why: intra- = within vascul/o = vessel -ar = pertaining to
Review: Yes ◯　No ◯

33. The term **abdominocentesis** means:
   A. surgical puncture of the abdomen.
   B. swelling of the abdomen.
   C. dilation of the abdomen.
   D. suturing of the abdomen.

Answer: **A**
Why: abdomin/o = pertaining to the abdomen -centesis = to puncture
Review: Yes ◯　No ◯

34. The suffix -**stomy** means:
   A. to cut into.
   B. surgical repair.
   C. surgical removal.
   D. to form a new opening.
   E. to suture an opening.

Answer: **D**
Why: -stomy = to make a new opening
Review: Yes ◯　No ◯

35. The term **stenosis** means:
   A. softening.
   B. dilation.
   C. spasm.
   D. narrowing.

Answer: **D**
Why: sten/o = narrow -osis = condition
Review: Yes ◯　No ◯

36. **Cardiomegaly** is a term that means:
   A. rupture of the heart.
   B. hardening of the heart tissue.
   C. inflammation of the heart.
   D. occlusion of heart vessels.
   E. enlargement of the heart.

Answer: **E**
Why: cardi/o = heart -megaly = large or enlargement
Review: Yes ◯　No ◯

37. The term **lymphadenitis** means:
   A. inflammation of lymph fluid.
   B. inflammation of adrenal glands.
   C. infection of the spleen.
   D. inflammation of the lymph glands/ nodes.

Answer: **D**
Why: lymph/o = pertaining to lymph aden/o = pertaining to a gland -itis = inflammation
Review: Yes ◯　No ◯

38. A term meaning *rupture of the uterus* is:
   A. metrorrhea.
   B. metrorrhexis.
   C. menorrhagia.
   D. meatorrhaphy.
   E. metritis.

Answer: **B**
Why: metr/o = related to the uterus -rrhexis = rupture of a body part; another term with the same meaning is hysterorrhexis
Review: Yes ◯　No ◯

39. The microscopic examination of cells is called:
   A. cytoscopy.
   B. cystoscope.
   C. cythemia.
   D. cystotomy.

Answer: **A**
Why: cyt/o = cell -scopy = to study or examine
Review: Yes ◯　No ◯

40. The prefix meaning *between* is:
  A. extra-.
  B. intra-.
  C. inter-.
  D. supra-.
  E. infra-.

Answer: **C**
Why: inter- = between, in the midst
Review: Yes ○   No ○

41. The term used for surgical removal of a blood clot is:
  A. hematectomy.
  B. hemolysis.
  C. thrombolysis.
  D. thrombectomy.

Answer: **D**
Why: thromb/o = clot, blood clot -ectomy = surgical removal, to excise
Review: Yes ○   No ○

42. The term meaning *hemorrhage from an artery* is:
  A. arteriosclerosis.
  B. arteriorrhagia.
  C. arteriorrhaphy.
  D. arteriolysis.
  E. arteriotomy.

Answer: **B**
Why: arteri/o = artery -rrhagia = hemorrhage, to burst forth
Review: Yes ○   No ○

43. The term meaning *destruction of a stone* is:
  A. lithogenesis.
  B. litholysis.
  C. lithiasis.
  D. lithotomy.

Answer: **B**
Why: lith/o = stone, calculus -lysis = destruction
Review: Yes ○   No ○

44. The term meaning *below the lungs* is:
  A. subpulmonary.
  B. infrapulmonary.
  C. interpulmonary.
  D. interthoracic.
  E. intercostal.

Answer: **A**
Why: sub- = beneath, under pulmon/o = lungs -ary = pertaining to
Review: Yes ○   No ○

45. The term **cholecystitis** means inflammation of the:
  A. gallbladder.
  B. liver.
  C. adrenal glands.
  D. kidneys.

Answer: **A**
Why: chol/e = bile (gall) cyst/o = bladder, sac -itis = inflammation
Review: Yes ○   No ○

46. The term **stomatomycosis** means a condition of:
  A. fungus in the mouth.
  B. mucus in the mouth.
  C. fungus in the stomach.
  D. mucus in the stomach.
  E. inflammation of the mouth.

Answer: **A**
Why: stomat/o = mouth, opening myc/o = fungus -osis = condition
Review: Yes ○   No ○

47. The term for inflammation of the gums and tongue is:
  A. gingivoglossitis.
  B. stomatitis.
  C. glossopharyngitis.
  D. glossostomatitis.

Answer: **A**
Why: gingiv/o = gum tissue gloss/o = tongue -itis = inflammation
Review: Yes ◯   No ◯

48. The term meaning *incision of the abdominal wall* is:
  A. abdominocentesis.
  B. laparectomy.
  C. laparotomy.
  D. peritonitis.
  E. gastrotomy.

Answer: **C**
Why: lapar/o = abdomen, abdominal wall -tomy = incision into
Review: Yes ◯   No ◯

49. The term meaning *behind the peritoneum* is:
  A. subperitoneal.
  B. retroperitoneal.
  C. subabdominal.
  D. intraperitoneal.

Answer: **B**
Why: retro- = located behind, backward peritone/o = pertaining to the peritoneum -al = pertaining to
Review: Yes ◯   No ◯

50. The term meaning *surgical repair of the hands* is:
  A. chiromegaly.
  B. dactylomegaly.
  C. chiroplasty.
  D. dactyloplasty.
  E. dactylitis.

Answer: **C**
Why: chir/o = pertaining to the hand -plasty = surgical repair, plastic surgery
Review: Yes ◯   No ◯

51. A term meaning *stretching of the stomach* is:
  A. gastrectasia.
  B. gastralgia.
  C. gastrorrhagia.
  D. gastroplasty.

Answer: **A**
Why: gastr/o = stomach -ectasia = dilation, stretching
Review: Yes ◯   No ◯

52. The term meaning *take away pain or free from pain* is:
  A. algesia.
  B. analgesia.
  C. angina.
  D. anesthesia.
  E. dysplasia.

Answer: **B**
Why: an- = without -algesia = sensation of pain
Review: Yes ◯   No ◯

53. The term meaning *inflammation of the brain* is:
  A. meningitis.
  B. cephalalgia.
  C. encephalitis.
  D. encephalomeningitis.

Answer: **C**
Why: en- = within cephal/o = head -itis = inflammation
Review: Yes ◯   No ◯

54. The word root **dactyl/o** means:
   A. ear.
   B. foot.
   C. hand.
   D. eye.
   E. finger.

Answer: **E**
Why: dactyl/o = digit, finger or toe
Review: Yes ○   No ○

55. The term **dyskinesia** means:
   A. painful knee.
   B. difficult movement.
   C. deformed spine.
   D. curved spine.

Answer: **B**
Why: dys- = difficult, painful kinesi/o = movement, motion -ia = pertaining to
Review: Yes ○   No ○

56. The term meaning *increased heart rate (pulse)* is:
   A. tachycardia.
   B. bradycardia.
   C. hyperpnea.
   D. hypoxia.
   E. arrhythmia

Answer: **A**
Why: tachy- = rapid, fast cardi/o = pertaining to the heart -ia = pertaining to
Review: Yes ○   No ○

57. The term meaning *on one side* is:
   A. medial.
   B. bilateral.
   C. transverse.
   D. unilateral.

Answer: **D**
Why: uni- = one later/o = side -al = pertaining to
Review: Yes ○   No ○

58. The term **cyanosis** means:
   A. lack of oxygen.
   B. swelling of the feet.
   C. bluish condition.
   D. condition of red cells.
   E. obstructed airway.

Answer: **C**
Why: cyan/o = blue, discoloration -osis = condition of
Review: Yes ○   No ○

59. The term **antipyretic** means:
   A. increased temperature.
   B. bacteria-reducing.
   C. fever-reducing.
   D. decreased pus formation.

Answer: **C**
Why: anti- = against pyret/o = relating to fever -ic = pertaining to
Review: Yes ○ No ○

60. The suffix meaning *the study of* is:
   A. -logist.
   B. -graphy.
   C. -logy.
   D. -scopy.
   E. -osis.

Answer: **C**
Why: -logy = study of, knowledge
Review: Yes ○   No ○

61. The term **cytology** means:
   A. person who studies cells.
   B. study of the bladder.
   C. measuring bladder contents.
   D. study of cells.

Answer: **D**
Why: cyt/o = cell -logy = study of
Review: Yes ○   No ○

62. The term **leukopenia** means:
    A. increased platelets.
    B. decreased white cells.
    C. enlarged red cells.
    D. increased thrombocytes.
    E. increased white count.

Answer: **B**
Why: leuk/o = white (cells) -penia = decrease, lack of
Review: Yes ○   No ○

63. The term meaning *thickening (hardening) of the arteries* is:
    A. phlebectasia.
    B. arteriorrhagia.
    C. arteriosclerosis.
    D. phlebotomy.

Answer: **C**
Why: arteri/o = artery scler/o = thickening, hardening -osis = condition of
Review: Yes ○   No ○

64. The prefix **ab-** means:
    A. against.
    B. before.
    C. toward.
    D. uneven.
    E. away from.

Answer: **E**
Why: ab- = away from, absent
Review: Yes ○   No ○

65. The prefix **peri-** means:
    A. middle.
    B. side.
    C. below.
    D. around.

Answer: **D**
Why: peri- = around, about
Review: Yes ○   No ○

66. The term **neuralgia** means:
    A. tumor of nerve cells/fibers.
    B. surgical removal of nerve fibers.
    C. pain in the nerves.
    D. numbness of nerves.
    E. twitching of nerves.

Answer: **C**
Why: neur/o = nerve, nerve cell -algia = pain
Review: Yes ○   No ○

67. The term **cervicofacial** pertains to the:
    A. neck and arm.
    B. face and neck.
    C. spine and pelvis.
    D. face and scalp.

Answer: **B**
Why: cervic/o = neck, neck of an organ facial = pertaining to the face
Review: Yes ○   No ○

68. A term meaning *destruction of kidney tissue* is:
    A. renopathy.
    B. nephropexy.
    C. nephralgia.
    D. pyelitis.
    E. nephrolysis.

Answer: **E**
Why: nephr/o = kidney -lysis = destruction, breakdown
Review: Yes ○   No ○

69. The term **posteromedial** pertains to:
    A. upper back.
    B. lower back.
    C. middle back.
    D. toward the back.

Answer: **C**
Why: poster/o = back, backside medi/o = the middle -al = pertaining to
Review: Yes ○   No ○

70. The term **osteoarthropathy** means:
    A. bone inflammation.
    B. inflammation of joints.
    C. condition of swollen joints.
    D. disease of joints and bones.
    E. infection of the bones.

Answer: **D**
Why: oste/o = bone arthr/o = joint -pathy = disease process, disease
Review: Yes ⭕   No ⭕

71. The term **orchidectomy** means:
    A. surgical removal of a testicle.
    B. incision into the scrotum.
    C. undescended testicle.
    D. excision of the scrotum.

Answer: **A**
Why: orchid/o = relating to the testicle -ectomy = surgical removal
Review: Yes ⭕   No ⭕

72. The term **adenoma** means:
    A. benign tumor.
    B. malignant tumor.
    C. tumor of a gland.
    D. pituitary disease.
    E. abnormal growth.

Answer: **C**
Why: aden/o = gland -oma = tumor
Review: Yes ⭕   No ⭕

73. The term **mammoplasty** means:
    A. surgical reconstruction of the breast.
    B. excision of breast tumor.
    C. X-ray exam of the breasts.
    D. biopsy of breast tissue.

Answer: **A**
Why: mamm/o = breast -plasty = plastic surgery, surgical reconstruction
Review: Yes ⭕   No ⭕

74. The term **adrenomegaly** means:
    A. pathology of a gland.
    B. destruction of tissue.
    C. enlargement of the adrenal gland(s).
    D. condition of the thyroid.
    E. inflammation of a gland.

Answer: **C**
Why: adren/o = adrenal gland(s) -megaly = enlargement
Review: Yes ⭕   No ⭕

75. The term **gynecopathy** means:
    A. study of female reproductive system.
    B. specialist who studies women's diseases.
    C. inflammation of female organs.
    D. any disease of the female reproductive system.

Answer: **D**
Why: gynec/o = female -pathy = any disease process
Review: Yes ⭕   No ⭕

76. A term meaning *an ingrown nail* is:
    A. onychectomy.
    B. onychalgia.
    C. onychitis.
    D. onychocryptosis.
    E. onychorrhea.

Answer: **D**
Why: onych/o = fingernail or toenail crypt/o = hidden, concealed (ingrown) -osis = any condition of
Review: Yes ⭕   No ⭕

77. The term meaning *excision of fatty tissue* is:
    A. lipolysis.
    B. lipoma.
    C. lipectomy.
    D. lipoidosis.

Answer: **C**
Why: lip/o = fat, fatty tissue -ectomy = surgical removal, excision
Review: Yes ⭕   No ⭕

78. The term meaning *rupture of a vein* is:
  A. phleborrhagia.
  B. phlebopexy.
  C. phlebectasia.
  D. phleborrhexis.
  E. phlebitis.

Answer: **D**
Why: phleb/o = vein -rrhexis = rupture
Review: Yes ◯   No ◯

79. The term **duodenoscopy** means:
  A. examination of the colon.
  B. inspection of the duodenum with a scope.
  C. make a new opening into the duodenum.
  D. incision into the colon.

Answer: **B**
Why: duoden/o = duodenum, part of small intestine -scopy = to examine or inspect using an endoscope
Review: Yes ◯   No ◯

80. A term meaning *a painful tendon* is:
  A. tendonitis.
  B. tenotomy.
  C. tenodynia.
  D. tendoplasty.
  E. tenorrhaphy.

Answer: **C**
Why: ten/o = tendon, connects muscle to bone -dynia = pain
Review: Yes ◯   No ◯

81. The term **dacryocystitis** means:
  A. excision of a tear sac.
  B. protrusion of a lacrimal sac.
  C. pain in a lacrimal sac.
  D. inflammation of a tear sac.

Answer: **D**
Why: dacry/o = tear (lacrimal) cyst/o = sac, bladder -itis = inflammation of
Review: Yes ◯   No ◯

82. The term **intracerebral** means:
  A. between the spine and brain.
  B. within the spinal cord.
  C. beneath the meninges.
  D. within the main part of the brain.
  E. between the meninges.

Answer: **D**
Why: intra- = within cerebr/o = cerebrum, main part of the brain -al = pertaining to
Review: Yes ◯   No ◯

83. The term meaning *condition of fungus of the nails* is:
  A. dermatomycosis.
  B. onychomycosis.
  C. dermatosis.
  D. onychitis.

Answer: **B**
Why: onych/o = finger or toe nail myc/o = fungus -osis = any condition
Review: Yes ◯   No ◯

84. The term meaning *death of tissue or bone* is:
  A. necrosis.
  B. necropsy.
  C. necrophilia.
  D. necrotomy.
  E. necrectomy.

Answer: **A**
Why: necr/o = death, dead cells or tissue -osis = any condition
Review: Yes ◯   No ◯

85. The term meaning *passing from front to rear* is:
  A. anterosuperior.
  B. anteroexternal.
  C. anteroinferior.
  D. anteroposterior.

Answer: **D**
Why: anter/o = anterior, front, before poster/o = back, rear
Review: Yes ◯   No ◯

86. The term **aplasia** means:
  A. decreased plasma.
  B. lack of formation.
  C. difficulty breathing.
  D. without pulse.
  E. painful breathing.

Answer: **B**
Why: a- = without, not -plasia = development, formation
Review: Yes ◯   No ◯

87. The term **endocarditis** means:
  A. infection of the heart valves.
  B. heart attack.
  C. inflammation of the inside lining of the heart.
  D. aneurysm within the heart.

Answer: **C**
Why: endo- = inside, innermost cardi/o = heart -itis = inflammation of
Review: Yes ◯   No ◯

88. The term **pyeloplasty** means:
  A. surgical repair of the renal pelvis.
  B. plastic surgery of the kidney.
  C. incision into the kidney.
  D. excision of the renal pelvis.
  E. surgical repair of the pelvis.

Answer: **A**
Why: pyel/o = pelvis, renal pelvis -plasty = surgical repair
Review: Yes ◯   No ◯

89. The term meaning *below normal temperature* is:
  A. hypoxia.
  B. hypotensive.
  C. hypothermia.
  D. hypotrophy.

Answer: **C**
Why: hypo- = below, sub, less than normal therm/o = temperature -ia = pertaining to
Review: Yes ◯   No ◯

90. The term **hysterorrhaphy** means:
  A. rupture of the uterus.
  B. removal of the cervix.
  C. suturing of the uterus.
  D. surgical fixation of the cervix.
  E. incision into the cervix.

Answer: **C**
Why: hyster/o = uterus -rrhaphy = suturing, sewing
Review: Yes ◯   No ◯

91. The term **proctorrhagia** means
  A. rupture of the rectum.
  B. fissure of the anus.
  C. inflammation of the rectum.
  D. hemorrhage from the rectum.

Answer: **D**
Why: proct/o = rectum and anus -rrhagia = hemorrhage, burst forth
Review: Yes ◯   No ◯

92. The term for *disease of the retina* is:
  A. renopathy.
  B. retinitis.
  C. retinoplasty.
  D. renography.
  E. retinopathy.

Answer: **E**
Why: retin/o = retina of the eye -pathy = disease process
Review: Yes ◯   No ◯

93. The term meaning herniation of the meninges is:
  A. meningomyelocele.
  B. myelocele.
  C. meningocele.
  D. encephalocele.

Answer: **C**
Why: mening/o = meninges -cele = herniation, protrusion
Review: Yes ◯   No ◯

94. The term meaning *suppression of menses* is:
    A. menstruation.
    B. menorrhagia.
    C. menorrhea.
    D. menostasis.
    E. dysmenorrhea.

Answer: **D**
Why: men/o = menstruation, menses -stasis = control, suppress
Review: Yes ○   No ○

95. The term meaning *across the chest* is:
    A. anterolateral.
    B. transverse.
    C. transthorax.
    D. anterothoracic.

Answer: **C**
Why: trans- = across, cross over thorax = pertaining to the chest
Review: Yes ○   No ○

96. The term meaning *excessive formation of cells or tissue* is:
    A. hyperphasia.
    B. hyperplasia.
    C. hypertonic.
    D. hyperopia.
    E. hypotonic.

Answer: **B**
Why: hyper- = excessive, more than normal -plasia = formation
Review: Yes ○   No ○

97. The term **pyogenesis** means:
    A. growth of cells.
    B. formation of pus.
    C. production of bile.
    D. origin of a fever.

Answer: **B**
Why: py/o = pus -genesis = beginning, formation
Review: Yes ○   No ○

98. The term **hemiplegia** means:
    A. inflammation of the lower legs.
    B. moving one half of the body.
    C. paralysis of upper body.
    D. paralysis of one half of the body.
    E. paralysis of one leg.

Answer: **D**
Why: hemi- = half, one half -plegia = pertaining to paralysis
Review: Yes ○   No ○

99. The term **nasopharyngeal** means pertaining to:
    A. nose and sinuses.
    B. mouth and throat.
    C. nose and throat.
    D. mouth and sinuses.

Answer: **C**
Why: nas/o = nose pharyng/o = pharynx, throat -al = pertaining to
Review: Yes ○   No ○

100. The term **neurotripsy** means:
    A. removal of a nerve.
    B. surgical crushing of a nerve.
    C. suturing of a nerve.
    D. paralysis of a nerve.
    E. rupture of a nerve.

Answer: **B**
Why: neur/o = nerve, nerve cell -tripsy = surgically crushing
Review: Yes ○   No ○

101. Select the correct spelling of the term:
    A. Hemmorrhoid
    B. Hemorrhoid
    C. Hemmorhoid
    D. Hemorhoid
    E. Hemorroid

Answer: **B**
Review: Yes ○   No ○

102. Scraping of a body cavity is:

    A.   curretage.

    B.   currettage.

    C.   curetage.

    D.   curettage.

Answer: **D**

Review: Yes ◯   No ◯

CRITICAL THINKING CASE REVIEW

Mr. Valdez is scheduled for a lithotripsy of his right kidney. The physician explained common side effects of the procedure are blood in the urine and pain for which he gave the patient a prescription.

1. The kidneys are located in the back of the body which is referred to as:

    A.   dorsal.

    B.   distal.

    C.   lateral.

    D.   inferior.

    E.   caudal.

Answer: **A**

Why: Dorsal refers to the backside of the body

Review: Yes ◯   No ◯

2. The lithotripsy is a medical procedure that:

    A.   requires an opening into the abdomen.

    B.   crushes stones.

    C.   visualizes the problem through a scope.

    D.   repairs the kidney.

Answer: **B**

Why: "Litho" refers to stone and "tripsy" to crushing

Review: Yes ◯   No ◯

3. The procedure is being done for:

    A.   cholylithiasis.

    B.   polynephritis.

    C.   neuritis.

    D.   nephrolithiasis.

    E.   stomatitis.

Answer: **D**

Why: "Nephron" refers to kidney; "lith" refers to stones, and "iasis" refers to abnormal.

Review: Yes ◯   No ◯

4. The prescription given to Mr. Valdez for pain is an:

    A.   antibiotic.

    B.   anesthetic.

    C.   antiemetic.

    D.   analgesic.

Answer: **D**

Why: "a" refers to absence of; "algia" refers to pain; "ic" refers to condition of

Review: Yes ◯   No ◯

5. The doctor advised Mr. Valdez that one of the side effects of the lithotripsy is:

    A.   hematuria.

    B.   hematocrit.

    C.   ureteritis.

    D.   cystitis.

    E.   thrombitis.

Answer: **A**

Why: The side effect is blood in the urine; "hemo/hemat" refers to blood, and "uria" refers to urine.

Review: Yes ◯   No ◯

Anatomy and Physiology

Review Tip:

"Anatomy and Physiology" is the most demanding chapter. Be sure to study all the figures and tables!! The national exams generally contain at least two questions on each body system. The endocrine system, with the glands and hormones, tends to be the most difficult. Remember, during the exam, do not spend too much time on any one question. At least one question will require you to know the order of structures such as the order that urine flows from the body or the order of the vertebrae or the parts of the large (or small) intestines. Schedule your study time by body system and reward yourself when you finish this grueling chapter!

OVERVIEW

Knowledge of anatomy and physiology is a foundation for many areas of medical assisting and medical administrative specialization. It is used in both administrative (e.g., insurance billing and coding) and clinical practice (e.g., patient assessment). With a solid understanding of the structure and function of body parts, you will be able to analyze questions and to solve problems.

Anatomy—the study of body structure

Physiology—the study of body function

Pathology—the study of abnormal changes in body structure or function, usually caused by disease

BODY ORDERING

Living things are arranged from simple to complex. Figure 6-1 demonstrates the order of the structures that make up the human body.

- Chemicals—atoms and molecules
- Cells—structural and functional units of life

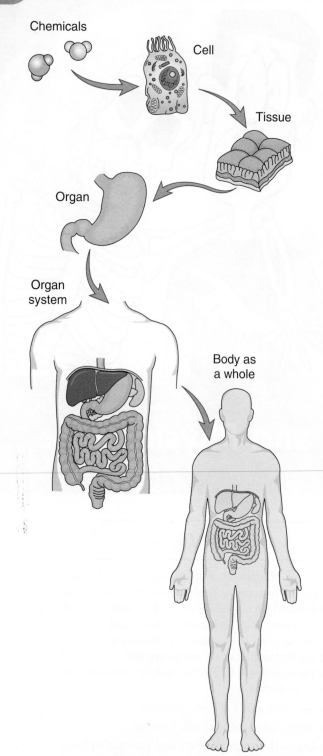

Chemicals

Cell

Tissue

Organ

Organ
system

Body as
a whole

FIGURE 6-1 Body ordering. (Reprinted with permission from Cohen BJ, Wood DL. *Memmler's the Human Body in Health and Disease.* 9th Ed. Philadelphia: Lippincott Williams & Wilkins, 2000.)

■ Tissues—groups of cells with similar structures and functions (such as connective tissue)

■ Organ—group of tissues working together to perform a function (e.g., kidney)

■ Systems—group of organs working together to perform a set of related functions

  • Integumentary system—skin and related structures that contain and protect

  • Skeletal system—bones and related structures that support

  • Muscular system—muscles and related structures that accommodate movement

  • Nervous system—nerves and related structures that receive stimuli and initiate responses

  • Sensory system—sensory neurons and special sense organs that detect the environment and changes

  • Endocrine system—glands and related structures that produce hormones

  • Cardiovascular system—heart and blood vessels that circulate blood to transport nutrients and remove waste from tissues

  • Lymphatic system—lymph, lymph nodes, and related organs that protect against and fight disease

  • Respiratory system—lungs and related structures that transport oxygen (O_2) and remove carbon dioxide (CO_2)

  • Digestive system—mouth, esophagus, stomach, intestines, liver, gallbladder, and pancreas, which ingest and process food and eliminate solid waste products

  • Urinary system—kidneys, ureters, bladder, and urethra, which remove nitrogen-type waste and regulate water balance

  • Reproductive system—gonads (ovaries or testes) and related sex organs and structures that reproduce the species

■ Body (organism)—group of systems working together to maintain life

ANATOMIC DESCRIPTORS

The national exams contain several questions related to the location of specific organs and other anatomic structures. Directional terms of the body help describe and locate these structures.

Body Directions and Planes

Figure 6-2 shows the imaginary planes dividing the body: the **frontal** (or coronal) **plane**, the **sagittal plane**, and the **transverse** (or horizontal) **plane**. The body is in anatomic position—upright, face forward, and arms down and slightly away from the sides with palms forward and feet and legs parallel. Other important descriptors of body directions are: **superior** (cranial or cephalic), **anterior** (ventral), **posterior** (dorsal), **inferior** (caudal), **proximal, distal, medial,** and **lateral.**

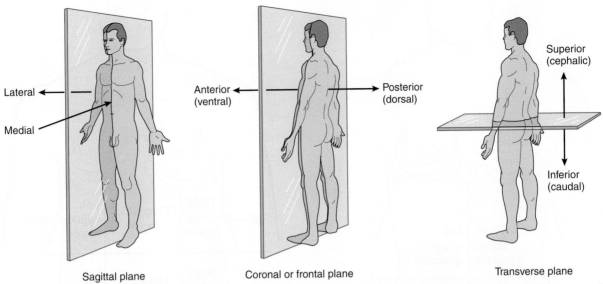

FIGURE 6-2 Body planes and directions. (Reprinted with permission from Willis MC. *Medical Terminology: A Programmed Learning Approach to the Language of Health Care.* Baltimore: Lippincott Williams & Wilkins, 2002.)

Body Cavities

The locations of organs are usually described as being in a specific body cavity or space. Directional terms (e.g., posterior, anterior, inferior) are used to determine the position in relation to other organs also found in that cavity. Figure 6-3 illustrates the following body cavities:

■ Cranial cavity—contains the brain

■ Spinal cavity—contains the spinal cord; runs continuously from the brain stem in the cranial cavity to the end of the spinal cord

■ Thoracic cavity—contains the heart, lung, and large blood vessels; it is separated from the abdominal cavity by the diaphragm; within the thoracic cavity lies the mediastinum, a smaller cavity between the lungs that contains the heart and large blood vessels

■ Abdominal cavity—contains the stomach, most of the intestines, the kidneys, liver, gallbladder, pancreas, and spleen; it is separated from the thoracic cavity (superior) by the diaphragm and from the pelvic cavity (inferior) by an imaginary line across the top of the hip bones

■ Pelvic cavity—contains the urinary bladder, rectum, and internal organs of the male/female reproductive systems; it is separated from the abdominal cavity (superior) by an imaginary line between the hip bones

Abdominal Quadrants and Regions

The abdomen is divided into four quadrants (right upper, left upper, right lower, and left lower) and nine regions

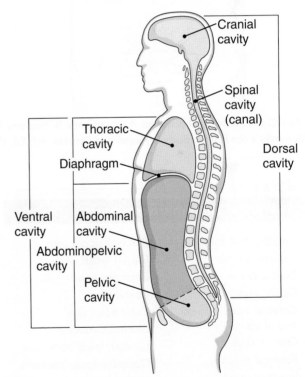

FIGURE 6-3 Body cavities. (Reprinted with permission from Cohen BJ, Wood DL. *Memmler's the Human Body in Health and Disease.* 9th Ed. Philadelphia: Lippincott Williams & Wilkins, 2000.)

(right hypochondriac, epigastric, left hypochondriac, right lumbar, umbilical, left lumbar, right iliac, hypogastric, and left iliac), as shown in Figure 6-4. Box 6-1 lists additional anatomic descriptors used to locate or describe the location of many body structures.

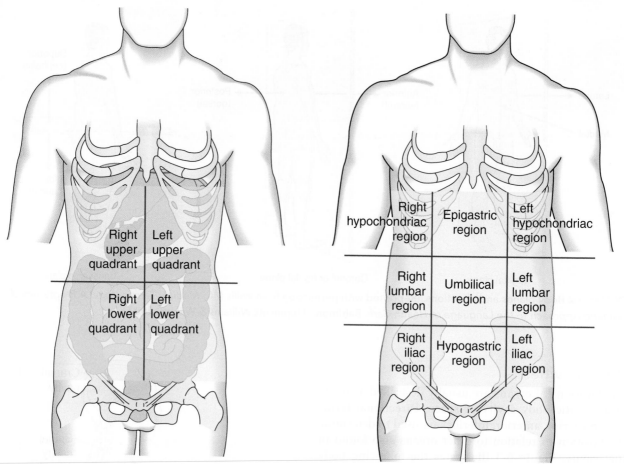

FIGURE 6-4 Abdominal divisions. **A.** Quadrants. **B.** Regions. (Reprinted with permission from Cohen BJ, Wood DL. *Memmler's the Human Body in Health and Disease.* 9th Ed. Philadelphia: Lippincott Williams & Wilkins, 2000.)

BOX 6-1

Additional anatomic descriptors

Antebrachial: forearm

Axillary: armpit

Buccal: cheek

Celiac: abdominal

Cervical: neck or lower end of uterus

Cranial: skull

Femoral: thigh

Inguinal: groin

Mammary: breast

Ophthalmic: eyes

Palmar: palm

Pectoral: chest

Plantar: sole of foot

Sacral: lower spine

Umbilical: navel

Antecubital: area anterior to elbow

Brachial: upper arm

Carpal: wrist

Cephalic: head

Costal: ribs

Cutaneous: skin

Gluteal: buttocks

Lumbar: lower back area

Occipital: lower posterior area of head

Otic: ears

Patellar: kneecap

Pedal: foot

Popliteal: back of knee

Tarsal: ankle

Vertebral: spine

BASIC BODY PROCESSES

For the body to grow, repair itself, and maintain equilibrium, certain processes must occur. Metabolism, fluid balance, and homeostasis are basic processes that take place or begin at the cell level.

Metabolism

Metabolism is energy transformation in living cells. This transformation occurs in two metabolic processes:

- Anabolism—builds up and repairs cells
- Catabolism—breaks down cells

Fluid Balance

Fluid balance is the regulation of the amount and composition of the body's fluids. The two major divisions of body fluid are given below:

- Extracellular fluid—body fluid outside the cell
- Intracellular fluid—body fluid inside the cell

The concentration of the fluid affects fluid movement and balance. The three basic solution concentrations are:

- Isotonic solution—this has the same concentration as intracellular fluid and moves in and out of the cell at the same rate; normal saline (0.9% salt) and 5% dextrose are examples of manufactured isotonic solutions

- Hypotonic solution—less concentrated than intracellular fluid, it results in excess fluid entering the cell and may cause the cell to rupture

- Hypertonic solution—more concentrated than intracellular fluid, it draws fluid away from the cell and causes the cell to shrink

Homeostasis

Homeostasis is the equilibrium or health of the body as measured by established norms for blood pressure, heart rate, temperature, respiratory rate, and other indicators.

BODY COMPOSITION

As previously noted, the body has an ordering of structures from simple to complex. Each type of structure (such as cells or tissues) has its own components or pieces, which are described in this section.

CELLS

Cells vary in size, shape, and function, but most cells contain the same basic components. Some of these components are shown in Figure 6-5.

- Cell (plasma) membrane—thin outermost layer of the cell; regulates what enters and leaves the cell

- Cytoplasm—colloidal substance (protoplasm) found in the cell; holds other structures in place

- Nuclear membrane—thin layer surrounding the nucleus

- Nucleus—located in the center of the cell; controls cell activity and contains genetic material (DNA)

- Nucleolus—small structure(s) in nucleus; holds ribonucleic acid (RNA) and ribosomes essential for protein formation

- Centriole—rod-shaped material in the cytoplasm that begins cell division

- Cilia (singular *cilium*)—hairlike processes on the cell surface that move foreign particles along the cell surface

- Flagella (singular *flagellum*)—whiplike processes on the cell surface; accommodate cell movement

Cell Division

Cell division occurs when one cell splits into two identical cells. The process is:

- Interphase—DNA duplicates and chromosomes double

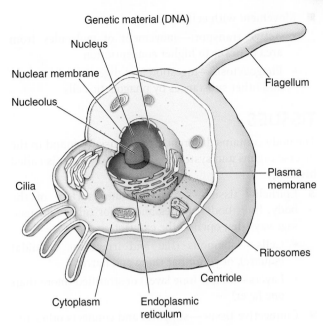

FIGURE 6-5 Basic human cell with select structures.

- Mitosis—also referred to as cell division; comprises four phases:
  - Prophase—centrioles move to opposite ends of the cell, forming two poles; they stretch filaments between them, resembling longitudes on a globe
  - Metaphase—chromosomes line up along an equator-type line along centriole filaments
  - Anaphase—duplicated chromosomes separate, and one of each begins to move toward the opposite centriole or pole
  - Telophase—nucleus divides in the center, forming two distinct cells

Cellular Movement of Substances

The maintenance of homeostasis and fluid balance and the process of metabolism require constant movement of nutrients into the cell and the elimination of waste products from the cell. The movement occurs at the cell or plasma membrane. It is semipermeable, meaning it allows passage of some substances but not others. The types of movement are categorized either as not requiring or requiring cell energy.

- Movement without cellular energy
  - Diffusion—movement of molecules from area of higher to lower concentration
  - Osmosis—water diffusion (movement from area of higher to lower concentration) through a semipermeable membrane
  - Filtration—process of pushing water with dissolved materials through one side of a membrane; an example is kidney filtration

■ Movement with cellular energy
  • Active transport—movement of molecules from area of lower to higher concentration
  • Phagocytosis—ingestion and digestion of bacteria and other substances by phagocytic cells

TISSUES

The body contains different types of **tissues** found in the diverse organs and systems. The study of tissue is called **histology**.

■ Epithelial tissue—forms the outer surface of the body; lines body cavities and major tubes and passageways that open to the exterior
  • Cells—squamous (flat and irregular), cuboidal (square), or columnar (long and narrow)
  • Layers—simple (one layer) or stratified (more than one layer)
■ Connective tissue—supports and connects other tissues and structures
  • Soft—areolar, adipose
  • Fibrous—tendons, ligaments, capsules, fascia
  • Hard—cartilage, bone
  • Liquid—blood, lymph
■ Muscle tissue—produces movement
  • Skeletal muscle—moves muscle and bone (voluntary)
  • Cardiac muscle—forms the heart (involuntary)
  • Smooth muscle—forms visceral organs (involuntary)
■ Nerve tissue—composed of neurons (nerve cells); provides networks to carry impulses

MEMBRANES

Membranes are thin sheets of tissue that line and protect body structures.

Epithelial Membranes

■ Serous membranes—secrete watery fluid
  • Parietal membranes—line body cavities
  • Visceral membranes—cover internal organs (pleura and pericardium are examples)
■ Mucous membranes—secrete mucus and line tubes or spaces open to the exterior
■ Cutaneous membrane—the skin

Connective Tissue Membranes

■ Synovial membranes—line joint cavities
■ Meninges—surround the brain and spinal cord and are composed of three layers
■ Fascia membranes—separate or bind muscles and permit movement of the skin
■ Other connective tissue membranes:

• Pericardium—surrounds heart
• Periosteum—surrounds bone
• Perichondrium—surrounds cartilage

BODY SYSTEMS

The chapter overview describes a *system* as a group of organs working together to perform a set of related functions. The human body comprises 12 interrelated systems and is described in detail in this section.

INTEGUMENTARY SYSTEM

Integumentary comes from the Greek word *integument*, meaning "cover." The **integumentary system** is the largest system in the body.

Functions of the Integumentary System

■ Protects against infection and other "invaders" (e.g., radiation)
■ Assists with prevention of dehydration
■ Controls body temperature
■ Receives sensory information
■ Eliminates waste products
■ Produces vitamin D

Components of the Integumentary System

■ Skin—the largest organ; external covering of the body (Fig. 6-6)
  • Epidermis ("epi" refers to above or outer)—the surface layer of the skin that contains strata (sublayers),

FIGURE 6-6 Cross-section of skin. (Reprinted with permission from Cohen BJ, Wood DL. *Memmler's the Human Body in Health and Disease.* 9th Ed. Philadelphia: Lippincott Williams & Wilkins, 2000.)

melanin (pigment giving the skin its color), and keratin (protein that thickens skin and makes skin waterproof)

- Dermis—the deeper layer of the skin that contains nerves, blood vessels, collagen, and other skin structures or appendages. Collagen is a fibrous protein found in the dermis, connective tissues, tendons, and ligaments. It is sometimes referred to as the body's glue, providing strength and flexibility.

■ Appendages—structures located in the dermis that perform special functions
- Sweat glands—coiled tubes located in the dermis that produce and transport sweat to help regulate body temperature and remove waste
- Ceruminous glands—structures located in the ear that secrete cerumen (earwax) for protection
- Sebaceous glands—structures connected to hair follicles located in the dermis that secrete sebum to lubricate skin and hair
- Hair—structures composed primarily of dead keratinized tissue that cover most of the body
- Nails—hard, keratinized structures located on tips of fingers and toes
- Subcutaneous tissue—layer of tissue below the dermis composed of adipose and elastic fibers that connects the dermis to muscle surfaces

Common Diseases and Disorders of the Integumentary System

■ Burns—tissue damage from exposure to heat, chemicals, or electricity
- First degree (superficial)—involves the epidermis; has a red appearance with minimal or no edema
- Second degree (partial thickness)—involves the epidermis and part of dermis; has a blistered red appearance with edema
- Third degree (full thickness)—involves epidermis, entire dermis, and often the underlying tissues; has a pale white or charred appearance with broken skin and edema

■ Carcinoma—skin cancer
- Basal cell carcinoma—malignant disease of the basal cell layer of skin
- Squamous cell carcinoma—malignant disease of the squamous cell layer of skin; more likely to metastasize than basal cell
- Melanoma—highly malignant nevus (mole)

Other common diseases and disorders of the integumentary system appear in Box 6-2.

SKELETAL SYSTEM

The **skeletal system** is the framework of the body. The human skeleton is composed of **206 bones**, cartilage, and ligaments.

BOX 6-2

Common skin diseases and disorders

Abrasion—scrape
Acne—inflammation of sebaceous glands
Albinism—abnormal absence of pigment in skin, hair, and eyes
Alopecia—baldness
Avulsion—tearing away from body structure
Cyst—a sac containing a liquid
Decubitus—bedsore; ulceration resulting from pressure and poor circulation
Dermatitis—inflammation of the skin characterized by pruritus (itching), erythema (redness), and lesions
Eczema—form of dermatitis with a combination of vesicles and dry, leathery patches
Eschar—scab
Excoriation—abrasion (scrape) of the epidermis
Fissure—furrow, crack, groove, or crevice
Furuncle—boil
Herpes simplex—cold sore or fever blister caused by the herpes simplex virus
Herpes zoster (shingles)—painful vesicles along peripheral nerve tracts caused by the herpes zoster virus, which also causes varicella (chicken pox)
Impetigo—bacterial infection, usually around the mouth and nose, caused by staphylococci or streptococci; dry to crusty vesicles
Lesion—abnormal change in localized tissue caused by injury or disease
Macule—small spot or colored area (such as a freckle)
Nevus (mole)—raised congenital spot on skin surface
Papule—pimple
Pediculosis—infestation with lice
Psoriasis—chronic inflammatory skin disease characterized by scaly red patches on body surface
Pustule—pus- or lymph-filled vesicle
Scleroderma—disease causing thickened, rigid skin
Tinea corporis—ringworm; fungal infection
Tinea pedis—athlete's foot; fungal infection
Ulcer—open lesion on the skin or mucous membrane
Urticaria—hives
Verruca—wart
Vesicle—blisterlike sac on the skin
Vitiligo—skin disease with white milky patches surrounded by normal pigmentation
Wheal—round, elevated skin lesion with white center and red periphery

Functions of the Skeletal System

- Provides frame and strength to the body
- Produces body movement
- Provides protection for organs (e.g., the skull protects the brain)
- Serves as storehouse for calcium (Ca) salts
- Produces blood cells in the bone marrow

Components of the Skeletal System

- Bone—hard connective tissue impregnated with a Ca substance (206 bones in the adult skeleton)
- Cartilage—firm connective tissue found primarily in joints, thorax walls, larynx, airway passages, and ears
- Ligaments—bands of fibrous connective tissue that connect the articulating ends of bones to facilitate or limit movement; **do not confuse ligaments with tendons, which connect muscle to bone**
- Joints—areas where two or more bones come together or articulate, such as the knee, shoulder, and neck (see Box 6-3, which describes joint movements)

BOX 6-3

Joint movements

Abduction—moving away from the body midline, e.g., spreading the arms (the opposite of adduction)

Adduction—moving toward the body midline, e.g., bringing the arms to the sides (the opposite of abduction)

Circumduction—drawing an imaginary circle with a body structure, e.g., the arms

Eversion—turning wrists or ankles outward, away from the body such as turning the foot away from the body (the opposite of inversion)

Inversion—turning inside out, such as turning the heels out so toes face each other (the opposite of eversion)

Extension—bringing the limbs or phalanges toward a straight position such as opening the fingers of a closed hand (the opposite of flexion)

Hyperextension—extreme or abnormal extension, usually resulting in injury (e.g., dislocated finger)

Flexion—bending such as closing the fingers of the hand (the opposite of extension)

Dorsiflexion pointing the toes up

Plantar flexion—pointing toes downward, which flexes the arch of the foot (e.g., en pointe dancing in ballet)

Rotation—turning on an axis, such as turning the head to indicate "No"

Organization of the Skeletal System

The major bones are illustrated in Figure 6-7. These bones are divided into the axial segment and the appendicular segment.

Axial Skeleton

The **axial** segment of the skeleton consists of the bones of the skull, spine, and chest.

- Cranium—skull (Fig. 6-8)
  - Frontal—forehead
  - Parietal—sides and top
  - Temporal—lower sides
  - Mastoid process—lower portion of the temporal bone
  - Styloid process—projection inferior to the external ear
  - Zygomatic process—upper cheek
  - Occipital—base of the skull, contains the foramen magnum (the opening in the skull that connects the spinal cord to the brain)
  - Sphenoid—bat-shaped, lateral eye orbits
  - Ethmoid—bony area between the nasal cavity and the orbits
- Facial—14 bones form the face (major bones are listed in Fig. 6-8)
  - Nasal—2 bones that form the bridge of the nose
  - Zygomatic—arch of the cheek
  - Mandible—lower jaw
  - Maxilla—upper jaw
- Vertebral column (spine)—26 vertebrae (bones) that cover the spinal cord (Fig. 6-9)
  - Cervical vertebrae (7 vertebrae)—neck bones; the first is called the *atlas* (supports the head); the second is called the *axis* (pivot for the head)
  - Thoracic vertebrae (12 vertebrae)—chest; attaches to the posterior portion of ribs
  - Lumbar vertebrae (5 vertebrae)—small of back; heavier and larger than other vertebrae
  - Sacrum (one vertebra)—posterior of bony pelvis located between the 2 hip bones
  - Coccyx (one vertebra)—tailbone
- Thorax—rib cage
  - Ribs—12 pair of bones that make up the thorax; the bars of the cage
  - Sternum—breast bone that, with the ribs, protects the heart
    - Manubrium—top of the breast bone that joins with the clavicle and first ribs
    - Xiphoid process—small tip at the lower end of the sternum

FIGURE 6-7 Human skeleton. (Reprinted with permission from Willis MC. *Medical Terminology: A Programmed Learning Approach to the Language of Health Care*. Baltimore: Lippincott Williams & Wilkins, 2002.)

Appendicular Skeleton

The **appendicular skeleton** consists of the bones of the upper and lower extremities and the girdles attaching them to the axial skeleton portion.

- Shoulder girdle
  - Clavicle—collar bone, which joins the sternum at the anterior and the scapula laterally
  - Scapula—shoulder blade
- Upper extremities—arms, hands, fingers, and thumbs
  - Humerus—upper arm (largest arm bone)

- Radius—lateral bone of forearm (in anatomic position, thumb side)
- Ulna—medial bone of forearm (in anatomic position)
- Carpals—the 8 bones that make up the wrist
- Metacarpals—the 5 bones of the palm of the hand
- Phalanges—fingers (3 bones each) and thumbs (two bones each)
- Pelvic girdle—attaches lower extremities to axial skeleton
  - Ilium—superior wing-shaped portions of hip bones

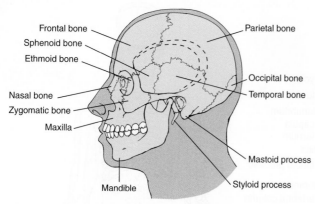

FIGURE 6-8 The adult skull. (Reprinted with permission from Oatis CA. *Kinesiology: The Mechanics and Pathomechanics of Human Movement.* Baltimore: Lippincott Williams & Wilkins, 2003.)

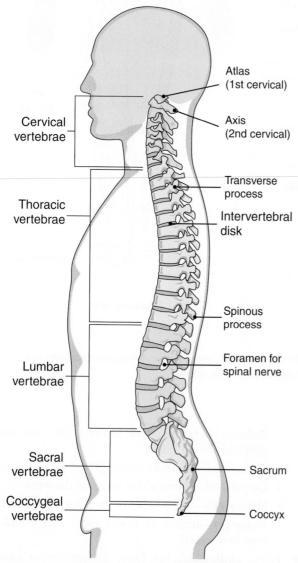

FIGURE 6-9 Adult vertebral column. (Reprinted with permission from Cohen BJ, Wood DL. *Memmler's the Human Body in Health and Disease.* 9th Ed. Philadelphia: Lippincott Williams & Wilkins, 2000.)

- Ischium—inferior portion of hip bones that supports weight when sitting
- Pubis—anterior union of the hip bones

■ Lower extremities—legs, feet, and toes
- Femur—thigh bone; **the body's largest, longest, and strongest bone**
- Patella—kneecap
- Tibia—shin bone
- Fibula—smaller leg bone, lateral to tibia
- Tarsals—the 7 ankle and foot bones (largest is the calcaneus, or heel bone)
- Metatarsals—the 5 foot bones
- Phalanges—toe bones (3 bones each), great toes (2 bones each)

Common Diseases and Disorders of the Skeletal System

■ Congenital or developmental disorders—skeletal abnormalities resulting from birth defects or occurrences during the developmental stages
- Cleft palate—congenital deformity caused by a malunion of the maxilla, leaving an opening in the roof of the mouth (palate)
- Spina bifida—congenital deformity caused by malformation of vertebrae that exposes the spinal column
- Scoliosis—abnormal lateral curvature of the vertebral column
- Kyphosis (hunchback)—an excessive curvature in the thoracic portion of the vertebral column
- Lordosis (swayback)—excessive curvature in the lumbar portion of the vertebral column

Note: Know the differences between scoliosis, kyphosis, and lordosis.

- Rickets—structural deformities of the bone resulting from lack of vitamin D

■ Arthritis—inflammation of the joints
- Osteoarthritis—degenerative joint disease resulting in deformities and chronic pain; usually occurs as part of the aging process, but excessive joint use (such as long-distance running) and trauma are also contributory factors
- Rheumatoid arthritis—inflammation and overgrowth of synovial membranes and joint tissues characterized by swelling of joints, usually occurring in young adults
- Gout—inflammation and pain, usually of the great toes or thumbs, caused by accumulation of uric acid crystals; the highest incidence occurs in late-middle-aged men
- Septic arthritis—serious bloodstream bacterial infection attacking the joints; common pathogens are *Streptococcus, Staphylococcus,* and tuberculosis

| Closed | Open | Greenstick | Impacted | Comminuted | Spiral | Colles |

FIGURE 6-10 Types of fractures.

- Fractures—a break or rupture in the bone; Figure 6-10 illustrates some of the following types of fractures:
  - Simple—closed fracture with no open wound
  - Compound—open fracture with an external wound
  - Greenstick—incomplete break or a bending of the bone, usually in children
  - Impacted—broken ends of the bone are forced into each other
  - Comminuted—splintering or crushing of the bone with several fragments
  - Spiral—fracture caused by a twisting motion
  - Colles—displaced fracture of the distal radius, proximal to the wrist
- Neoplasms—tumors
  - Malignant—cancerous tumors (e.g., osteosarcoma, osteochondroma)
  - Nonmalignant—benign tumors such as cysts
- Osteomyelitis—inflammation of the bone or marrow caused by pathogens
- Osteoporosis—porous, brittle bones resulting from low levels of Ca salts; common in menopausal women

MUSCULAR SYSTEM

The **muscular system** contains approximately 650 muscles that make up the general form of the body.

Functions of the Muscular System

- Produces body movement through chemical reactions at cellular level
- Maintains body posture and alignment
- Protects bones and internal organs
- Generates heat

Muscle Traits

- Excitability—receive and respond to a stimulus
- Contractility—shorten (often associated with the body movement of flexion)
- Extensibility—stretch or lengthen (associated with the body movement of extension)
- Elasticity—return to original length after shortening or lengthening

Types of Muscle Tissues

- Smooth muscle—forms the walls of hollow organs, blood vessels, and respiratory passages; moves substances through the systems (involuntary); striated
- Skeletal muscle—attached to bones, moves muscle and bones (voluntary)
- Cardiac muscle—forms the wall of heart, creates pumping action of the heart (involuntary); striated

Components of the Muscular System

- Muscles—tissue made up of contractile fibers that effect movement of organs and body parts; Figure 6-11 illustrates anterior and posterior muscles
- Tendons—**connective tissue that attaches muscle directly to the periosteum (covering) of the bone**
- Aponeurosis—broad sheet that attaches muscle to muscle or muscle to select bones, such as the skull
- Synapses—neuromuscular junctions transmitting messages from the nerves that stimulate muscles to act

Body Mechanics

- Lever—bone acts as fixed bar moving around a pivot
- Fulcrum—joint acts as pivot to the bone
- Force—muscle contracts and pulls bone

Common Diseases and Disorders of the Muscular System

- Muscular dystrophy—progressive weakening of muscles that leads to paralysis; may be congenital
- Myasthenia gravis—progressive neuromuscular disease characterized by great muscle weakness and fatigue that results from poor adenosine triphosphate (ATP) production; may be an autoimmune disorder

FIGURE 6-11 The muscular system. A. Anterior. B. Posterior. (Reprinted with permission from Cohen BJ, Wood DL. *Memmler's the Human Body in Health and Disease.* 9th Ed. Philadelphia: Lippincott Williams & Wilkins, 2000.)

- Tendonitis—inflammation of the tendon
- Sprain—overstretching of the ligament
- Strain—overstretching of the tendon
- Atrophy—wasting of muscle, often resulting from nonuse

NERVOUS SYSTEM

The **nervous system** is the coordinating agent of the body. Similar to a command post and communication center, it carries messages to and from points and decides on actions and responses.

Functions of the Nervous System

- Regulates body functions and processes
- Communicates stimuli and responses throughout the body
- Generates thoughts, sensations, emotions, and perceptions

Organization of the Nervous System

- Central nervous system (CNS)—brain and spinal cord; integrates sensory information and responses
- Peripheral nervous system (PNS)—nerves originating in the brain and spinal cord that extend outside the CNS and transmit sensory information and responses
  - Somatic nervous system—transmits sensory information to skeletal muscle; voluntary
  - Autonomic nervous system—transmits sensory information to smooth and cardiac muscles (visceral) and glands; involuntary
    - Sympathetic nervous system—prepares the body for stressful situations (i.e., "fight or flight")
    - Parasympathetic nervous system—returns the body to rest and replenishment of energy
  - Afferent (sensory) division of systems—transmits information to the brain
  - Efferent (motor) division of systems—transmits information from the brain to organs and other body structures

Components of the Nervous System

- Neurons—nerve cells, the structural and functional units of the nervous system
  - Dendrites—neuron fibers conducting impulses *to* the cell body
  - Axons—neuron fibers conducting impulses *away from* the cell body
  - Myelin sheath—fatty material that covers and protects neuron fibers; speeds conduction
- Nerves—bundles of neurons that conduct impulses and connect to the brain and spinal cord

- Neuroglia—nonconducting cells that support and protect nervous tissue
- Synapses—neuromuscular junctions (gaps) between neurons
- Neurotransmitters—chemicals released by the axons that stimulate the next cell to continue the transmission of the impulse; the **three main neurotransmitters are acetylcholine, epinephrine, and norepinephrine**
- Meninges—3 layers of connective tissue covering and completely enclosing the brain and spinal cord
  - Dura mater—outer layer, thickest and toughest of the meninges; from the Latin *mater*, meaning "mother"
  - Arachnoid—middle layer, attached to deepest meninges by weblike fibers with space for movement of cerebral spinal fluid; from the Latin *arachnoid*, meaning "spider"
  - Pia mater—innermost layer, attached directly to nervous tissue of brain and spinal cord
- Cerebrospinal fluid (CSF)—clear fluid that flows through the brain and spinal cord and into the subarachnoid spaces of the meninges; cushions and supports nervous tissue and transports nutrients and waste products from the cells
- Brain—organ acting as the primary center for regulating and coordinating body functions and activities (Fig. 6-12); divided into right and left hemispheres
  - Lobes—5 areas of the brain located in each hemisphere; each lobe has a corresponding bone that protects it
    - Frontal—controls speech and voluntary muscle movement
    - Parietal—contains the sensory area and interprets impulses from skin (e.g., pain, heat); also estimates distance, size, and shapes
    - Temporal—interprets sound (auditory sense) and smell (olfactory sense); also associated with personality, behavior, emotion, and memory
    - Occipital—interprets sight
    - Insula—believed to be associated with visceral functions
  - Cerebrum—**largest part of the brain**, divided into right and left hemispheres by the longitudinal fissure; contains auditory, visual, gustatory, and olfactory areas and areas of higher mental faculties
  - Cerebellum ("little brain")—involved in synergic control of skeletal muscles and coordination of voluntary muscular movements; connected to the cerebrum, brain stem, and spinal cord by the pons

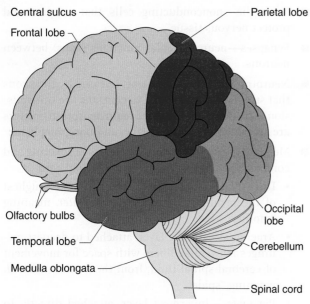

Central sulcus — Parietal lobe
Frontal lobe
Olfactory bulbs
Temporal lobe
Medulla oblongata
Occipital lobe
Cerebellum
Spinal cord

FIGURE 6-12 Surfaces of the brain. (Reprinted with permission from Willis MC. *Medical Terminology: A Programmed Learning Approach to the Language of Health Care.* Baltimore: Lippincott Williams & Wilkins, 2002.)

- Pons—area where nerves cross, resulting in nerves located on one side of the brain controlling the opposite side of the body; connects the cerebellum with the nervous system
- Medulla oblongata—portion of the brain connecting with the spinal cord; contains centers for control of heartbeat, respiratory rate, and blood pressure
- Midbrain—connects the pons and cerebellum with the cerebrum; functions as relay for certain eye and ear reflexes
- Diencephalon—located between the cerebral hemispheres and the brain stem; **contains the thalamus and hypothalamus**
  - Thalamus—located midbrain in the diencephalon, serves as relay for sensory and motor signals
  - Hypothalamus—located in the diencephalon, contains nerve cells that assist with maintenance of water balance, fat and sugar metabolism, secretion of endocrine glands, and regulation of body temperature by linking the nervous system to the endocrine system via **the pituitary gland located just below the thalamus, just above the brain stem**
- Ventricles—**cavities or spaces** in the brain and spinal cord where CSF is formed, filtered, and circulated
■ Cranial nerves (see Box 6-4)—12 pairs of nerves located in the cranium that control sensory, special sensory, somatic motor, and visceral motor impulses; these nerves are identified by Roman numerals

---

BOX 6-4

Cranial nerves

I.   **O**lfactory nerve—transmits smells from the nasal mucosa to the brain

II. **O**ptic nerve—transmits vision from the eye to the brain

III. **O**culomotor nerve—facilitates contraction of many of the eye muscles

IV. **T**rochlear nerve—innervates eyeball muscles

V.   **T**rigeminal nerve—composed of three branches that innervate the face, transmitting sensory (pain, temperature, touch), motor (muscles of mastication), and lingual (taste) impulses

VI. **A**bducens nerve— innervates the lateral rectus muscle; responsible for abduction of the eye (outward movement)

VII. **F**acial nerve—controls facial expressions; combines with the fibers of the trigeminal nerve providing the sense of taste to the anterior two-thirds of the tongue

VIII. **A**uditory nerve—also known as the vestibulocochlear or acoustic nerve; transmits impulses for hearing and equilibrium

IX. **G**lossopharyngeal nerve—contains sensory and motor fibers that supply the posterior tongue, pharynx, and parotid gland (largest salivary gland); controls swallowing

X.   **V**agus nerve—the longest cranial nerve supplying organs in the thoracic and abdominal cavities; innervates glands that produce digestive juices and other secretions

XI. **A**ccessory nerve—divides into two branches, cranial and spinal; the cranial branch innervates the muscles of the larynx, and the spinal branch innervates two muscles of the neck, the sternocleidomastoid and the trapezius.

XII. **H**ypoglossal nerve—transmits impulses to control the muscles of the tongue

A pneumonic used to remember the 12 pairs of cranial nerves is given below:

On **O**ld **O**lympus **T**iny **T**ops **A** **F**in **A**nd **G**erman **V**iewed **A**mber **H**ops

---

■ Spinal cord—continuous tubelike structure located within the spinal vertebrae that extends from the occipital bone to the coccyx (review order of vertebrae in Figure 6-9); contains ascending and descending nerve tracts that carry transmissions to and from the brain

■ Spinal nerves—31 pairs of nerves arising from the spinal cord, with extending branches to the body parts

■ Ganglia (singular *ganglion*)—small, raised areas of gray matter, located outside the CNS, that contain cells of neurons

Common Diseases and Disorders of the Nervous System

Brain or Spinal Cord

- Trauma—injuries as a result of blunt or penetrating force (e.g., gunshot and knife wounds, motor vehicle accidents, diving accidents)
- Neoplasms—malignant and benign tumors
- Paralysis—loss of movement and sensation to a body part or area because of disease or trauma
  - Hemiplegia—paralysis of one side of body
  - Paraplegia—paralysis of the trunk or lower extremities
  - Quadriplegia—paralysis of all extremities and usually the trunk

Brain and Cranial Nerves

- Alzheimer disease—degenerative disorder of the brain beginning with dementialike symptoms and progressing to a nonfunctioning of neuron fibers that prevents communication between cells for ordinary tasks (e.g., swallowing) and leads to death; etiology is unknown
- Bell palsy—unilateral facial muscle paralysis (drooping of eye and mouth) resulting from dysfunction of cranial nerve VII
- Cerebral palsy—loss of mental function or sensation and control of movement resulting from birth injury or defect
- Cerebrovascular accident (CVA)—stroke; occlusion or hemorrhage of vessel(s) in the brain that results in impairment of mental functions or paralysis
- Concussion—mild head injury (MHI) or mild traumatic brain injury (MTBI) resulting in subtle or more serious physical, cognitive, or emotional symptoms
- Dementia—irrecoverable deterioration of mental functions that begins with memory loss and progresses to excitability, defective judgment, delusions, and loss of control of body functions; multiple causes (e.g., alcohol abuse, epilepsy, strokes, lesions)
- Encephalitis—inflammation of the brain
- Epilepsy—abnormal electrical activity of the brain that results in seizures; multiple causes, such as head trauma, high fevers, disease processes, poisoning, or overdose
- Hydrocephalus—accumulation of CSF in the brain caused by an obstruction that results in mounting pressure and destruction of brain tissue
- Narcolepsy—uncontrollable episodes of falling asleep, also known as sleep epilepsy
- Parkinson disease—chronic progressive neurologic disease characterized by fine tremors and muscle weakness and rigidity; etiology believed to be associated with low dopamine production; repeated concussions may be a precursor
- Transient ischemic attack (TIA)—ministrokes; temporary episodes of impaired neurologic function resulting from decreased blood flow to the brain

Spinal Cord and Nerves

- Amyotrophic lateral sclerosis (ALS or Lou Gehrig disease)—progressive disease of the motor neurons that causes muscle atrophy and weakness
- Herpes zoster—shingles; an infection caused by the herpes zoster virus (the same virus that causes varicella), resulting in blisterlike lesions and pain along the nerve trunks
- Multiple sclerosis—progressive inflammation and hardening of the myelin sheath in the nervous system
- Neuritis—inflammation of the nerve
- Poliomyelitis—vaccine-preventable disease that attacks the gray matter of the spinal cord; paralysis or partial paralysis may occur
- Sciatica—neuritis and associated pain of the sciatic nerve and its branches

SENSORY SYSTEM

The sensory system is closely aligned with the nervous system and serves to protect the body by recognizing the environment and detecting changes. These functions allow the nervous system to transmit stimuli, determine responses, and send reactive messages.

General Senses

General or somatic sensors are located throughout the body.

- Pressure—receptors in skin and internal organs
- Temperature—receptors in skin and internal organs
- Touch—receptors in skin and internal organs
- Position/orientation—receptors in muscles, tendons, and joints
- Pain—receptors in skin, internal organs, muscles, tendons, and joints

Special Senses

The special senses are sight, hearing, smell, and taste. The components of these senses are located in specific organs and structures.

Vision (Sight)

Figure 6-13 illustrates the following structures of the eye; Box 6-5 lists common diseases and disorders of the eye.

- Eye—organ containing receptors for sight
  - Sclera—white outer coat of eye
    - Cornea—anterior transparent cover of sclera; focuses light rays

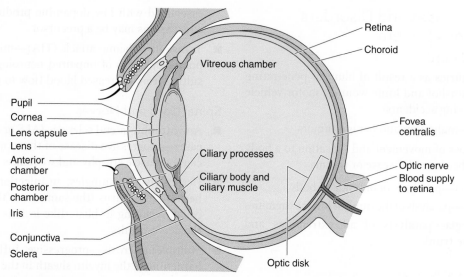

FIGURE 6-13 The eye. (Reprinted with permission from Willis MC. *Medical Terminology: A Programmed Learning Approach to the Language of Health Care*. Baltimore: Lippincott Williams & Wilkins, 2002.)

BOX 6-5

Common diseases and disorders of the eye

Astigmatism—impaired vision from irregular curve of cornea; image focuses improperly on retina; may be mild to severe; usually corrected with glasses or contact lenses

Cataract—cloudy or opaque lens; usually corrected by surgery

Conjunctivitis—inflammation of the conjunctiva caused by infection or irritation

Diabetic retinopathy—damage to the retina in diabetic patients resulting from hemorrhage of vessels; usually progressive and related to the control of the person's diabetes

Exophthalmia—protrusion of the eyeballs, usually resulting from endocrine disorder

Glaucoma—disease causing damage to optic nerve from increased intraocular pressure; often results in blindness if uncontrolled

Hyperopia—farsightedness; a condition in which distant objects can be seen more clearly than closer objects

Macular degeneration—progressive, abnormal growth of blood vessels or other materials in retina; usually leads to blindness, although laser surgery may slow process

Myopia—condition of nearsightedness; can see objects close by but not far away

Presbyopia— type of farsightedness; most common eye condition associated with aging

Strabismus—inability of both eyes to simultaneously focus on a subject; known as "lazy eye" or as being "cross-eyed"

- Choroid—middle layer of the eye between sclera and retina
  - Iris—colored portion of eye; regulates amount of light entering eye
  - Pupil—hole in the middle of the iris
- Retina—innermost layer of the eye; contains photoreceptors
  - Rods—function in dark, recognize shades of gray; located throughout the retina
  - Cones—function in light, recognize color; located throughout the retina
  - Optic disk—blind spot, area where the optic nerve exits the eye
- Chambers
  - Anterior—between the lens and cornea; contains aqueous humor (clear, watery fluid that maintains the slight curve of the cornea)
  - Posterior—between the lens and the retina; contains vitreous humor (gelatinlike fluid that maintains shape of eyeball) and some aqueous humor
- Lens—transparent refractory structure between the iris and vitreous humor

■ Accessory structures
- Eyebrows and lashes—help protect against foreign objects entering the eye
- Eyelids—moisturize eyes, also protect against foreign objects
- Lacrimal structures—glands and ducts that secrete and drain **tears, which help to prevent infection** and remove foreign bodies

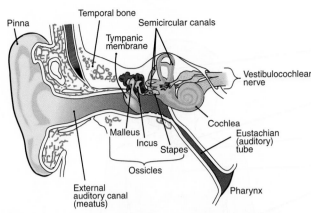

FIGURE 6-14 The ear. (Reprinted with permission from Cohen BJ, Wood DL. *Memmler's the Human Body in Health and Disease.* 9th Ed. Philadelphia: Lippincott Williams & Wilkins, 2000.)

- Conjunctiva—mucous membrane lining of the eyelid
- Optic nerve—second cranial nerve; carries visual impulses from the rods and cones to the brain

Hearing (Auditory Sense)

Figure 6-14 illustrates the following structures of the ear; Box 6-6 lists common diseases and disorders of the ear.

- Ear—sense organ for hearing and equilibrium
- Outer ear
  - Pinna (auricle)—external ear; directs waves to the canal
  - External auditory canal—tubelike opening or meatus from the pinna to the tympanic membrane

---

BOX 6-6

Common diseases and disorders of the ear

Deafness—partial or complete hearing loss; many causes, such as trauma, disease, nerve damage

Ménière disease—chronic disturbance in labyrinth, resulting in dizziness, loss of equilibrium, and deafness; unknown cause; treatment is palliative (attempting to provide relief for signs and symptoms)

Otitis media—infection of middle ear; most common in infants and toddlers; usually treated with antibiotics

Otosclerosis—partial deafness resulting from bone growth involving the ossicles; may be improved by surgery

Tinnitus—ringing in the ears

Vertigo—dizziness

  - Ceruminous glands—glands in the beginning of the ear canal that produce cerumen (earwax) to protect the internal ear structures
  - Tympanic membrane (eardrum)—boundary between external and middle ear canals; vibrates to transmit sound waves to inner ear
- Middle ear—contains three auditory (hearing) ossicles (bones) that amplify sound from the tympanic membrane and transmit to fluid in inner ear
  - Malleus (hammer)—first ossicle
  - Incus (anvil)—second ossicle
  - Stapes (stirrup)—third ossicle
- Eustachian tube—connects the middle ear with the throat and pharynx; equalizes pressure on the tympanic membrane
- Inner ear (labyrinth)—contains vestibule, semicircular canal, and cochlea, with receptors for hearing and balance
  - Vestibule—middle section of the inner ear that involves balance
  - Semicircular canal—curved passageway in the inner ear that detects motion and regulates balance
  - Cochlea—snail-shaped tube that contains the receptor for hearing

Smell (Olfactory Sense)

- Nasal cavity
  - Olfactory epithelium—contains receptors for smell
  - Olfactory nerve—first cranial nerve leading from olfactory center in the temporal lobe of the brain to olfactory sensors in epithelium

Taste (Gustatory)

- Tongue
  - Glossal papillae—taste receptors, or taste buds, located on the tongue that sense bitter, sour, sweet, and salty tastes
  - Cranial nerves—facial and glossopharyngeal cranial nerves associated with taste

ENDOCRINE SYSTEM

The endocrine system contains glands producing regulatory chemicals or hormones (Fig. 6-15). This system, in conjunction with the nervous system, regulates and coordinates other body systems. The nervous system communicates to the endocrine system the need for hormone adjustments resulting from environmental changes. The hormones are secreted into the bloodstream and carried to target cells where the reactions occur. **The term *endocrine* comes from the Greek word *endon*, meaning "within" (because the secretions are within the gland).**

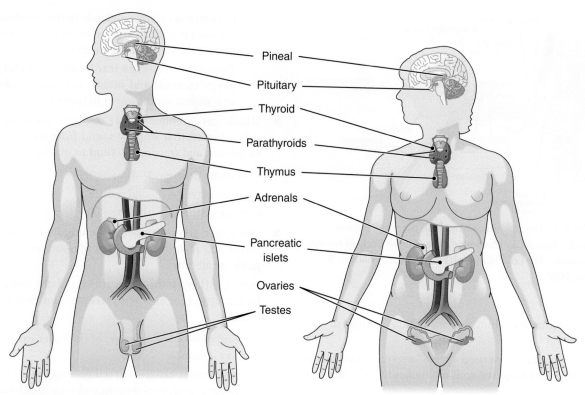

FIGURE 6-15 Endocrine glands. (Reprinted with permission from Cohen BJ. *Medical Terminology*. 4th Ed. Philadelphia: Lippincott Williams & Wilkins, 2003.)

Table 6-1 summarizes the endocrine glands and their hormones and functions. Other glands, called *exocrine glands* secrete externally or into ducts. These glands and hormones will be discussed with the appropriate systems. Examples are salivary glands, mammary glands, sweat glands, and Bartholin glands.

Functions of the Endocrine System

- Regulates growth, metabolism, reproduction, and behavior
- Coordinates and stimulates many body functions by secreting and sending hormones to specific cells

Common Diseases and Disorders of the Endocrine System

Pineal Gland

- Seasonal affective disorder (SAD)—overproduction of melatonin during long periods of darkness (winter), resulting in depression

Anterior Pituitary Gland

- Dwarfism—decreased production of growth hormone (GH) that results in abnormally small size
- Giantism—overproduction of GH that results in abnormally large size

- Acromegaly—overproduction of GH after puberty that results in wide, large face, hands, and feet

Thyroid Gland

- Goiter—enlarged thyroid
- Hypothyroidism—underactivity of the thyroid
  - Cretinism—hypothyroidism; decreased secretion of thyroxine in infants that results in impaired physical and mental development
  - Myxedema—atrophy of the thyroid in adults that results in decreased secretion of thyroxine, causing forms of physical and mental decline
- Hyperthyroidism—overactivity of the thyroid
  - Graves disease—hyperthyroidism; increased secretion of thyroxine characterized by goiter, exophthalmia (bulging eyes), weight loss, extreme nervousness, and rapid metabolism

Parathyroid Gland

- Tetany—spasms resulting from low blood Ca

Adrenal Cortex Gland

- Addison disease—hyposecretion of cortisol by the adrenal cortex, resulting in muscle atrophy, tissue weakness, and skin pigmentation

TABLE 6-1 ▸ Endocrine glands, hormones, and select functions

Gland and Location	Hormones and Select Functions
Pineal gland Descends from the roof of the diencephalon	Melatonin—regulates sexual development and sleep/wake cycles
Pituitary gland ("Master gland") Just below the hypothalamus in the brain	
Anterior pituitary (adenohypophysis)	Growth hormone (GH)—promotes growth of bone and soft tissue Thyroid-stimulating hormone (TSH)—stimulates thyroid to produce thyroid hormones Adrenocorticotropic hormone (ACTH)—stimulates adrenal cortex to produce hormones for stress and water/electrolyte balance Follicle-stimulating hormone (FSH)—stimulates secretion of estrogen and growth of testes; promotes development of sperm cells Luteinizing hormone (LH)—causes development of corpus luteum in females and stimulates secretion of testosterone in males Prolactin—stimulates female breast development and milk secretion
Posterior pituitary (neurohypophysis)	Vasopressin or antidiuretic hormone (ADH)—increases reabsorption in kidney and stimulates blood vessels to contract Oxytocin—increases uterine contractions and causes breast milk secretion
Thyroid gland Covers the larynx; butterfly-shaped	Thyroid hormone (thyroxine, T_4; T_3)—increases metabolic rate; necessary for normal cell growth Calcitonin—reduces plasma calcium concentrations
Parathyroid glands Four small bodies located bilateral and dorsal to the thyroid	Parathyroid hormone (PTH)—increases calcium level in blood
Thymus gland Upper part of the chest behind the sternum	Thymosin—stimulates production of T cells, facilitating immunity
Adrenal glands On the top of each kidney	
Adrenal cortex	Aldosterone—regulates sodium and potassium levels Cortisol (glucocorticoid)—increases blood glucose and assists in stress Androgens—stimulate development of secondary sex characteristics
Adrenal medulla	Epinephrine—increases heart rate and blood pressure Norepinephrine—aids neurotransmission
Pancreas In the epigastric region of the abdomen, behind the stomach	Both an endocrine and exocrine gland Insulin (endocrine)—decreases sugar levels Glucagon (endocrine)—increases sugar levels Pancreatic juice (exocrine)—aids in digestion, transported to the duodenum
Gonads (sex glands) *Ovaries (female)* On either side of the uterus; almond-shaped glands	Estrogens—stimulate growth of breasts, uterus, and secondary sex characteristics Progesterone—prepares and maintains the uterine lining for pregnancy
Testes (male) In the scrotal sac below the penis	Testosterone—stimulates development of sex characteristics and sperm

■ Cushing syndrome—overproduction of cortisol by the adrenal cortex, resulting in round face, excessive weight gain, thin skin, and high blood glucose

Pancreas

■ Diabetes mellitus—most common endocrine disorder; low production of insulin, resulting in cells retaining sugar

• Insulin-dependent diabetes mellitus (IDDM)—type 1 diabetes

• Non–insulin-dependent diabetes mellitus (NIDDM)—type 2 diabetes

CARDIOVASCULAR SYSTEM

The **cardiovascular** (or circulatory) **system** pumps blood, carrying life-sustaining O_2 and other substances throughout the body. The primary components are blood, blood vessels, and the heart.

Functions of the Cardiovascular System

■ Transports O_2, nutrients, and other needed substances to body tissues

■ Assists in removal of body wastes

■ Regulates acidity (pH) of body fluids

■ Assists in regulating body temperature

Components of the Cardiovascular System

Blood

Blood is the connective tissue containing cells and fluid in a viscous consistency that circulates in vessels throughout the body. Blood cells are formed by a process called **hematopoiesis** by which undifferentiated stem cells give rise to all blood cells. They do not originate in the bloodstream. A simple hematopoiesis model during development is found in Figure 6-16. Bone marrow, the spleen, the liver, and thymus are involved in blood cell production.

■ Plasma—liquid portion of blood (55%)

• Albumin—the most abundant plasma protein; maintains osmotic pressure

• Fibrinogen—the smallest amount of plasma protein; assists in the coagulation (clotting) process

• Globulin—plasma protein used for gamma globulin

• Serum—clear, liquid portion of blood that remains after the blood clots

■ Cellular components of blood (45%)

• Erythrocytes—red blood cells (RBCs); in the adult are formed in bone marrow and contain hemoglobin to carry O_2; **mature cells do not have a nucleus**

• Leukocytes—white blood cells (WBCs); fight infection

• Platelets (thrombocytes)—cell fragments; function in coagulation

Blood Vessels

Blood vessels are the arteries, veins, and capillaries that carry blood throughout the body.

■ Arteries (Fig. 6-17)—blood vessels throughout the body that carry oxygenated blood (brighter red) away from the heart; **the exception is the pulmonary artery which carries deoxygenated blood to the lungs**

■ Veins (Fig. 6-18)—blood vessels throughout the body that contain valves and carry deoxygenated blood (darker red) toward the heart; **the exception is the pulmonary vein that carries oxygenated blood from the lungs back to the heart**

■ Capillaries—small blood vessels connecting veins and arteries

Heart

The heart is the body's pump, a fist-sized muscular organ composed of three layers and an outer covering.

■ Endocardium—inner layer

■ Myocardium—middle layer

■ Epicardium—outer layer

■ Pericardium—outer fibrous sac that covers and protects the heart

■ Chambers—four heart chambers: two superior and two inferior

• Right atrium (plural *atria*)—superior chamber that receives deoxygenated blood from the systemic vessels

• Left atrium—superior chamber that receives oxygenated blood from the pulmonary veins

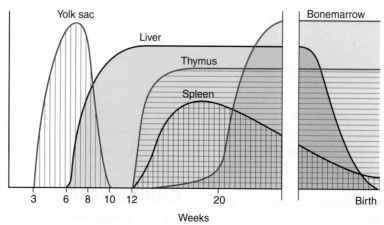

FIGURE 6-16 A schematic diagram of hematopoiesis during development.

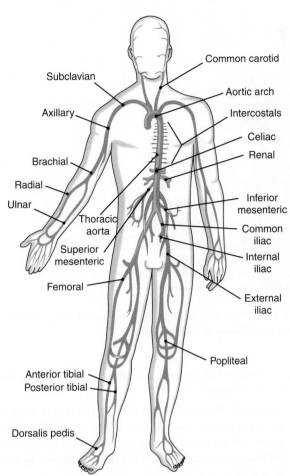

FIGURE 6-17 Major arteries. (Reprinted with permission from Cohen BJ, Wood DL. *Memmler's the Human Body in Health and Disease.* 9th Ed. Philadelphia: Lippincott Williams & Wilkins, 2000.)

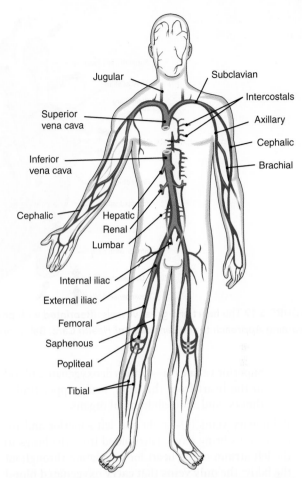

FIGURE 6-18 Major veins. (Reprinted with permission from Cohen BJ, Wood DL. *Memmler's the Human Body in Health and Disease.* 9th Ed. Philadelphia: Lippincott Williams & Wilkins, 2000.)

- Right ventricle—inferior chamber that pumps blood to the lungs
- Left ventricle—inferior chamber that pumps blood to the body tissues

■ Valves—flaplike structures that open and close, allowing blood to flow through the heart in one direction

- Atrioventricular valves (AV)—located between each atrium and ventricle; their closing prevents backflow of blood into the atria
  - Tricuspid valve (3 flaps)—AV valve located between the right atrium and ventricle
  - Mitral valve (bicuspid; 2 flaps)—AV valve located between the left atrium and ventricle
- Semilunar valves (SL)—located between the ventricles and the pulmonary artery and aorta; their closing prevents backflow of blood into the ventricles
  - Aortic valve—located between the left ventricle and the aorta

  - Pulmonary valve—located between the right ventricle and the pulmonary artery

■ Great vessels of the heart—Figure 6-19 identifies structures and demonstrates how blood flows through the heart

- Aorta—largest body artery; consists of 3 parts: ascending, aortic arch, and descending
- Coronary arteries (right and left)—supply blood to the myocardium of the heart; significant blockage of these arteries results in myocardial infarction (MI; heart attack)
- Pulmonary artery—only artery that carries deoxygenated blood; transports blood from the heart to the lungs to be oxygenated
- Vena cava—**largest body vein**; has inferior and superior branches
  - Inferior vena cava—brings deoxygenated blood to the heart from the lower extremities, pelvis, and some abdominal organs

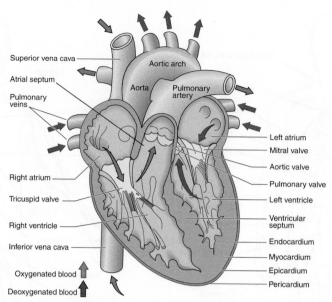

FIGURE 6-19 The heart and great vessels. (Reprinted with permission from Willis MC. *Medical Terminology: A Programmed Learning Approach to the Language of Health Care*. Baltimore: Lippincott Williams & Wilkins, 2002.)

- ○ Superior vena cava—brings deoxygenated blood to the heart from the head, neck, upper limbs, thorax, and some abdominal organs
- ■ Pulmonary veins (4)—right and left superior and inferior veins bring oxygenated blood from the lungs to the left atrium of the heart for circulation throughout the body; **the only veins that carry oxygenated blood**

The Cardiac Cycle

The main function of the cardiovascular system is to circulate blood (Fig. 6-20). The major portion of this function is accomplished through the pumping of the heart in a rhythmic cycle of contraction and relaxation called the *cardiac cycle.*

- ■ Atrial systole (**contraction**)—the atria contract, forcing blood into ventricles through the tricuspid and mitral valves, which close at the end of the contraction
- ■ Ventricular diastole (**relaxation**)—the ventricles relax, filling with blood from the atria
- ■ Ventricular systole (**contraction**)—the ventricles contract, forcing blood through the SL valves to the aorta and pulmonary artery
- ■ Atrial diastole (**relaxation**)—the atria relax, filling with blood from the vena cava and pulmonary veins
- ■ Cycle repeats beginning with atrial systole

Cardiac Conduction

The heart is stimulated to contract through a series of electrical impulses or signals located throughout the heart itself. The impulses are carried or relayed through a group of structures that make up the conduction system (Fig. 6-21). These conduction paths, with the cardiac cycle, produce the electrocardiogram, which will be discussed in Chapter 20.

- ■ Sinoatrial (SA) node—located in the upper wall of the right atrium, the **SA node is the pacemaker of the heart** and initiates a normal heartbeat and rate of **60 to 80 beats per minute (sinus rhythm)**; it causes the atria to contract
- ■ AV node—located in the atrial septum at the lower right, the AV node picks up the impulse or signal from the SA node that causes the atria to contract; if the SA node fails, the AV node may initiate the impulse; the resulting heart rate is slower, at 40 to 60 beats per minute
- ■ Bundle of His—specialized cells in the ventricular septum, carrying the impulse from the AV node; should the SA and AV nodes fail, the bundle of His may initiate the impulse; the resulting heart rate is 20 to 40 beats per minute
- ■ Bundle branches—2 branches extending from the bundle of His that carry the impulse down the ventricular septum
- ■ Purkinje fibers—smaller fibers arising from the bundle branches that carry the impulse to the ventricular walls, causing them to contract

Common Diseases and Disorders of the Cardiovascular System

Diseases and Disorders of the Blood

- ■ Anemia—abnormally low hemoglobin or RBCs, decreasing O_2 supply to the tissues; anemia has many causes and types; main symptoms are fatigue and weakness
  - • Aplastic anemia—anemia that results from bone marrow damage decreasing the production of RBCs

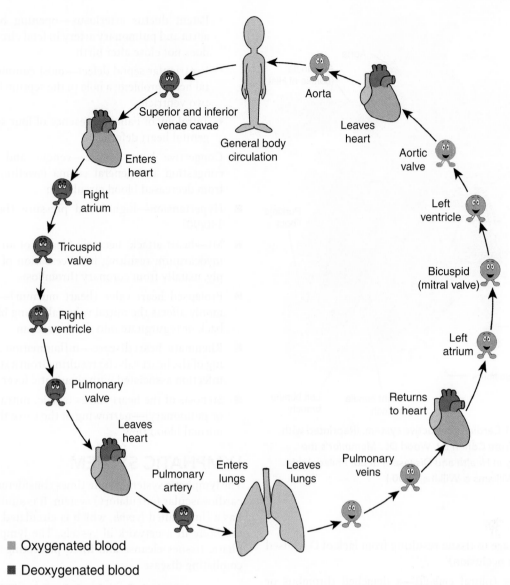

- Oxygenated blood
- Deoxygenated blood

FIGURE 6-20 Blood circulation through the body.

- Pernicious anemia—anemia that results from **vitamin B₁₂** deficiency
- Sickle cell anemia—chronic inherited disease found in Africans and their descendants, causing the hemoglobin cell to mutate its shape
- Leukemia—type of malignancy; rapid and abnormal development of leukocytes (WBCs) in spleen, bone marrow, and lymph nodes
- Hemophilia—genetic bleeding disorder; deficiency of specific clotting factors that results in abnormal bleeding, especially into the joints, from minor trauma; the causative gene is transmitted from mother to sons

Diseases and Disorders of the Blood Vessels

- Aneurysm—genetic or traumatic weakness of a blood vessel wall demonstrated by a "bubble" or

outpouching caused by pressure of blood; an abdominal aortic aneurysm is called an *AAA* or *triple A*
- Arteriosclerosis—hardening of the artery and loss of elasticity resulting from thickening of the vessel wall
  - Atherosclerosis—most common form of arteriosclerosis, with irregular fatty deposits on artery wall (plaque) that result in narrowing and occlusion of vessel; may cause MIs, CVAs, gangrene, and other disorders associated with blood vessel blockage

Note: The difference between atherosclerosis and arteriosclerosis is a highly probable exam question.

  - Coronary artery disease (CAD)—arteriosclerosis or atherosclerosis-type process of the coronary arteries, usually leading to myocardial ischemia

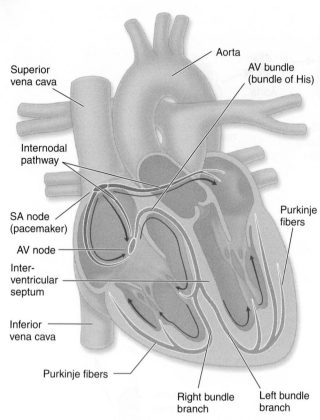

Superior vena cava

Aorta

AV bundle (bundle of His)

Internodal pathway

SA node (pacemaker)

AV node

Inter-ventricular septum

Inferior vena cava

Purkinje fibers

Purkinje fibers

Right bundle branch

Left bundle branch

FIGURE 6-21 Cardiac conductive system. (Reprinted with permission from Cohen BJ, Wood DL. *Memmler's the Human Body in Health and Disease.* 9th Ed. Philadelphia: Lippincott Williams & Wilkins, 2000.)

(damage to tissue resulting from lack of O₂ caused by an occlusion)

- Embolus (plural *emboli*)—a detached thrombus or other substance that occludes a vessel

- Thrombophlebitis—inflammation of a vein with clots

- Thrombus (plural *thrombi*)—an attached blood clot located within the cardiovascular system

Diseases and Disorders of the Heart

- Angina pectoris—severe constricting chest pain resulting from lack of blood supply to the heart; associated with CAD

- Arrhythmias—abnormal heart rhythms
  - Bradycardia—slow heart rate
  - Tachycardia—fast heart rate
  - Flutters—rapid, coordinated heartbeats
  - Fibrillation—rapid, uncoordinated contractions of the heart (may be atrial or ventricular)
  - Heart blocks—interruption of the heart's electrical conduction

- Congenital heart disease—disorder present at birth

- Patent ductus arteriosus—opening between the aorta and pulmonary artery in fetal circulation that does not close after birth
- Ventricular septal defect—most common congenital heart problem; a hole in the septum between the two ventricles
- Tetralogy of Fallot—presence of four specific congenital heart defects

- Congestive heart failure—venous and pulmonary congestion and general edema (swelling) resulting from decreased blood circulation

- Hypertension—high blood pressure (beginning at 140/90)

- MI—heart attack; necrosis (death) of an area in the myocardium resulting from cessation of blood supply, usually from coronary thrombosis

- Prolapsed heart valve (heart murmur)—most commonly affects the mitral valve, allowing blood to leak back or regurgitate into the left atrium

- Rheumatic heart disease—inflammation and hardening of the heart valve(s) resulting from a streptococcal infection associated with rheumatic fever

- Stenosis of the heart valves (aortic, mitral, tricuspid, or pulmonary)—narrowing of the valve that prevents normal blood flow

LYMPHATIC SYSTEM

The lymphatic system is sometimes considered part of the cardiovascular (circulatory) system. It is similar in that it has a fluid called *lymph*, which is circulated throughout the body in a network of vessels. The lymph and lymphatic tissues cleanse and filter, protecting against and combating disease.

Functions of the Lymphatic System

- Defends against disease
- Assists in developing immunities
- Returns excess interstitial fluid to the blood

Components of the Lymphatic System

- Lymph—clear fluid resembling blood plasma that contains some RBCs and WBCs and lymphocytes
- Lymphocytes—white cells that protect the body against infection and aid in establishing immunity
- Lymph vessels—similar to veins, they carry lymph and contain valves and lymph nodes
  - Lymph capillaries—microscopic vessels
  - Lymphatic ducts (2)—narrow tubular channels carrying lymph to the bloodstream
    - Thoracic duct—the larger lymph duct; it drains the entire body except the right side above the diaphragm

○ Right lymphatic duct—the smaller lymph duct; it drains the right side of the body above the diaphragm

■ Lymph nodes—oval-shaped fibrous capsules that filter and cleanse the lymph as it enters the blood

■ Tonsils—3 pairs of masses of lymphoid tissue that filter foreign organisms entering the body through the mouth or nose and assist in the formation of white cells

  • Palatine tonsils—located on each side of the soft palate, these lymph masses are the ones commonly referred to as the "tonsils"

  • Pharyngeal tonsils—adenoids; located on upper pharynx

  • Lingual tonsils—located at back of tongue

■ Spleen—organ located in the **upper left hypochondriac region of the abdomen under the diaphragm** dome; contains lymph tissue; cleanses blood, destroys old RBCs, produces RBCs before birth, and reserves blood in case of emergencies (e.g., hemorrhage)

■ Thymus—gland, considered part of the endocrine system, that produces thymosin, which is necessary for T cell production and the function of lymphocytes in fighting disease

Common Diseases and Disorders of the Lymphatic System

■ Splenomegaly—enlarged spleen, associated with certain infectious diseases

■ Lymphoma—benign or malignant tumor of lymph tissue

  • Hodgkin disease—chronic malignant lymphoma(s) with enlarged spleen; treated by chemotherapy and radiation; generally seen in young men

  • Non-Hodgkin lymphoma—widespread malignant disease in lymph tissues; responds poorly to therapy; generally seen in older adults

■ Acquired immunodeficiency syndrome (AIDS)—decreased immunity resulting from infection with the human immunodeficiency virus (HIV); leaves patient susceptible to opportunistic diseases

■ Mononucleosis (mono)—acute infectious disease caused by Epstein–Barr virus, resulting in lymph tissue involvement, including enlarged spleen; generally seen in young adults

Overview of Immunity

Immunity is the individual's resistance to specific diseases or disorders, usually by developing or acquiring the corresponding antibody to that disease or disorder. Immunity is a function of the lymphatic system. The national exams often contain questions concerning active and passive immunity, which are described in Box 6-7.

BOX 6-7

Types of immunity

Immunity—resistance or the condition of not being susceptible to a disease

Active Immunity

Long-term immunity—produced by the body's own production of antibodies

■ **Natural active immunity**—acquired from exposure to disease-causing organisms

■ **Artificial active immunity**—acquired from immunization with killed or attenuated organisms, toxins, or recombinant DNA

Passive Immunity

Short-term immunity—produced by introducing antibodies manufactured outside the body

■ **Natural passive immunity**—acquired from maternal antibodies while in the uterus or breast-feeding

■ **Artificial passive immunity**—acquired from immunization with antibodies or globulins of disease-causing organisms

---

Additional Terms Associated With Immunity

■ Antigen—a substance (e.g., bacteria/viruses, bacterial/viral toxins, foreign blood cells) when introduced into the body, causes the formation of antibodies

■ Antibody—a substance produced in the body in response to the presence of an antigen; antibodies enhance activities of leukocytes and produce globulins, protecting the body against further assault from the specific antigen

■ Phagocytosis—ingestion of bacteria and particles by phagocytes (a form of leukocyte)

■ Globulins—the fraction of the blood serum protein associated with antibodies; vaccination with globulins produces passive immunity

■ Immunization (vaccination)—protection from communicable diseases by administration of living attenuated agents (e.g., measles), killed organisms (e.g., pertussis), inactivated toxins (e.g., tetanus), or recombinant DNA (e.g., hepatitis B); Box 6-8 identifies common vaccine-preventable diseases; also, refer to Chapter 24.

RESPIRATORY SYSTEM

The **respiratory system** is a group of body structures (Fig. 6-22) responsible for breathing or ventilation. The process involves taking in O_2, which is needed to sustain human cells, and giving off CO_2, which is the waste product of respiration.

BOX 6-8

Common vaccine-preventable diseases

Diphtheria
Haemophilus influenzae b
Hepatitis A
Hepatitis B
Herpes zoster (shingles)
Human papillomavirus
Influenza (select strains)
Measles
Meningitis (select strains)
Mumps
Pertussis (whooping cough)
Pneumonia (select strains)
Polio
Rotavirus
Rubella (German measles)
Tetanus (lockjaw)
Varicella (chicken pox)

Functions of the Respiratory System

■ Obtains O_2 and other gases from the external environment

■ Delivers gases to the blood (diffusion)

■ Removes CO_2, a waste product of respiration, from the cells

■ Transports CO_2 to the external environment

Components of the Respiratory System

Respiratory Center

The respiratory center is the bundled nerve cells, located in the medulla oblongata and pons of the brain, controlling breathing and responding to changing levels of O_2 and CO_2 in the blood.

Upper Respiratory Tract

The upper respiratory tract is the passageway for gases. It is composed of the following:

■ Nose—projection on the face that warms and moistens air as it enters the body; contains cilia and hair to prevent foreign particles and some bacteria from entering the respiratory system

■ Pharynx (throat)—passageway from nose to larynx

■ Larynx (voice box)—organ between the pharynx and trachea containing the vocal cords, which vibrate to produce speech

■ Epiglottis—flaplike structure that covers the larynx during swallowing

Lower Respiratory Tract

The lower respiratory tract is composed of the following:

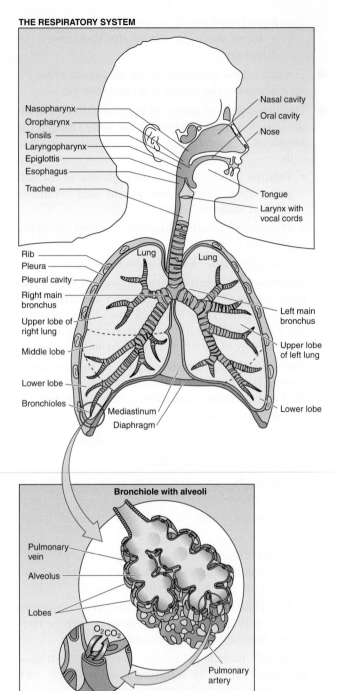

THE RESPIRATORY SYSTEM

FIGURE 6-22 The respiratory system. (Reprinted with permission from Willis MC. *Medical Terminology: A Programmed Learning Approach to the Language of Health Care.* Baltimore: Lippincott Williams & Wilkins, 2002.)

■ Trachea—tube branching into 2 bronchi, which lead into the lungs

■ Bronchi (singular *bronchus*)—tubes from the trachea entering the lungs that subdivide into 2 more branches in the lungs

  • Bronchioles—smaller branches of the bronchi

  • Alveoli (singular *alveolus*)—air sacs at the ends of the bronchioles **where the exchange of gases occurs**

- Lungs (2)—main organ of the respiratory system, located in the thoracic cavity; distributes and exchanges gases
  - Right lung—contains 3 lobes
  - Left lung—contains 2 lobes
  - Pleura—lung linings containing pleural fluid to protect lungs and reduce friction during respiration
- Thorax—cavity containing the lungs
- Diaphragm—**muscle tissue separating thoracic and abdominal cavities** that contracts and expands during respiration, allowing lungs to fill and empty air

Additional Respiratory System Terms

- Cheyne–Stokes respiration—irregular breathing pattern of slow and shallow, then rapid and deep respirations, with pauses for 20 to 30 seconds; frequently occurs before death
- Inspiration (inhalation)—bringing air into lungs; the diaphragm contracts, increasing the size of the thoracic cavity and allowing air to enter the lungs
- Expiration (exhalation)—releasing air from the lungs; the diaphragm relaxes, decreasing the size of the thoracic cavity and pushing air out
- External respiration—exchange of O_2 and CO_2 in the lungs and capillaries
- Internal respiration—exchange of O_2 and CO_2 between the capillaries and the tissue cells
- Pulmonary—referring to the lungs
- Rales—sometimes referred to as rhonchi; a crackling breath sound resulting from increased secretions in the bronchi
- Stridor—high-pitched breath sounds resembling wind, caused by partial obstruction of air passages
- Wheeze—squeaking or whistling breath sound, usually caused by narrowed tracheobronchial airways, as in asthma

Common Diseases and Disorders of the Respiratory System

- Asthma—episodic chronic respiratory disorder resulting from constricted bronchi, associated with allergens, infection, pollutants, cold air, exercise, or stress; characterized by wheezing and low O_2 levels
- Atelectasis—decreased or absence of air in part or in all of the lung and alveoli resulting from collapse of these structures
- Bronchitis—chronic or acute inflammation of the bronchi
- Carcinoma (cancer)—malignant tumor of lung or other areas of respiratory system
- Chronic obstructive pulmonary disease (COPD)—usually progressive respiratory system disorder with irreversible obstruction of air exchange in the bronchi, alveoli, and lungs; emphysema is a form of COPD
- Croup—acute viral infection, usually in infants, characterized by barking cough
- Cystic fibrosis—a genetic disorder that produces abnormally thick mucous secretions blocking and impairing the bronchi, pancreatic and bile ducts, and intestines
- Emphysema—a form of COPD characterized by irreversible loss of elasticity in alveoli that impedes respiration
- Legionnaires disease—a type of pneumonia caused by the *Legionella pneumophila* bacteria
- Pertussis (whooping cough)—a vaccine-preventable bacterial infection (*Bordetella pertussis*) producing a "whoop" coughing sound; may be fatal in infants
- Pharyngitis—sore throat, inflammation of the pharynx
- Pleurisy—inflammation of the pleura
- Pneumonia—viral or bacterial infection causing inflammation of the lungs
- Pneumothorax—partial or complete collapse of the lung(s) resulting from air in the pleural cavity
- Pulmonary edema—fluid accumulation in the lungs, often associated with congestive heart failure
- Tuberculosis—an infectious bacterial disease characterized by tubercles in the tissue; the lung is the most common disease site

DIGESTIVE SYSTEM

The **digestive system** consists of the digestive tract, or alimentary canal, and its accessory organs, including the liver, pancreas, and gallbladder (Fig. 6-23). These organs take food and process it into usable energy for the body's growth, maintenance, and survival. The nutrients are absorbed and circulated, and the solid waste is eliminated.

Functions of the Digestive System

- Digestion—physical and chemical processes changing food into simple nutrients to be used by the cells for energy and building materials
- Absorption—the transfer of the products of digestion into the blood and lymph for circulation
- Elimination—excretion of the solid waste products of digestion in the form of feces

Components of the Digestive System

Digestive Tract

The digestive tract, or alimentary canal, is the system of tubelike organs in which digestion occurs; it begins at the mouth and ends at the anus.

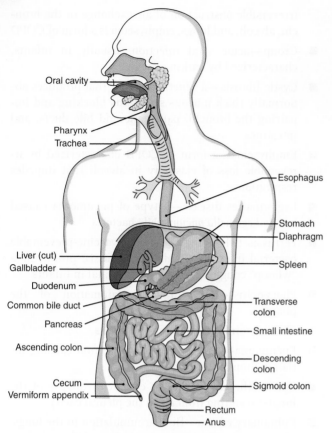

FIGURE 6-23 The digestive system. (Reprinted with permission from Cohen BJ, Wood DL. *Memmler's the Human Body in Health and Disease.* 9th Ed. Philadelphia: Lippincott Williams & Wilkins, 2000.)

■ Mouth (oral cavity)—orifice in the lower face where food enters the body; chewing (mastication) and mixing with saliva occurs, forming a bolus
  • Salivary glands (exocrine glands)—three pair of glands located in the mouth that secrete saliva to moisten food and to begin the chemical breakdown of carbohydrates (starches and sugars)
  • Teeth—hard dentine structures located in the upper and lower jaws used for chewing (mastication); adults have 32 teeth
■ Pharynx (throat)—this organ is part of the respiratory system and also allows masticated food to pass from the mouth to the esophagus
■ Esophagus—tube from the pharynx to the stomach
■ Stomach—J-shaped organ between the esophagus and the duodenum that produces a churning action, mixing food with gastric acids and enzymes as part of digestion; also stores food
  • Mesentery—composed of 2 layers of peritoneum that lie on the walls of the peritoneal cavity connecting the intestines to the wall of the abdomen
■ Small intestine—longest portion of digestive tract; all digestion of fats, proteins, and carbohydrates takes

place here and the absorption of nutrient products into the blood
  • Duodenum—upper portion of the small intestine, separated from the stomach by the pyloric sphincter; food mixed with gastric acid moves into it and mixes with bile from the gallbladder and other digestive juices from the pancreas; absorption of vitamins, minerals, and other nutrients begin here
  • Jejunum—middle portion of the small intestine; absorption of proteins, fats, and fat-soluble vitamins A, D, E, and K takes place here
  • Ileum—lower portion of the small intestine, opening into the cecum and responsible for absorption of vitamin B_{12}; malabsorption of B_{12} results in pernicious anemia
  • Villi (singular *villus*)—tiny projections in the small intestine lining where absorption of nutrients occurs
■ Large intestine—the final organ of the digestive tract, it connects to the small intestine by the ileum and ends at the anus; manufactures vitamins K and B; absorbs fluids and electrolytes; forms, stores, and excretes feces
  • Cecum—upper portion of the large intestine; contains the appendix; receives undigested food and absorbs fluids and salt that remain after intestinal digestion
  • Colon—largest portion of large intestine; divided into four parts
    ○ Ascending colon—portion of colon vertically positioned along right side of abdominal cavity; receives liquid waste from the small intestine; absorbs excess water to help solidify and mixes with bacteria to break down fibers
    ○ Transverse colon—portion of colon positioned horizontally and bridging the ascending and descending colons; continues the fermentation and movement of feces
    ○ Descending colon—portion of colon vertically positioned along the left side of the abdominal cavity; its primary function is to store feces to be emptied into the sigmoid and the rectum
    ○ Sigmoid—lower S-shaped portion of colon connected to the descending colon and the rectum
  • Rectum—the lower portion of the large intestine, connecting the sigmoid to the anus and containing the reflexes for defecation
  • Anus—the final portion of the digestive tract, where feces are excreted
    ○ Internal sphincter—involuntary-control sphincter located in the anus
    ○ External sphincter—voluntary-control sphincter located in the anus

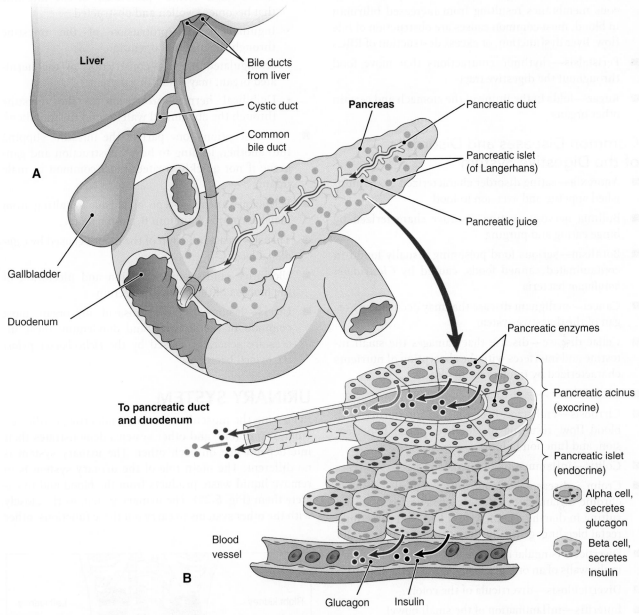

FIGURE 6-24 The pancreas with exocrine and endocrine functions.

Note: The exams generally contain questions requiring knowledge of the different portions and correct ordering of the large and small intestines.

Accessory Digestive Organs

The organs outside the digestive tract that are involved in the digestive system functions are as follows:

- Liver—largest gland in the body, located in the upper right portion of the abdominal cavity; produces bile, detoxifies blood, removes bilirubin, manufactures plasma protein involved in the production of pro-thrombin and fibrinogen, and aids metabolism

- Pancreas—an endocrine gland located behind the stomach producing pancreatic juice, which is transported to the duodenum to aid in digestion, and **insulin and glucagon, which regulate carbohydrate metabolism. Refer to** Figure 6-24.

- Gallbladder—pear-shaped sac located on the inferior surface of the liver; stores bile to aid in digestion and fat absorption; **bile is carried from the gallbladder to the duodenum via the common bile duct**

Additional Digestive System Terms

- Enzymes—proteins that act as catalysts increasing the speed of digestion; each enzyme is specific to a certain type of food and reaction

- Hepatic—referring to the liver

- Jaundice—yellowing of skin, white of eyes, and mucous membranes resulting from increased bilirubin in blood; most common causes are obstruction of bile flow, liver dysfunction, or excess destruction of RBCs
- Peristalsis—rhythmic contractions that move food throughout the digestive tract
- Rugae—folds in the lining of the stomach and certain other organs

Common Diseases and Disorders of the Digestive System

- Anorexia—eating disorder characterized by a diminished appetite and aversion to food
- Bulimia nervosa—eating disorder characterized by binge eating and purging
- Botulism—serious food poisoning, usually found in contaminated canned foods, caused by *Clostridium botulinum* bacteria
- Cancer—malignant disease that may occur in any organ of the digestive system
- Celiac disease—disease that damages the small intestine and interferes with the absorption of nutrients characterized by intolerance to gluten
- Cholelithiasis—gallstones
- Cirrhosis—end-stage liver disease interfering with blood flow, resulting in jaundice, portal hypertension, and function failure
- Colitis—inflammation of the colon
- Crohn disease—inflammatory bowel disease; chronic inflammatory disease of ileum or colon resulting in diarrhea, pain, weight loss, and sometimes rectal bleeding; generally affects young female adults
- Diverticula (singular *diverticulum*)—abnormal pouches in the walls of an organ, usually found in the colon
- Diverticulosis—diverticula of the colon
- Enteritis—inflammation of the small bowel
- Gastroesophageal reflux disease (GERD)—backflow of stomach acids into the esophagus due to an incompetent esophageal sphincter, resulting in burning and discomfort; can lead to ulcers
- Giardiasis—infectious diarrhea caused by *Giardia lamblia*, which is found in contaminated water
- Hemorrhoids—inflammation and dilation of veins in rectum and anus
- Hepatitis—acute or chronic inflammation of the liver; there are at least eight types of identified hepatitis (A, B, C, D, E, F, G, H), with different causes and prognoses
- Hernia—protrusion of an organ or part of an organ through the wall normally containing it; the intestine is the most common organ to herniate
  - Hiatal hernia—protrusion of the stomach into the diaphragm

- Incarcerated hernia—protrusion of the intestine that becomes swollen and obstructed
- Inguinal hernia—protrusion of the intestine through the inguinal opening
- Strangulated hernia—constriction of the herniated organ; may result in gangrene
- Umbilical hernia—protrusion of the intestine through the abdominal wall around the umbilicus
- Intussusception—one part of the intestine slipping into another, leading to bowel obstruction and gangrene if not quickly treated; most common in male infants
- Pernicious anemia—type of anemia resulting from malabsorption of vitamin B_{12} in the ileum
- Thrush—yeast infection of the mouth caused by *Candida albicans*
- Ulcerative colitis—inflammation and ulceration of the mucosa of the colon and rectum
- Ulcers—lesions of the mucosa of any organ; most common in the stomach and duodenum; these ulcers are generally caused by the *Helicobacter pylori* (*H. pylori*) bacteria

URINARY SYSTEM

Reviewing the muscular, nervous, endocrine, cardiovascular, respiratory, and other systems demonstrates their interdependence on each other. The urinary system is no different. The main role of the **urinary system** is to remove liquid waste products from the blood and to excrete them (Fig. 6-25). The urinary system works closely with the other systems to carry out these functions; other

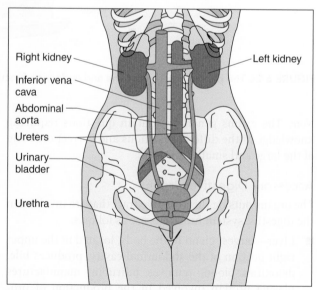

FIGURE 6-25 The urinary system. (Reprinted with permission from Willis MC. *Medical Terminology: A Programmed Learning Approach to the Language of Health Care.* Baltimore: Lippincott Williams & Wilkins, 2002.)

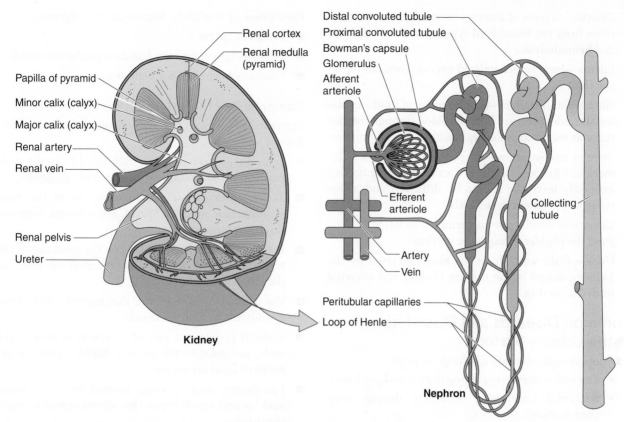

Kidney

Nephron

FIGURE 6-26 Longitudinal section of the kidney and enlarged nephron. (Reprinted with permission from Willis MC. *Medical Terminology: A Programmed Learning Approach to the Language of Health Care.* Baltimore: Lippincott Williams & Wilkins, 2002.)

functions are listed in the next section with the male reproductive system.

Functions of the Urinary System

■ Excretes nitrogen waste products and excess water and salts from the blood in the form of urine

■ Assists the liver in detoxification

■ Assists in maintaining pH balance

■ Assists in maintaining blood volume

Components of the Urinary System

Kidneys

The kidneys are two muscular, bean-shaped organs located in the back of the abdominal cavity that filtrate, reabsorb selected substances, and excrete urine; Figure 6-26 illustrates the anatomy of the kidney and an enlarged nephron.

■ Cortex—outer layer

■ Medulla—inner layer

• Renal pyramids—triangular wedges in the medulla containing nephrons

○ Nephrons—group of microscopic coiled tubules (more than 1 million in each kidney) located in

the renal pyramids that filter blood and form urine; the main structures are collecting tubules and glomerulus (plural: glomeruli) network of blood capillaries (enclosed in Bowman's capsule) and arterioles; the bottom of the paperclip-shaped segment of the nephron is called the loop of Henle

○ Calices (singular *calix*)—group of renal pyramid points **forming the renal pelvis, where urine collects**; also spelled *calyces* (singular *calyx*)

Ureters

The **ureters** are 2 slim tubes that carry urine from the kidneys to the urinary bladder.

Urinary Bladder

The **urinary bladder** is a saclike organ behind the symphysis pubis that temporarily stores urine.

Urethra

The **urethra** is the tube that takes urine from the bladder out of the body through the opening called the urinary meatus.

Additional Urinary System Terms

■ Dehydration—water deficit

- Dialysis—a form of osmosis removing certain impurities from the blood (two types: **peritoneal dialysis** and **hemodialysis**)
- Edema—local or generalized excess retention of tissue fluid
- Glomerular filtration—the movement of fluid and materials under pressure from the blood through the glomerular membrane; the beginning of urine formation
- Tubular reabsorption—the process that follows glomerular filtration; the filtered water and other needed materials leave the tubule by diffusion and active transport to enter tissue fluids
- Urination—voiding or micturition; discharge of urine from the bladder through the urethra
- Urine—fluid waste from the blood secreted by the kidneys; stored in the urinary bladder and excreted from the urethra

Common Diseases and Disorders of the Urinary System

- Enuresis—involuntary discharge of urine
  - diurinal enuresis- occurring during waking hours
  - nocturnal enuresis - occurring during sleep (bed-wetting)
- Glomerulonephritis—acute or chronic inflammation of the kidney glomeruli; symptoms include edema, blood and protein in the urine, and possible uremia
- Hydronephrosis—distention of the renal pelvis resulting from obstructed flow of urine
- Hypospadias—congenital disorder in which the male urethra opens on the underside of the penis
- Incontinence—inability to retain urine, semen, or feces
- Nephrolithiasis (renal calculi)—kidney stones
- Polycystic kidney disease—familial disorder producing cysts in the kidney tubules and leading to kidney failure
- Pyelonephritis—inflammation and pyogenic infection of the renal pelvis
- Renal failure—acute or chronic loss of kidney function resulting in buildup of nitrogen waste in the body
- Uremia—high levels of nitrogen waste in the body

REPRODUCTIVE SYSTEMS

The male and female each has a different **reproductive system**. The male sperm uniting with the female ovum results in the formation of a new and distinct human. The function of reproductive systems is to perpetuate the human species.

Male Reproductive System

The male of the human species is characterized by having an X and a Y chromosome.

Functions of the Male Reproductive System

- Produces sperm
- Deposits sperm into the female reproductive canal
- Produces hormones for male sex characteristics

Components of the Male Reproductive System

Figure 6-27 illustrates the components of the male reproductive system.

- Scrotum—external pouch suspended from the male perineum that contains the testes and epididymis
- Testes (testicles)—2 glandular organs in the male scrotum that produce sperm, some semen (seminal fluid), and testosterone
- Epididymis—2 coiled tubules on the posterior of the testes that store and carry sperm from the testes to the vas deferens
- Vas deferens (vas)—tubule that carries sperm from epididymis to seminal vesicles
- Seminal vesicles—a pair of accessory glands in the male, posterior to the urinary bladder, that secrete nutrient fluid for sperm
- Ejaculatory duct—passage formed by the seminal vesicles and vas deferens that allows semen to enter the urethra
- Prostate gland (exocrine gland)—donut-shaped gland around the male urethra at the bladder neck that secretes alkaline fluid to protect sperm
- Cowper gland (exocrine gland)—2 small glands located at the base of the penis that secrete lubricant during intercourse

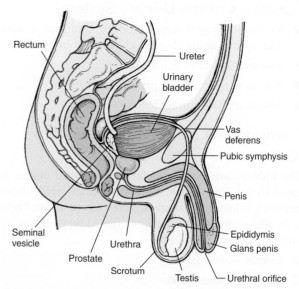

FIGURE 6-27 The male reproductive system. (Reprinted with permission from *Stedman's Medical Dictionary.* 27th Ed. Baltimore: Lippincott Williams & Wilkins, 2000.)

- Penis—external male sex organ that contains the urethra; during sexual arousal, it becomes engorged with blood and firm and erect, allowing entry to the female vagina where the sperm is ejected (ejaculated)
  - Glans penis—acorn-shaped head of penis
  - Prepuce—foreskin; a fold of skin covering the glans penis

Additional Male Reproductive System Terms

- Circumcision—surgical removal of foreskin
- Gamete—male (sperm) or female (ovum) reproductive cell
- Genitalia—external sex organs
- Spermatozoa—sperm
- Vasectomy—male sterilization procedure; tying off or removing part or all of vas deferens

Common Diseases and Disorders of the Male Reproductive System

- Benign prostatic hyperplasia (BPH)—nonmalignant enlargement of the prostate
- Cancers of the male reproductive system—malignancies, usually in the testes or prostate
- Cryptorchidism—failure of testes to descend into the scrotum
- Hypospadias—congenital anomaly; the male urethra opens on the posterior of the penis
- Impotence—inability of the male to achieve erection or ejaculation
- Orchiditis (also spelled orchitis)—inflammation of the testes
- Phimosis—inability to retract the foreskin over the glans penis because of tightness of the skin
- Priapism—abnormal, painful, prolonged penile erection, usually resulting from spinal cord injury or disease

Female Reproductive System

The female of the human species is characterized by two X chromosomes.

Functions of the Female Reproductive System

- Produces ova (eggs) for fertilization
- Carries and nurtures developing fetus
- Gives birth
- Provides food source for newborn
- Produces hormones for female sex characteristics, reproduction, and lactation

Components of the Female Reproductive System

Figure 6-28 depicts the components of the female reproductive system.

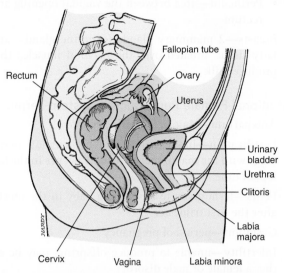

FIGURE 6-28 The female reproductive system. (Reprinted with permission from *Stedman's Medical Dictionary.* 27th Ed. Baltimore: Lippincott Williams & Wilkins, 2000.)

- Ovaries—2 female sex glands located in the pelvis that form ova (the female egg or germ cell) and secrete estrogen
- Uterus—female organ located in pelvic cavity between the oviducts and the vagina; it houses and nourishes the growing fetus and placenta
  - Fundus—upper region of the uterus
  - Body—large central area of the uterus
  - Cervix—lower uterine region opening to the vagina
  - Endometrium—lining of the uterus that sloughs off during menstruation; provides nourishment and protection during pregnancy
- Fallopian tubes (oviducts)—canals that pick up ova released by the ovaries and carry them to the uterus; location of fertilization of the ova by the sperm
- Vagina—part of the birth canal; muscular tube connecting the cervix of the uterus to the external female genitalia
- Vulva—external female genitalia
  - Mons pubis—soft pad over the symphysis pubis
  - Labia majora—two large folds covering the vaginal opening, extending from the mons pubis to the perineum
  - Labia minora—two small folds of skin inside the labia majora
  - Clitoris—small nodule of erectile tissue located in the superior junction of the labia majora; contributes to sexual arousal
  - Bartholin glands (exocrine glands)—glands at the vaginal opening that provide lubrication during sexual intercourse

- • Perineum—area between the vaginal opening and rectum
- ■ Breasts—2 mammary glands (exocrine glands) and fatty tissue situated over the pectoral muscles that produce milk

Additional Female Reproductive System Terms

- ■ Antepartum—time before delivery
- ■ Fertilization—impregnation of the female's ovum (egg) with the male's sperm; usually occurs in the fallopian tube
- ■ Fetus—term given to developing baby in the uterus after the first trimester
- ■ Gestation—period of pregnancy
- ■ Infertility—unable to produce offspring; may be either a female or male disorder
- ■ Menarche—first female menses; usually occurs between 9 and 15 years of age
- ■ Menopause—cessation of menses and female reproduction as a result of aging or surgical removal of the ovaries or uterus
- ■ Menstrual cycle—an approximately 28-day phase beginning with menstruation, followed by the thickening of the endometrium; midcycle, ovulation occurs, followed by secretion of progesterone by the corpus luteum to prepare the uterus for a fertilized ovum; if pregnancy does not occur, the cycle repeats
- ■ Menstruation (menses)—shedding of the endometrium of the uterus in the form of vaginal bleeding when pregnancy does not occur, usually every 28 days
- ■ Neonatal—first 30 days after birth
- ■ Ovulation—release of an ovum (egg) from the follicle into the ovarian tube resulting from cyclical hormonal function
- ■ Papanicolaou smear (Pap smear)—test for cervical cancer that involves microscopically examining cervical scrapings
- ■ Parturition—process of delivery; giving birth
- ■ Placenta—oval vascular structure in the uterus during pregnancy that supplies nutrients to the fetus
- ■ Pregnancy—gestation; period of fetal development in the uterus from fertilization to birth, usually lasting 40 weeks

Common Diseases and Disorders of the Female Reproductive System

- ■ Abortion—termination of pregnancy before fetal viability; may be spontaneous (naturally occurring) or medically/surgically induced
- ■ Abruptio placentae—premature separation of the placenta
- ■ Amenorrhea—absence of menstrual flow

- ■ Carcinomas—malignancies of the female reproductive system that most commonly occur in the breasts, ovaries, uterus, and cervix
- ■ Eclampsia—toxemia of pregnancy with high blood pressure, albuminuria, oliguria, seizures, and sometimes coma and death
- ■ Ectopic pregnancy (extrauterine)—implantation of fertilized ovum outside the uterus, most commonly in the fallopian tubes
- ■ Endometriosis—condition caused by abnormal location of endometrium tissue outside the uterus; causes pain and, sometimes, cyst formation
- ■ Fibroids—nonmalignant tumors of the uterus
- ■ Menorrhagia—painful menses
- ■ Miscarriage—spontaneous abortion; natural interruption of a pregnancy before the seventh month
- ■ Pelvic inflammatory disease (PID)—inflammation of the pelvic cavity organs resulting from widespread infection
- ■ Placenta previa—implantation of the placenta in the lower uterus
- ■ Premenstrual syndrome (PMS)—irritability, bloating, and depression preceding menses

Sexually Transmitted Diseases

Sexually transmitted diseases (STDs) or infections (STIs) affect both males and females. The act of intercourse results in passing and intermingling of body secretions between the sexual partners. These secretions may contain pathogens that are then sexually transmitted from one person to another. The more sexual partners a person has, the higher the risk of becoming infected.

- ■ AIDS—decreased immunity resulting from infection with HIV; leaves victim susceptible to opportunistic diseases
- ■ Chlamydia—caused by *Chlamydia trachomatis*; the most prevalent STD; symptoms are frequently undetected and result in female PID; babies born to mothers with chlamydia are at risk for chlamydial pneumonia
- ■ Genital herpes—viral infection of the male and female genital tracts' mucous membranes with painful lesions; incurable and may lead to cervical cancer in women; newborns become infected through the female birth canal
- ■ Genital warts—infection caused by human papillomaviruses; a potential cause of cervical cancer
- ■ Gonorrhea—contagious inflammation of the genital mucous membrane of either sex, caused by *Neisseria gonorrhoeae*
- ■ HIV—the virus causing AIDS
- ■ Syphilis—chronic STD resulting in lesions (chancres) that may spread to the bone and other body systems; disease may be congenital

TERMS

ANATOMY AND PHYSIOLOGY REVIEW

The following list reviews the terms discussed in this chapter, *as well as other important terms that you may see on the exam.*

abduction moving away from the body midline (the opposite of adduction) (e.g., spreading the arms)

abortion termination of pregnancy before viability; may be spontaneous (naturally occurring) or medically/surgically induced

abruptio placentae premature separation of the placenta

absorption the transfer of the products of digestion into the blood and lymph for circulation

acquired immunodeficiency syndrome (AIDS) decreased immunity resulting from infection with the human immunodeficiency virus (HIV), leaving victim susceptible to opportunistic diseases

acromegaly overproduction of the growth hormone after puberty, resulting in wide, large face, hands, and feet

active transport movement of molecules from area of lower to area of higher concentration

Addison disease hyposecretion of cortisol by the adrenal cortex, resulting in muscle atrophy, tissue weakness, and skin pigmentation

adduction moving toward the body midline (the opposite of abduction) (e.g., bringing the arms to the sides)

adrenal glands endocrine glands located on top of each kidney; refer to Table 6-1 for functions

alveoli (singular *alveolus*) air sacs at the ends of the bronchioles where the exchange of gases occurs

Alzheimer disease degenerative disorder of the brain beginning with dementialike symptoms and progressing to a nonfunctioning of neuron fibers that prevents communication between cells for ordinary tasks (such as swallowing), which results in death; etiology is unknown

amenorrhea absence of menstrual flow

amyotrophic lateral sclerosis (ALS) progressive disease of the motor neurons, causing muscle atrophy and weakness; also known as *Lou Gehrig disease*

anabolism phase of metabolism in which cells are built or repaired

anaphase third phase of mitosis; duplicated chromosomes separate, and one of each begins to move toward opposite centrioles or poles

anatomy the study of body structure

anemia abnormally low hemoglobin or red blood cells, decreasing oxygen supply to the tissues; many causes and types; the main symptoms are fatigue and weakness

aneurysm congenital or traumatic weakness of the vessel wall demonstrated by a "bubble" or outpouching caused by pressure of blood; an abdominal aortic aneurysm is also called *AAA* or *triple A*

angina pectoris severe constricting chest pain from lack of blood supply to the heart; associated with coronary artery disease

anorexia diminished appetite and aversion to food

antepartum time before delivery

anterior in front (ventral)

antibody a substance produced in the body in response to the presence of an antigen;

antigen a substance (e.g., bacteria/viruses, bacterial/viral toxins, foreign blood cells) that causes the formation of antibodies

anus the final portion of the digestive tract, where feces are excreted

aorta the largest body artery; consists of three parts: ascending, aortic arch, and descending

aponeurosis broad sheet of muscle fibers attaching muscle to muscle or muscle to select bones, such as the skull

appendicular skeleton consists of the bones of the upper and lower extremities and the girdle attaching them to the axial skeleton.

arrhythmias abnormal heart rhythms

arteriosclerosis hardening of the arteries and loss of elasticity resulting from thickening of the vessel wall

arthritis inflammation of the joints

asthma an episodic chronic respiratory disorder resulting from constricted bronchi; associated with allergens, infection, pollutants, cold air, exercise, or stress; characterized by wheezing and low oxygen levels

astigmatism impaired vision resulting from irregular curve of cornea;

atelectasis a decrease or absence of air in part or all of the lung and alveoli, resulting in a collapse of these structures

atherosclerosis the most common form of arteriosclerosis; irregular fatty deposits on arterial wall result in narrowing and occlusion of vessel;

atrioventricular (AV) node located at the lower right of the atrial septum, it picks up the impulse or signal from the sinoatrial (SA) node that causes atrial contraction;

axial skeleton consists of the bones of the skull, spine, and chest

Bell palsy unilateral facial muscle paralysis (drooping of eye and mouth) resulting from dysfunction of the seventh cranial nerve

benign prostatic hyperplasia (BPH) nonmalignant enlargement of the prostate

bile a substance produced by the liver and stored in the gallbladder that aids in digestion and fat absorption

body organism; a group of systems working together to maintain life

body cavities spaces within the body that house internal organs

botulism serious food poisoning, usually found in contaminated canned foods, caused by *Clostridium botulinum* bacteria

brain an organ acting as the primary center for regulating and coordinating body functions and activities;

bronchi (singular *bronchus*) tubes from trachea entering the lungs that subdivide into two more branches in the lungs

bronchioles smaller branches of the bronchi

bronchitis chronic or acute inflammation of the bronchi

Bulimia nervosa eating disorder characterized by binge eating and purging

bundle branches 2 branches extending from the bundle of His in the heart that carry the electrical impulse down the ventricular septum

bundle of His specialized cells in the cardiac ventricular septum that carry the electrical impulse from the atrioventricular (AV) node; should the sinoatrial and AV nodes fail, the bundle of His may initiate the impulse;

cardiovascular system the body system containing the heart and blood vessels to circulate blood, transport nutrients, and remove waste from tissues

carpals 8 wrist bones

cartilage firm but often flexible connective tissue found primarily in joints, thorax walls, larynx, and airway passages and ears

catabolism the phase of metabolism in which cells are broken down

cataract a cloudy or opaque lens that impairs sight; usually corrected by surgery

caudal the location near the sacral region of the spinal column

cecum the upper portion of the large intestine; contains the appendix

celiac disease damages the small intestine and interferes with the absorption of nutrients characterized by intolerance to gluten

cells the structural and functional units of life

central nervous system (CNS) made up of the brain and spinal cord; integrates sensory information and responses

centriole rod-shaped material in the cytoplasm that begins cell division

cerebellum "little brain"; portion of the brain involved in synergic control of skeletal muscles and coordination of voluntary muscular movements; connected to the cerebrum, brain stem, and spinal cord by the pons

cerebral palsy loss of mental function, sensation, or control of movement resulting from birth injury or defect

cerebrospinal fluid (CSF) clear fluid that flows through the brain and spinal cord and into the subarachnoid spaces of the meninges; it cushions and supports nervous tissue and transports nutrients and waste products from the cells

cerebrovascular accident (CVA) stroke; occlusion or hemorrhage of vessel(s) in the brain, resulting in impairment of mental functions or paralysis or both

cerebrum the largest part of the brain, divided into right and left hemispheres by the longitudinal fissure;

Cheyne–Stokes respiration an irregular breathing pattern of slow and shallow, then rapid and deep respirations, with pauses for 20 to 30 seconds; frequently occurs before death

chlamydia the most prevalent sexually transmitted disease, caused by *Chlamydia trachomatis*

cholelithiasis gallstones

chronic obstructive pulmonary disease (COPD) a usually progressive respiratory system disorder with irreversible obstruction of air exchange in the bronchi, alveoli, and lungs; emphysema is a form of COPD

cilia hairlike processes that trap and move foreign particles

circumcision surgical removal of foreskin

circumduction drawing an imaginary circle with a body structure (e.g., the arms)

cirrhosis end-stage liver disease with interference with blood flow, resulting in jaundice, portal hypertension, and liver failure

clavicle collar bone joining the sternum at the anterior and the scapula laterally

cochlea snail-shaped tube in ear containing receptor for hearing

colitis inflammation of the colon

collagen a fibrous protein found in the dermis, connective tissues, tendons, and ligaments; it is sometimes referred to as the body's glue, providing strength and flexibility

Colles fracture displaced fracture of the distal radius, proximal to the wrist

colon largest portion of large intestine; divides into four parts: ascending colon, transverse colon, descending colon, and sigmoid

concussion mild head injury (MHI) or mild traumatic brain injury (MTBI) resulting in subtle or more serious physical, cognitive, or emotional signs and symptoms

congestive heart failure (CHF) venous and pulmonary congestion and general edema (swelling) resulting from decreased blood circulation

conjunctivitis inflammation of the conjunctiva caused by infection or irritation

coronary artery disease (CAD) arteriosclerosis or atherosclerosis of the coronary arteries, usually leading to myocardial ischemia (damage to tissue)

Cowper glands 2 small glands located at the base of the penis that secrete lubricant during intercourse

cranial location associated with the head

cretinism hypothyroidism; decreased secretion of thyroxine in infants resulting in failure of physical and mental development

Crohn disease chronic inflammatory disease of ileum or colon resulting in diarrhea, pain, weight loss, and sometimes rectal bleeding;

croup acute viral infection, usually in infants, characterized by barking cough

cryptorchidism failure of testes to descend into the scrotum

Cushing syndrome overproduction of cortisol by the adrenal cortex, resulting in round face, overweight, thin skin, and high blood glucose

cystic fibrosis a genetic disorder producing abnormally thick mucous secretions that block and impair the bronchi, pancreatic and bile ducts, and intestines

cytoplasm colloidal substance (protoplasm) found in the cell; holds other structures in place

dendrites neuron fibers conducting impulses to the cell body

dermis deeper layer of skin containing nerves, blood vessels, and other skin structures or appendages

diabetes mellitus most common endocrine disorder; low production of insulin, resulting in cells retaining sugar; two types: insulin-dependent diabetes mellitus (type 1 diabetes) and non–insulin-dependent diabetes mellitus (type 2 diabetes)

diabetic retinopathy damage to the retina in diabetic patients from hemorrhage of vessels;

dialysis a form of osmosis that removes certain impurities from the blood (two types: peritoneal and hemodialysis)

diaphragm muscle tissue separating thoracic and abdominal cavities that contracts and expands during respiration, allowing lungs to fill and empty air

diastole relaxation portion of the cardiac cycle

diffusion movement of molecules from area of higher to lower concentration

digestion physical and chemical processes changing food into simple nutrients to be utilized by the cells for energy and building materials and into solid waste to be eliminated from the body

digestive system body system containing mouth, esophagus, stomach, intestines, rectum, liver, gallbladder, and pancreas; the system ingests and processes food and eliminates solid waste products

distal away from the origin of a structure

diverticula (singular *diverticulum*) abnormal pouches in the walls of an organ, usually the colon

diverticulosis diverticula of the colon

dorsal posterior; in back

dorsiflexion pointing the toes up

duodenum upper portion of small intestine, separated from the stomach by the pyloric sphincter

dwarfism decreased growth hormone, resulting in abnormally small size

eclampsia toxemia of pregnancy, with high blood pressure, albuminuria, oliguria, seizures, and sometimes coma

ectopic pregnancy extrauterine pregnancy; implantation of fertilized ovum outside the uterus, most commonly in the ovarian tubes

ejaculatory duct passage formed by the seminal vesicles and vas deferens allowing semen to enter the urethra

elimination excretion of the solid waste products of digestion in the form of feces

embolus (plural *emboli*) a detached thrombus or other substance occluding a vessel

emphysema a form of chronic obstructive pulmonary disease that impedes respiration; characterized by irreversible loss of elasticity in alveoli

endocardium inner layer of the heart

endocrine system body system containing glands and related structures that produce and secrete hormones into the bloodstream or into its own surrounding tissues.

endometriosis condition caused by endometrium tissue located outside the uterus that causes pain and, sometimes, cyst formation

enteritis inflammation of the small intestine

enucleation removal of the eyeball

enuresis involuntary discharge of urine

enzymes proteins that act as catalysts to increase the speed of digestion;

epicardium outer layer of the heart

epidermis surface layer of skin containing strata and melanin

epididymis 2 coiled tubules on the posterior of the testes that store and carry sperm from the testes to the vas deferens

epiglottis flaplike structure covering larynx during swallowing

epilepsy abnormal electrical activity of the brain resulting in seizure;

erythrocytes red blood cells (RBCs); contain hemoglobin to carry oxygen; mature cells do not have a nucleus

esophagus tube from the pharynx to the stomach

eustachian tube connects middle ear with throat and pharynx; equalizes pressure on tympanic membrane

eversion turning wrists or ankles outward, away from the body (the opposite of inversion)

exocrine gland a gland that excretes its product through a duct to an environment external to itself or into the bloodstream

exophthalmia protrusion of the eyeballs, usually resulting from an endocrine disorder

expiration exhalation; letting air out of the lungs;

extension bringing the limbs or phalanges toward a straight position (the opposite of flexion)

extracellular fluid body fluid outside the cell

fallopian tubes oviducts; canals leading from the ovaries to the uterus where fertilization of the ova by the sperm occurs

femur thigh bone; the body's largest, longest, and strongest bone

fertilization impregnation of the female ovum (egg) with the male sperm

fetus term given after the first trimester to a developing baby in the uterus

fibroids nonmalignant tumors of the uterus

fibula smaller lower leg bone, lateral to tibia

filtration process of moving fluid containing dissolved particles through a membrane; an example is kidney filtration

flagella whiplike processes on the cell surface; accommodate cell movement

flexion bending (the opposite of extension), such as closing the fingers of the hand

fluid balance the regulation of the amount and composition of the body's fluids

frontal plane imaginary line or cut of the body made in line with the ears and then down the middle of the body, resulting in a front and a back portion; also called *coronal plane*

gallbladder pear-shaped sac located on the inferior surface of the liver; stores bile to aid in digestion and fat absorption

gamete male (sperm) or female (ovum) reproductive cell

ganglion marked swelling of gray matter, located outside the central nervous system, containing cells of neurons

gastroesophageal reflux disease (GERD) backflow of stomach acids into the esophagus due to an incompetent esophageal sphincter, resulting in burning and discomfort; can lead to ulcers

genital herpes painful and incurable viral infection of the male or female genital tract's mucous membrane;

genitalia external sex organs

genital warts infection caused by the human papillomavirus; believed to be a precursor of female cervical cancer

gestation period of pregnancy

giantism overproduction of the growth hormone, resulting in abnormally large size

giardiasis infectious diarrhea caused by *Giardia lamblia* in contaminated water

glans penis acorn-shaped head of penis

glaucoma a disease of the eye characterized by increased intraocular pressure; causes damage to optic nerve; often results in blindness

globulins the fraction of the blood serum protein associated with antibodies; vaccination with globulins produces passive immunity

glomerular filtration the movement of fluid and materials under pressure from the blood through the kidney's glomerular membrane; the beginning of urine formation

glomerulonephritis acute or chronic inflammation of the kidney glomeruli;

glomeruli networks of blood capillaries enclosed in Bowman capsule

goiter enlarged thyroid

gonorrhea contagious inflammation of the genital mucous membrane of either sex, caused by *Neisseria gonorrhoeae*

gout inflammation and pain, usually of the great toes or thumbs, caused by accumulation of uric acid crystals;

Graves disease hyperthyroidism; increased secretion of thyroxine; characterized by goiter, exophthalmia (bulging eyes), weight loss, extreme nervousness, and rapid metabolism

hematopoiesis the process by which undifferentiated stem cells give rise to all other blood cells; the process *by* which cells that produce blood are generated

hemodialysis a form of dialysis that removes blood via a catheter placed directly into a vein; the blood then circulates through a dialysis machine to remove impurities

hemophilia genetic bleeding disorder involving a deficiency of specific clotting factors and resulting in excessive bleeding, especially into the joints

hemorrhoids inflammation and dilation of veins in rectum and anus

hepatic referring to the liver

hepatitis acute or chronic inflammation of the liver;

hernia protrusion of an organ or part of an organ through the wall normally containing it; intestine is the most common organ to herniate

herpes zoster shingles; infection caused by the herpes zoster virus forming blister-type lesions and producing pain along the nerve trunks

histology study of tissues

homeostasis equilibrium or health of the body as measured by established norms for blood pressure, heart rate, temperature, respiration rate, and other indicators

human immunodeficiency virus (HIV) the virus causing acquired immunodeficiency syndrome

human papillomavirus (HPV) the virus associated with genital warts and cervical cancer

humerus upper arm bone

hydrocephalus accumulation of cerebrospinal fluid in the brain caused by an obstruction and resulting in mounting pressure and destruction of brain tissue

hydronephrosis distention of the renal pelvis resulting from obstructed flow of urine

hyperextension extreme or abnormal extension, usually resulting in injury

hyperopia farsightedness; a condition in which distant objects can be seen more clearly than closer objects

hypertension high blood pressure (beginning at 140/90)

hyperthyroidism overactivity of the thyroid

hypertonic solution fluid more concentrated than intracellular fluid; it draws fluid away from the cell and causes the cell to shrink

hypospadias congenital disorder; the male urethra opens on the underside of the penis

hypothalamus located in the diencephalon, the hypothalamus contains nerve cells assisting in maintenance of water balance, fat and sugar metabolism, secretion of endocrine glands, and regulation of body temperature

hypothyroidism underactivity of the thyroid

hypotonic solution fluid less concentrated than intracellular fluid; it results in excess fluid entering the cell and may cause the cell to rupture

ileum lower portion of the small intestine, opening into the cecum

ilium superior wing-shaped portion of hip bones

immunity the individual's ability to resist specific diseases or disorders, usually by acquiring the corresponding antibody

immunization vaccination; protection from communicable diseases by administration of living attenuated agents (e.g., measles), killed organisms (e.g., pertussis), inactivated toxins (e.g., tetanus), or recombinant DNA (e.g., hepatitis B)

impotence inability of the male to achieve erection or ejaculation

incontinence inability to retain urine, semen, or feces

incus anvil; second ossicle (bone) of the middle ear

inferior below

infertility inability to produce offspring; may be either a female or male disorder

inspiration inhalation; bringing air into lungs;

integumentary system the largest system of the body, it contains skin, glands, hair, nails, blood vessels, and nerves to protect against infection and other "invaders"; assists with prevention of dehydration; controls body temperature; receives sensory information; eliminates waste products; and produces vitamin D

intracellular fluid body fluid inside the cell

intussusception one part of the intestine slipping into another, leading to bowel obstruction

inversion turning inside out (the opposite of eversion)

ischium inferior portion of hip bones supporting the body weight when sitting

isotonic solution with the same concentration as intracellular fluid, moves in and out of the cell at the same rate

jaundice yellow color of skin, white of eyes, and mucous membranes resulting from increased bilirubin in blood;

joints areas where 2 or more bones come together or articulate

keratin a protein in the epidermis that thickens and waterproofs the skin

kidneys two muscular, bean-shaped organs located in the back of the abdominal cavity that filtrate, reabsorb selected substances, and excrete urine

kyphosis hunchback; an excessive curvature in the thoracic portion of the vertebral column

labyrinth inner ear; contains vestibule, semicircular canal, and cochlea with receptors for hearing and balance

large intestine the final organ of the digestive tract; connects to the small intestine at the ileum; sections include cecum, colon, rectum; ends at the anus; manufactures vitamins K and B; absorbs fluids and electrolytes; forms, stores, and excretes feces

larynx voice box; organ between the pharynx and trachea containing vocal cords, which vibrate to produce speech

lateral away from midline, toward the side

Legionnaires disease a type of pneumonia caused by the *Legionella pneumophila* bacteria

leukemia type of malignancy characterized by rapid and abnormal development of leukocytes (white blood cells) in spleen, bone marrow, and lymph nodes

leukocytes white blood cells (WBCs); fight infection

ligaments bands of fibrous connective tissue connecting the articulating ends of bones to facilitate or limit movement

liver largest gland in the body, located in the upper right portion of the abdominal cavity; it produces bile, detoxifies blood, and aids metabolism

lordosis swayback; excessive curvature in the lumbar portion of the vertebral column

lungs two main organs of the respiratory system that are located in the thoracic cavity; they distribute and exchange gases

lymphatic system body system containing lymph, lymph nodes, and related organs to protect against and fight disease

macular degeneration progressive abnormal growth of blood vessels or other structures in the retina, usually leading to blindness

malleus hammer; first ossicle (bone) of the middle ear

mandible lower jaw bone

maxilla upper jaw bone

medial toward the middle or center

mediastinum small cavity within the thoracic cavity that lies between the lungs and contains the heart and large blood vessels

medulla oblongata portion of the brain connecting with spinal cord; contains centers for control of heartbeat, respirations, and blood pressure

melanin pigment giving the skin its color

membranes thin sheets of tissue that line and protect body structures

menarche first female menses; usually occurs between 9 and 15 years of age

meninges (singular meninx) three layers of connective tissue covering that completely enclose the brain and spinal cord

menopause cessation of menses and female reproduction from aging or surgical removal of the ovaries and uterus

menorrhagia painful menses

mesentery composed of 2 layers of peritoneum that lie on the walls of the peritoneal cavity connecting the intestines to the wall of the abdomen

menstrual cycle a phase lasting approximately 28 days, beginning with menstruation, followed by the thickening of the endometrium; midcycle, ovulation occurs, followed by secretion of progesterone by the corpus luteum to prepare the uterus for a fertilized ovum;

menstruation menses; the shedding of the endometrium of the uterus in the form of vaginal bleeding when pregnancy does not occur, usually in a 28-day cycle

metabolism energy transformation in living cells

metacarpals five bones that form the palm of the hand

metaphase second phase of mitosis; chromosomes line up along an equator-type line along centriole filaments

metatarsals the five foot bones

midbrain connects the pons and cerebellum with the cerebrum; functions as relay for certain eye and ear reflexes

mild head injury (MHI) concussion

mild traumatic brain injury (MTBI) concussion

miscarriage spontaneous abortion; a natural interruption of a pregnancy before the seventh month

mitosis cell division; comprises four phases: prophase, metaphase, anaphase, and telophase

mouth oral cavity; orifice in the lower face where food enters the body

multiple sclerosis progressive inflammation and hardening of the myelin sheath in the nervous system

muscular system body system that contains muscles and related structures that accommodate movement

myocardial infarction (MI) heart attack; necrosis (death) of an area in the myocardium resulting from cessation of blood supply, usually from coronary thrombosis

myocardium middle layer of the heart

myopia condition of nearsightedness; can see objects close by but not far away

myxedema atrophy of thyroid in adults, resulting in decreased secretion of thyroxine, causing forms of physical and mental decline

narcolepsy uncontrollable episodes of falling asleep; also known as sleep epilepsy

neonatal first 30 days after birth

nephrolithiasis (renal calculi) kidney stones

nephrons group of microscopic coiled tubules (more than 1 million in each kidney), located in the renal pyramids, that filter blood and form urine; main structures are collecting tubules, glomeruli, and arterioles; the bottom of the paperclip-shaped segment of the nephron is called the loop of Henle

nervous system body system containing nerves and related structures that receive stimuli and initiate responses

neurotransmitter chemical released by the axons that stimulates the next cell to continue the transmission of an impulse

nucleolus small structure in the cell nucleus that holds ribonucleic acid (RNA) and ribosomes essential for protein formation

nucleus located in the center of the cell; controls cell activity and contains genetic material (DNA)

orchiditis (also spelled orchitis) inflammation of the testes

organ group of tissues working together to perform a function, such as the kidney

osmosis water diffusion (movement from area of higher to lower concentration) through a semipermeable membrane

osmotic pressure the tendency of a higher-concentration solution to draw in water from a lower-concentration solution

osteoarthritis degenerative joint disease that results in deformities and chronic pain; usually occurs as part of the aging process

osteoblast cell that forms bone tissue

osteochondroma malignancy of the bone and cartilage

osteomyelitis inflammation of the bone or marrow caused by pathogens

osteoporosis porous, brittle bones resulting from low levels of calcium salts

osteosarcoma malignant tumor of the bone

otitis media infection of middle ear

ovaries 2 female endocrine sex glands (gonads) that secrete estrogen to stimulate growth of breasts, uterus, and secondary sex characteristics and form ova (the female gametes) and progesterone to prepare and maintain uterus in pregnancy;

ovulation release of an ovum (egg) from the follicle into the ovarian tube resulting from cyclical hormone function

pancreas an endocrine and exocrine gland located behind the stomach that produces pancreatic juice, and insulin and glucagon

Papanicolaou smear (Pap smear) test for cervical cancer that involves microscopically examining cervical scrapings

parasympathetic nervous system portion of the nervous system that returns the body to rest and replenishes energy

parathyroid gland one of 4 pea-sized glands located on or embedded in the thyroid that secrete parathyroid hormone, increasing blood levels of calcium

Parkinson disease chronic progressive neurologic disease characterized by fine tremors and muscle weakness and rigidity; etiology believed to be associated with low dopamine production

parturition process of delivery; giving birth

patella kneecap

patent ductus arteriosus (PDA) opening between the aorta and pulmonary artery in fetal circulation that does not close as it should after birth

pathology the study of abnormal changes in body structure or function, usually caused by disease

pelvic inflammatory disease (PID) inflammation of the pelvic cavity organs resulting from widespread infection

penis external male sex organ containing the urethra

peripheral nervous system (PNS) nerves outside the central nervous system originating from the brain and spinal cord; it transmits sensory information and responses

peristalsis rhythmic contractions that move food throughout the digestive tract

peritoneal dialysis a form of dialysis using the peritoneal membrane to filter wastes

pernicious anemia type of anemia resulting from malabsorption of vitamin B_{12} in the ileum

pertussis whooping cough; a vaccine-preventable bacterial infection caused by *Bordetella pertussis*,

phagocytosis ingestion and digestion of bacteria and other substances by phagocytic cells

phalanges fingers (3 bones each) and thumb (2 bones each); toes (3 bones each) and great toes (2 bones each)

pharyngitis sore throat; inflammation of the pharynx

pharynx throat; passageway from nose to larynx

phimosis inability to retract the foreskin over the glans penis because of tightness of the skin

physiology the study of body function

pineal gland endocrine gland located in the brain behind the hypothalamus that secretes melatonin, which regulates the body's sleep/wake cycles

pinna auricle; external ear; directs sound waves to the canal

pituitary endocrine gland located at the base of the brain, called "master gland" because of the number of hormones it secretes and functions it serves; Table 6-1 lists its functions

placenta oval vascular structure present in the uterus during pregnancy that supplies nutrients to the fetus

placenta previa abnormal implantation of the placenta in the lower uterus

plantar flexion pointing toes downward, which flexes the arch of the foot

plasma liquid portion of blood (55%)

platelets (thrombocytes) cell fragments; function in coagulation

pleura lung linings containing pleural fluid to protect lungs and reduce friction during respiration

pleurisy inflammation of the pleura

pneumonia viral or bacterial infection causing inflammation of the lungs

pneumothorax partial or complete collapse of the lung(s) resulting from air in the pleural cavity

polycystic kidney disease familial disorder producing cysts in the kidney tubules leading to kidney failure

pons area where nerves cross, resulting in nerves located on one side of the brain controlling the opposite side of the body; connects the cerebellum with the nervous system

pregnancy gestation; period of fetal development in the uterus from fertilization to birth, usually 40 weeks

premenstrual syndrome (PMS) irritability, bloating, and depression preceding menses

prepuce foreskin; a fold of skin on the penis covering the glans

presbyopia a form of farsightedness most common eye condition associated with aging

priapism abnormal, painful, prolonged penile erection, usually resulting from spinal cord injury or disease

prophase first stage of mitosis; centrioles move to opposite ends of the cell, forming two poles

prostate gland donut-shaped gland around the male urethra at the bladder neck that secretes alkaline fluid to protect sperm

proximal toward the origin of a structure

pubis anterior union of the hip bones

pulmonary edema fluid accumulation in the lungs, often associated with congestive heart failure

Purkinje fibers smaller fibers arising from the bundle branches located in the heart's conductive system that carry the electrical impulse to the ventricular walls, causing them to contract

pyelonephritis inflammation and pyogenic infection of the renal pelvis

radius lateral bone of forearm (in anatomic position)

rales crackling breath sound resulting from increased secretions in the bronchi; sometimes referred to as *rhonchi*

rectum the lower portion of the large intestine that contains the reflexes for defecation

renal failure acute or chronic loss of kidney function that results in buildup of nitrogen waste in the body

reproductive system body system containing gonads (ovaries or testes) and related sex-specific organs and structures to reproduce the species

respiratory system body system containing nose, pharynx, larynx, trachea, lungs, and related structures that transport oxygen and remove carbon dioxide

rheumatoid arthritis inflammation and overgrowth of synovial membranes and joint tissues characterized by swelling of joints

rotation turning on an axis, such as turning the head to indicate "no"

rugae folds in the lining of the stomach and some other organs

sagittal plane an imaginary line or cut through the body, bilaterally separating it into right and left halves

salivary glands three pairs of glands located in the mouth, secreting saliva that moistens food and begins the chemical breakdown of carbohydrates

scapula shoulder blade

scoliosis abnormal lateral curvature of the vertebral column

scrotum external pouch suspended from the male perineum containing the testes and epididymis

seminal vesicles a pair of accessory glands in the male, posterior to the urinary bladder, that secrete nutrient fluid for sperm

serum clear, liquid portion of blood that remains after the blood clots

sigmoid lower S-shaped portion of colon connected to the descending colon and the rectum

sinoatrial (SA) node located in the upper wall of the right atrium, it is the pacemaker of the heart

skeletal system body system containing bones and related structures to provide structural support

small intestine longest portion of digestive tract; digests fats, proteins, and carbohydrates and absorbs the nutrient products into the blood; contains 3 sections: duodenum, jejunum, and ileum

spermatozoa sperm

spina bifida congenital deformity exposing the spinal column, resulting from malformation of vertebrae

spinal cord continuous tubelike structure located within the spinal vertebrae extending from the occipital bone to the coccyx; it contains cerebrospinal fluid and ascending and descending nerve tracts that carry transmissions to and from the brain

stapes stirrup; third ossicle (bone) of the middle ear

stem cell an undifferentiated biologic cell that can differentiate into specialized cells

stomach J-shaped organ between the esophagus and the duodenum that produces a churning action that mixes food with gastric acids and enzymes as part of digestion; also stores food

strabismus inability of both eyes to simultaneously focus on a subject; commonly known as lazy eye or being cross-eyed

strata sublayers

stridor high-pitched breath sounds resembling wind; caused by a partial obstruction of air passages

superior above

sympathetic nervous system portion of the nervous system preparing the body for stressful situations ("fight or flight")

synapse neuromuscular junction between neurons

syphilis sexually transmitted disease resulting in lesions (chancre) that may spread to bone and other systems

systole contraction portion of the cardiac cycle

tarsals the 7 ankle and foot bones; the largest is the calcaneus, or heel bone

telophase final phase of mitosis; the nucleus divides in the center, forming two distinct cells

tendons connective tissue attaching muscle directly to the periosteum (covering) of the bone

testes male endocrine sex glands (gonads) that secrete testosterone and stimulate the development of male sex characteristics and sperm

tetany spasms caused by low blood calcium

thalamus located in the diencephalon, serves as relay for sensory input

thorax cavity containing lungs

thrombophlebitis inflammation of a vein with clots

thrombus (plural *thrombi*) a blood clot attached to a vessel wall

thrush yeast infection of the mouth caused by *Candida albicans*

tibia shin bone

tinnitus ringing in the ears

tissues group of cells with similar structures and functions

trachea tube branching into two bronchi leading into the lungs

transient ischemic attack (TIA) ministroke; temporary episode of impaired neurologic function resulting from decreased blood flow to the brain

transverse plane an imaginary line or cut through the body horizontally dividing it into superior and inferior sections

tuberculosis an infectious bacterial disease characterized by tubercles in the tissue; the lung is the most common disease site

tubular reabsorption the process that follows glomerular filtration; the filtered water and other needed materials leave the tubule by diffusion and active transport and enter tissue fluids

tympanic membrane eardrum; boundary between external and middle ear canals; vibrates, transmitting sound waves to inner ear

ulcerative colitis inflammation and ulceration of the mucosa of the colon and rectum

ulcers lesions of the mucosa of any organ; most common in the stomach and intestine

ulna medial bone of forearm (in anatomic position)

uremia high levels of nitrogen waste in the body

ureters 2 slim tubes that carry urine from the kidneys to the urinary bladder

urethra tube from the bladder that allows urine to leave the body

urinary bladder saclike organ behind the symphysis pubis that temporarily stores urine

urinary system body system containing kidneys, ureters, bladder, and urethra that removes nitrogen-type waste and regulates water balance

urination voiding or micturition; discharge of urine from the bladder

uterus female organ located in pelvic cavity from the oviducts to the vagina; houses and nourishes the growing fetus and placenta

vas deferens tubule carrying sperm from epididymis to seminal vesicles

vasectomy male sterilization procedure; tying off or removing part or all of vas deferens

vena cava largest body vein, with inferior and superior branches

vertebral column spine; 26 vertebrae (bones that cover the spinal cord)

vertigo dizziness

vestibule middle section of inner ear involving balance

villi (singular *villus*) tiny projections in the small intestine lining where absorption of nutrients occurs

wheeze squeaking or whistling breath sound, usually caused by narrowed tracheobronchial airways, as in asthma

xiphoid process small tip at the lower end of sternum

REVIEW QUESTIONS

All questions are relevant for the CMA (AAMA), RMA (AMT), and CMAS (AMT) exams.

1. The thoracic and abdominal cavities of the body are separated by the:
   A. ribs.
   B. stomach.
   C. diaphragm.
   D. peritoneum.

   Answer: **C**
   Why: The diaphragm is a dome-shaped muscle under the lungs that flattens during inhalation. This structure separates the thoracic cavity, which contain the lungs, from the abdomen.
   Review: Yes ○   No ○

2. The main tissue of the outer layer of the skin is:
   A. connective.
   B. adipose.
   C. mucosal.
   D. endothelial.
   E. epithelial.

   Answer: **E**
   Why: Epithelial tissue covers surfaces, such as skin. It also lines cavities and forms glands. Connective tissue supports and forms the framework of body parts. Adipose tissue contains cells that are able to store large amounts of fat. Mucosal tissue lines the tubes and other spaces that open to the outside of the body, for example, the lining of the nose.
   Review: Yes ○   No ○

3. The glands that are saclike in structure and produce oily secretions that lubricate the skin are:
   A. sebaceous.
   B. ceruminous.
   C. ciliary.
   D. mammary.

   Answer: **A**
   Why: Ceruminous glands are found in the ear canal and secrete cerumen, or earwax. Mammary glands are found in the breast and secrete breast milk. Ciliary glands are sweat glands found around the margin of the eyelids.
   Review: Yes ○   No ○

4. The portion of skeletal bone that manufactures blood cells is the:
   A. periosteum.
   B. red bone marrow.
   C. diaphysis.
   D. cartilage.
   E. epiphysis.

   Answer: **B**
   Why: Periosteum is the membrane covering the outside of bones. The diaphysis of a bone is the long, narrow shaft of the bone. The epiphysis is the end portion of a bone where the growth of the bone takes place. Cartilage is a tough, elastic, translucent material that covers the ends of the long bones. The red bone marrow is found in the center of bones and manufactures blood cells.
   Review: Yes ○   No ○

5. The structures that attach muscles to bones are:
   A. fascia.
   B. ligaments.
   C. tendons.
   D. cartilage.

   Answer: **C**
   Why: Fascia consists of fibrous bands or sheets that support organs and hold them in place. Ligaments are structures that connect bone to bone. Cartilage is a tough, elastic, translucent material that covers the ends of the long bones.
   Review: Yes ○   No ○

6. Nerve fibers are insulated and protected by a fatty material called:
   A. myelin.
   B. dendrites.
   C. neurons.
   D. axons.
   E. synapses.

Answer: **A**
Why: Neurons are the functional cells of the nervous system, and the axons and dendrites are the neuron fibers that conduct impulses away from and to cell bodies. A synapse is the contact point from one nerve cell to another nerve cell.
Review: Yes ○   No ○

7. The function of the lacrimal apparatus is to:
   A. refract light rays through the eye.
   B. assist in maintaining the shape of the cornea.
   C. produce tears to lubricate the eye.
   D. differentiate black-and-white vision.

Answer: **C**
Why: The lens of the eye is important in light refraction. Aqueous humor is a watery fluid that fills the eyeball in front of the lens and helps maintain the curve of the cornea. Rods and cones in the retinal layer are responsible for differentiating between black, white, and color.
Review: Yes ○   No ○

8. A bone that is part of the pelvic girdle is the:
   A. sphenoid.
   B. ethmoid.
   C. ischium.
   D. zygomatic.
   E. sternum.

Answer: **C**
Why: The sphenoid, ethmoid, and zygomatic are all bones of the skull. The sphenoid and ethmoid bones are part of the cranium, and the zygomatic is the cheekbone. The sternum is the chest bone.
Review: Yes ○   No ○

9. The cellular components of blood include:
   A. erythrocytes, leukocytes, and platelets.
   B. anticoagulants, antibodies, and electrolytes.
   C. plasma, serum, and hemoglobin.
   D. lipids, amino acids, and albumin.

Answer: **A**
Why: Cellular components include cells and cell fragments, including erythrocytes, leukocytes, and platelets. Lipids are fatty acids; anticoagulants found in the blood are clotting factors; electrolytes and amino acids are chemicals; and albumin is a form of protein. None of these substances are formed elements like cells.
Review: Yes ○   No ○

10. The chambers of the heart are the:
    A. septum and valves.
    B. endocardium and epicardium.
    C. apex and septum.
    D. ventricles and atria.
    E. AV node and SA node.

Answer: **D**
Why: The septum of the heart is a partition dividing the heart into two sides. The heart valves direct blood flow through the heart. Endocardium and epicardium are layers of heart. The apex of the heart refers to the region at the bottom tip of the heart. The SA and AV nodes are areas involved in the conduction cycle of the heart.
Review: Yes ○   No ○

11. An organ located in the left upper quadrant is the:
    A. thymus.
    B. spleen.
    C. appendix.
    D. liver.

Answer: **B**
Why: The thymus is located behind the sternum. The liver is in the right upper quadrant, and the appendix is in the right lower quadrant.
Review: Yes ○   No ○

12. An example of active immunity is:
   A. maternal antibodies passed through the uterus to the baby.
   B. immunization with antibodies.
   C. maternal antibodies acquired by the baby from breast milk.
   D. producing antibodies as a result of having a disease.
   E. injection of globulins of disease-causing organisms.

Answer: **D**

Why: Active immunity is obtained when the individual actually develops antibodies by having the disease or by injection of a killed or attenuated organism, forcing the body to produce antibodies. Passive immunity means that the antibodies are made outside of the body and are "passed" on to the person. The mother passing antibodies through her placenta or breast milk is an example of this type of immunity.
Review: Yes ○   No ○

---

13. The structure in the body also known as the voice box is the:
   A. pharynx.
   B. larynx.
   C. epiglottis.
   D. trachea.

Answer: **B**

Why: The pharynx is referred to as the throat. The epiglottis covers the larynx during swallowing to keep food and liquids out of the respiratory tract. The trachea is commonly called the windpipe.
Review: Yes ○   No ○

---

14. The wavelike movement that propels food through the digestive tract is called:
   A. osmosis.
   B. diffusion.
   C. metabolism.
   D. resorption.
   E. peristalsis.

Answer: **E**

Why: Diffusion is a process of movement of molecules from a higher concentration to a lower concentration. Metabolism is the combination of chemical processes resulting in growth and bodily functions within a living organism. Resorption is the loss of substance or bone. Osmosis is the movement of materials through a semipermeable membrane.
Review: Yes ○   No ○

---

15. The process that does not require oxygen for the breakdown of glucose is referred to as being:
   A. aerobic.
   B. anaerobic.
   C. catabolic.
   D. pyrogenic.

Answer: **B**

Why: Aerobic refers to a process that requires the presence of air or oxygen. The prefix *an-* at the beginning of a word means without air or oxygen. Pyrogenic means heat-producing, and catabolic refers to the process in which substances are metabolized into smaller substances (i.e., digestion of food).
Review: Yes ○   No ○

---

16. The term that means the body is in a state of equilibrium or balance is:
   A. anabolism.
   B. catabolism.
   C. homeostasis.
   D. metabolism.
   E. osmosis.

Answer: **C**

Why: Homeostasis is a state of equilibrium or health in the body. Metabolism is the body process of transforming energy in living cells. Anabolism is the building phase and catabolism is the breaking down phase of transforming energy. Osmosis is the process of water diffusing through a semipermeable membrane.
Review: Yes ○   No ○

---

17. The funnel-shaped basin that forms the upper end of the ureter is the:
   A. glomerulus.
   B. renal cortex.
   C. renal pelvis.
   D. Bowman capsule.

Answer: **C**

Why: The glomerulus and Bowman capsule are part of the nephron, the basic unit of the kidney. There are about 1 million nephrons in each kidney. The renal cortex is the outer portion of the kidney.
Review: Yes ○   No ○

18. In both males and females, the entire pelvic floor is called the:
   A. vestibule.
   B. peritoneum.
   C. fundus.
   D. pons.
   E. perineum.

Answer: **E**
Why: The vestibule refers to the area near the vaginal opening, and the fundus is the region in the top of the uterus, above the fallopian tube openings. The peritoneum is a membrane that lines the abdominal cavity. The pons is an area in the brain.
Review: Yes ○   No ○

19. A pregnancy that develops in a location outside the uterine cavity is referred to as:
   A. previa.
   B. miscarriage.
   C. abruptio.
   D. ectopic.

Answer: **D**
Why: The placenta is usually attached to the upper part of the uterus. Previa refers to the attachment of the placenta near the internal opening of the cervix. Abruptio refers to the premature separation of the placenta from the wall of the uterus. Miscarriage refers to a termination of pregnancy before the twentieth week of gestation, usually because of a problem with the conception or the womb environment.
Review: Yes ○   No ○

20. Which of the following body systems includes the thyroid and pituitary glands?
   A. Excretory
   B. Integumentary
   C. Endocrine
   D. Circulatory
   E. Nervous

Answer: **C**
Why: The excretory system refers to the kidneys and urinary tract. The integumentary system includes the skin, hair, nails, and sweat and sebaceous glands. The circulatory system refers to the veins and arteries. The nervous system includes the brain and nerves.
Review: Yes ○   No ○

21. The term **inguinal** pertains to what area or structure of the body?
   A. Intestines
   B. Bladder
   C. Groin
   D. Umbilicus

Answer: **C**
Why: The umbilicus is also known as the belly button or navel. The bladder is the internal organ that serves as a reservoir for urine. The intestines are in the abdomen. The groin or inguinal area is the region where the abdomen and thighs meet.
Review: Yes ○   No ○

22. The measure of acidity or alkalinity of a solution is called:
   A. acid.
   B. base.
   C. pH.
   D. buffer.
   E. neutral.

Answer: **C**
Why: An acid is a substance that can donate a hydrogen ion to another substance, and base refers to a substance that can receive a hydrogen ion. A buffer is a substance that tends to control the hydrogen ion concentration in a solution by adding or releasing hydrogen ions.
Review: Yes ○   No ○

23. A term that describes a solution that has the same concentration as cell fluids is:
   A. hypotonic.
   B. osmosis.
   C. isotonic.
   D. intercellular.

Answer: **C**
Why: Osmosis refers to the movement of a pure solvent, such as water, through a semipermeable membrane to equalize the solution's concentration. Hypotonic refers to a solution that is less concentrated than the fluids within a cell. Intercellular means between cells. The prefix *iso-* means equal or the same.
Review: Yes ○   No ○

24. The fibrous bands that support organs to hold them in place are:
   A. meninges.
   B. periosteum.
   C. fascia.
   D. synovia.
   E. tendons.

Answer: **C**
Why: Synovia is transparent, thick fluid found in joints. Meninges are the coverings of the brain and spinal cord. Periosteum is the covering of bones. Tendons are structures that attach muscle to bone.
Review: Yes ◯   No ◯

25. The membrane that surrounds the heart is the:
   A. endocardium.
   B. epicardium.
   C. mesocardium.
   D. pericardium.

Answer: **D**
Why: The prefix *peri-* means to surround, and the pericardium is the membrane or sac that surrounds the heart. The other choices refer to layers of heart muscle.
Review: Yes ◯   No ◯

26. The small tip of cartilage at the lower end of the sternum is the:
   A. zygomatic process.
   B. manubrium.
   C. styloid process.
   D. xiphoid process.
   E. ethmoid.

Answer: **D**
Why: The manubrium is the top part of the sternum. The zygomatic process is a bone in the upper cheek, and the ethmoid is a bone between the nasal cavity and orbits of the eye. The styloid process is the bony projection behind the ear.
Review: Yes ◯   No ◯

27. A major muscle in the body that assists in raising the arm away from the body is the:
   A. extensor carpi.
   B. biceps femoris.
   C. sartorius.
   D. deltoid.

Answer: **D**
Why: The extensor carpi muscles are located near the wrist in the forearm and assist in flexing and extending fingers. The biceps femoris muscle is one of the hamstring muscles and is found in the posterior thigh. The sartorius muscle is located in the leg.
Review: Yes ◯   No ◯

28. Cells that carry or transmit impulses toward the central nervous system are called:
   A. afferent neurons.
   B. efferent neurons.
   C. motor neurons.
   D. receptors.
   E. meninges.

Answer: **A**
Why: Motor neurons are also known as efferent neurons and carry impulses away from the central nervous system. Receptors are sensory nerve endings that respond to various kinds of stimulation. The meninges are the coverings of the brain and spinal cord.
Review: Yes ◯   No ◯

29. The space(s) in the brain where cerebrospinal fluid is formed is/are the:
   A. arachnoid.
   B. meninges.
   C. ventricles.
   D. lobes.

Answer: **C**
Why: The meninges are three layers surrounding the brain and spinal cord. The arachnoid is one of the meningeal layers. The lobes are divisions of the brain.
Review: Yes ◯   No ◯

30. Impulses from the receptors for smell are carried to the brain by the:
    A. proprioceptors.
    B. glossopharyngeal nerve.
    C. vestibulocochlear nerve.
    D. olfactory nerve.
    E. myelin sheath.

Answer: **D**
Why: Proprioceptors are receptors located in muscles, tendons, and joints that relay impulses that aid in judging position and changes in the locations of body parts in relation to each other. The glossopharyngeal nerve contains sensory fibers for taste and secretion of saliva. The vestibulocochlear nerve carries impulses for hearing and equilibrium. The myelin sheath is the fatty material that covers and protects neuron fibers.
Review: Yes ○   No ○

31. The hormone that is essential for growth is produced in the:
    A. parathyroid glands.
    B. adrenal glands.
    C. pituitary gland.
    D. thymus gland.

Answer: **C**
Why: The parathyroid glands secrete a hormone that regulates exchange of calcium between blood and bones. The adrenal glands secrete hormones whose primary functions are to increase blood pressure and heart rate and aid metabolism of carbohydrates, proteins, and fats. The thymus gland hormone promotes immunity.
Review: Yes ○   No ○

32. Which of the following represent layers of the heart?
    A. Atria and ventricles
    B. Ventricles and myocardium
    C. Epicardium and myocardium
    D. Endocardium and septum
    E. Septum and atria

Answer: **C**
Why: The atria and ventricles are chambers of the heart. The septum is the dividing wall of the right and left sides of the heart.
Review: Yes ○   No ○

33. The blood vessel that brings blood from the head, chest, and arms back to the heart is the:
    A. aorta.
    B. pulmonary vein.
    C. carotid artery.
    D. superior vena cava.

Answer: **D**
Why: The aorta, pulmonary vein, and carotid artery all carry blood away from the heart. The superior vena cava is a vein that carries blood back to the heart from the upper body.
Review: Yes ○   No ○

34. Which of the following is the proper sequence for the flow of blood in the body?
    A. Artery → vein → arteriole
    B. Venule → arteriole → capillary
    C. Vein → venule → capillary
    D. Capillary → arteriole → venule
    E. Artery → arteriole → capillary

Answer: **E**
Why: The sequence of blood flow through the body is from artery to arteriole to capillary, then to venule and vein. The artery and vein are larger vessels than arterioles and venules, and the capillaries are the smallest.
Review: Yes ○   No ○

35. The condition of inflammation of the lymphatic vessels is called:
    A. lymphoma.
    B. splenomegaly.
    C. lymphangitis.
    D. lymphocytopenia.

Answer: **C**
Why: Lymphoma refers to a tumor in the lymph tissue. Splenomegaly means enlargement of the spleen. Lymphocytopenia refers to a decrease in the number of lymphocytes in the blood.
Review: Yes ○   No ○

36. The lymphatic system includes the following organs and tissue *except*:
   A. hypothalamus.
   B. thymus.
   C. spleen.
   D. tonsils.
   E. adenoids.

Answer: **A**
Why: The hypothalamus is not a part of the lymphatic system, but is in the brain. It activates and controls the autonomic nervous system and aids in regulating body temperature, sleep, and appetite.
Review: Yes ○   No ○

37. The process in which white blood cells take in and destroy waste and foreign material is called:
   A. immunity.
   B. phagocytosis.
   C. hemolysis.
   D. leukocytosis.

Answer: **B**
Why: Hemolysis refers to destruction of red blood cells. Leukocytosis is an abnormal increase in the number of white blood cells. Immunity refers to a condition of being unaffected by a particular disease.
Review: Yes ○   No ○

38. The structure common to the respiratory and digestive systems is the:
   A. trachea.
   B. larynx.
   C. esophagus.
   D. pharynx.
   E. ileum.

Answer: **D**
Why: The larynx is known as the voice box, and the trachea is known as the windpipe. Both allow airflow in and out of the lungs. The esophagus transports food from the pharynx to the stomach. The pharynx transports both food to the digestive system and air to the respiratory system. The ileum is the lower part of the small intestine.
Review: Yes ○   No ○

39. An accumulation of air in the pleural space that may lead to collapse of the lung is called:
   A. hemothorax.
   B. thoracentesis.
   C. pleurisy.
   D. pneumothorax.

Answer: **D**
Why: Hemothorax refers to blood in the pleural space, and pneumothorax is an accumulation of air in the pleural space. Thoracentesis is a procedure in which a needle is inserted into the pleural space below the lung to remove fluid. Pleurisy refers to inflammation of the pleura, the covering or sac around each lung.
Review: Yes ○   No ○

40. The leaf-shaped cartilage that covers the opening of the larynx is the:
   A. epiglottis.
   B. soft palate.
   C. uvula.
   D. pharynx.
   E. villus.

Answer: **A**
Why: The pharynx is also known as the throat. The soft palate is the tissue that forms the back of the roof of the mouth; the uvula is the soft projection that hangs down from this area and is used in speech production. The epiglottis is the cartilage that guards the entrance of the trachea during swallowing so food will move into the esophagus, not the larynx and trachea. A villus is one of many tiny projections in the small intestine lining.
Review: Yes ○   No ○

41. Most of the digestive process occurs in the:
A. stomach.
B. large intestine.
C. small intestine.
D. esophagus.

Answer: **C**
Why: The esophagus is a muscular tube that transports food from the pharynx to the stomach. No digestion occurs in the esophagus. In the stomach, food is churned and mixes with digestive juices that begin to liquefy and break down food. The large intestine reabsorbs water and eliminates undigested waste. The small intestine secretes enzymes that digest proteins and carbohydrates. Digested food is absorbed through the walls of the small intestine.
Review: Yes ○   No ○

42. The lining of the stomach has many folds called:
A. diverticula.
B. rugae.
C. villi.
D. mesentery.
E. ulcers.

Answer: **B**
Why: Diverticula are the saclike bulges in the intestinal wall. Villi are the tiny fingerlike projections in the small intestine. Mesentery is a fold of peritoneum connecting the jejunum and the ileum with the dorsal wall of the abdomen. Ulcers are lesions of the mucosa of any organ.
Review: Yes ○   No ○

43. The first portion of the small intestine is the:
A. jejunum.
B. ileum.
C. duodenum.
D. pylorus.

Answer: **C**
Why: The pylorus is in the distal region of the stomach leading into the small intestine. The small intestine has three portions. The first is the duodenum, the second is the jejunum, and the third is the ileum.
Review: Yes ○   No ○

44. An accumulation of excessive fluid in the intercellular spaces is called:
A. acidosis.
B. alkalosis.
C. edema.
D. effusion.
E. osmosis.

Answer: **C**
Why: The condition that results from a decrease in the pH of body fluids is called acidosis; an increase in the pH of body fluids is alkalosis. Effusion refers to the fluid that escapes into a cavity or space.
Review: Yes ○   No ○

45. The kidneys are located in the:
A. retroperitoneal space.
B. renal pelvis.
C. dorsal cavity.
D. hypogastric region.

Answer: **A**
Why: Both the kidneys and ureters lie behind the peritoneum in the retroperitoneal space. The renal pelvis is the funnel-shaped basin that forms the upper end of the ureter. The dorsal cavity houses the brain and spinal cord, and the hypogastric region is the lowest area in the mid-abdomen.
Review: Yes ○   No ○

46. The term **hydronephrosis** means:
A. inability to retain urine.
B. involuntary discharge of urine.
C. inflammation and infection of the renal pelvis.
D. distention of the renal pelvis resulting from obstructed flow of urine.
E. excessive urine.

Answer: **D**
Why: Pyelonephritis is the term for inflammation and infection of the renal pelvis. Enuresis is the involuntary discharge of urine. Incontinence is the inability to retain urine. Polyuria is excessive urine.
Review: Yes ○   No ○

47. The sex glands of the male and female reproductive system are the:
  A. sperm and ova.
  B. prostate and uterus.
  C. testes and ovaries.
  D. penis and vagina.

Answer: **C**
Why: The sperm and ova are actually the sex cells of reproduction. The prostate is a gland that secretes a substance that enhances the motility of the sperm through the reproductive tract. The uterus is the structure in which the developing fetus grows to maturity. The penis and vagina are the structures that provide a transport system for sperm from the male to the female for fertilization of an ovum. The vagina is also the birth canal.
Review: Yes ○   No ○

48. Hematopoiesis is the:
  A. equilibrium of the body.
  B. generation of cells that produce blood.
  C. regulation of the body's fluids.
  D. energy transformation in cells
  E. solution drawing fluid away from cells.

Answer: **B**
Why: Hemostasis is the equilibrium of the body. Hematopoiesis is the process by which undifferentiated stem cells give rise to differentiated blood cells. Fluid balance is the goal in body fluid regulation; metabolism is the transfer of energy, and hypertonic is the type of solution that draws fluid away from cells.
Review: Yes ○   No ○

49. The largest artery in the body is the:
  A. superior vena cava.
  B. inferior vena cava.
  C. carotid artery.
  D. abdominal aorta.

Answer: **D**
Why: The superior and inferior vena cava are both veins. The carotid artery is in the neck and is smaller than the aorta.
Review: Yes ○   No ○

50. The term that refers to absence of menstrual flow in a woman of reproductive age is:
  A. menses.
  B. uremia.
  C. dysmenorrhea.
  D. menopause.
  E. amenorrhea.

Answer: **E**
Why: Menses refers to the normal menstrual period or flow. Dysmenorrhea is painful menstruation, and menopause is the term that means the total cessation of menstruation. Uremia is a condition of high levels of nitrogen waste in the body.
Review: Yes ○   No ○

51. The hormone produced by the embryonic cells of the fetus is:
  A. human chorionic gonadotropin hormone.
  B. adrenocorticotropic hormone.
  C. oxytocin.
  D. follicle-stimulating hormone.

Answer: **A**
Why: Adrenocorticotropic hormone, known as ACTH, and follicle-stimulating hormone, known as FSH, are hormones produced by the anterior pituitary gland. Oxytocin is produced by the posterior pituitary.
Review: Yes ○   No ○

52. A substance necessary for proper formation of a blood clot is:
  A. macrophage.
  B. lipid.
  C. hemoglobin.
  D. thrombin.
  E. albumin.

Answer: **D**
Why: Macrophages are a type of phagocyte that assist in disposing of foreign material in the blood. Lipids are fats and cholesterol. Hemoglobin is a protein that contains iron and allows oxygen to bond to red blood cells for transport through the bloodstream. Albumin is a protein found in the blood.
Review: Yes ○   No ○

53. The left atrioventricular (AV) valve in the heart is also known as the:
A. pulmonary valve.
B. aortic valve.
C. mitral valve.
D. tricuspid valve.

Answer: **C**
Why: The pulmonary and aortic valves are semilunar valves that are exit valves. AV valves are entrance valves and include the mitral and tricuspid valve. The tricuspid valve is on the right, and the mitral valve is on the left.
Review: Yes ○   No ○

54. The only artery in the body that carries deoxygenated blood is the:
A. superior vena cava.
B. aorta.
C. pulmonary artery.
D. coronary artery.
E. interior vena cava.

Answer: **C**
Why: The aorta and coronary arteries both carry oxygenated blood to supply the heart and body. The superior vena cava and inferior vena cava are veins, not arteries.
Review: Yes ○   No ○

55. A localized dilation resulting from weakness of a blood vessel wall is a(n):
A. embolus.
B. thrombus.
C. septal defect.
D. aneurysm.

Answer: **D**
Why: An embolus is a foreign object, air, gas, or a piece of blood clot circulating in the blood that may become lodged in a blood vessel. A thrombus is a blood clot. A septal defect is an abnormality, usually congenital, in the wall that divides the heart chambers.
Review: Yes ○   No ○

56. An example of a chronic obstructive pulmonary disease is:
A. asthma.
B. emphysema.
C. croup.
D. pleurisy.
E. pertussis.

Answer: **B**
Why: Asthma is characterized by recurring episodes of wheezing and coughing. Croup is caused by a viral infection, usually in infants. Pleurisy is inflammation of the pleura. Pertussis is known as whooping cough.
Review: Yes ○   No ○

57. A portion of the large intestine is the:
A. pylorus.
B. jejunum.
C. ileum.
D. sigmoid.

Answer: **D**
Why: The pylorus is the section of the stomach at the lowest end that connects to the duodenum. The jejunum and ileum are parts of the small intestine.
Review: Yes ○   No ○

58. A chronic degenerative disease of the liver is:
A. Crohn disease.
B. jaundice.
C. colitis.
D. cholecystitis.
E. cirrhosis.

Answer: **E**
Why: Crohn disease is a chronic inflammation of the intestine, usually the ileum. Colitis is inflammation of the colon, and jaundice is a condition of yellowing of the skin resulting from excess bilirubin in the blood caused by liver disorders. Cholecystitis is inflammation of the gallbladder.
Review: Yes ○   No ○

59. The tube that permits urine to pass from the bladder to the outside of the body is the:
A. urethra.
B. ureter.
C. renal pelvis.
D. urinary meatus.

Answer: **A**
Why: The urethra is the tube that extends from the kidney to the urinary bladder. The ureter is the tube carrying urine from the kidney to the bladder. The renal pelvis is the funnel-shaped portion of the kidney where urine collects in the kidney. The urinary meatus is not a tube, but rather is the external opening of the urethra to the outside of the body.
Review: Yes ○   No ○

60. The innermost layer of the uterus is the:
A. perineum.
B. myometrium.
C. endometrium.
D. peritoneum.
E. cervix.

Answer: **C**
Why: The perineum refers to the region between the vagina and rectum. The myometrium is the middle muscular layer of the uterus, and the peritoneum is the outer layer that envelopes the uterus. The cervix is the lower end of the uterus.
Review: Yes ○   No ○

61. The frontal or coronal plane of the body divides the body into:
A. right and left halves.
B. equal top and bottom halves.
C. unequal right and left sides.
D. front and rear.

Answer: **D**
Why: The transverse or horizontal plane divides the body into top and bottom halves. The sagittal plane divides the body into right and left sides but not necessarily equal halves. If divided into equal halves, it is called the midsagittal plane.
Review: Yes ○   No ○

62. The membrane attached to internal organs is the:
A. mucous membrane.
B. cutaneous membrane.
C. visceral layer.
D. parietal layer.
E. epithelial layer.

Answer: **C**
Why: The internal organs are the viscera, and the membrane surrounding them is the visceral layer. The mucous membranes line tubes and spaces open to the outside of the body. The cutaneous membrane is commonly known as the skin. The parietal layer is a serous membrane that is attached to the wall of a cavity or sac. The epithelial layer is the outer layer of the skin.
Review: Yes ○   No ○

63. The term that describes a disorder that breaks down tissues in a body system is:
A. degenerative.
B. infection.
C. metabolic.
D. neoplastic.

Answer: **A**
Why: Infection is an invasion of the body by pathogenic microorganisms. A metabolic disorder refers to a condition caused by disruption of the reactions involved in cellular metabolism in the body. Neoplastic refers to cancer or new growth.
Review: Yes ○   No ○

64. The study of the cause of any disease or of all factors that may be involved in the development of a disease is:
A. physiology.
B. anatomy.
C. histology.
D. incidence.
E. etiology.

Answer: **E**
Why: Physiology is the study of body function; anatomy is the study of body structure. Histology is the study of tissue. Incidence refers to the range of occurrence of a disease and its tendency to affect certain groups of individuals more than other groups.
Review: Yes ○   No ○

65. The chronic skin condition characterized by a red, flat area covered with silvery scales is:
   A. decubitus ulcer.
   B. urticaria.
   C. psoriasis.
   D. shingles.

Answer: **C**
Why: A decubitus ulcer, also known as a bedsore, is due to constant pressure on a part of the body, which impairs blood supply to the area of skin that is pressed between bone and the patient's bed. Urticaria, known as hives, appears as elevated red patches or wheals. Hives are usually a result of an allergic reaction. Shingles, caused by the herpes zoster virus, produces vesicle (blister)-type lesions.
Review: Yes ○   No ○

66. Which of the following is not one of the cranial bones?
   A. Frontal
   B. Parietal
   C. Ethmoid
   D. Temporal
   E. Maxilla

Answer: **E**
Why: The maxilla, the upper jaw bone, is part of the skull but is one of the facial bones.
Review: Yes ○   No ○

67. The bone that is part of the shoulder girdle and is between the sternum and the scapula is the:
   A. clavicle.
   B. humerus.
   C. ulna.
   D. manubrium.

Answer: **A**
Why: The humerus is the upper arm bone, and the ulna is the smaller medial bone of the forearm. The manubrium is the top portion of the sternum.
Review: Yes ○   No ○

68. The type of muscle responsible for producing peristalsis is:
   A. cardiac.
   B. skeletal.
   C. smooth.
   D. voluntary.
   E. diaphragmatic.

Answer: **C**
Why: Cardiac muscle is only found in the heart wall. Skeletal muscle is voluntary muscle attached to bones allowing movement of joints. Smooth muscle is involuntary and is found in the walls of internal organs and passageways such as the intestines, where peristalsis takes place. The term *diaphragmatic* refers to the diaphragm.
Review: Yes ○   No ○

69. The type of joint motion that allows movement away from the midline of the body, such as moving the arms straight out to the sides, is:
   A. circumduction.
   B. flexion.
   C. extension.
   D. abduction.

Answer: **D**
Why: Circumduction is movement in a circular pattern. Flexion is a bending motion decreasing the angle between bones, and extension is a straightening motion increasing the angle between bones.
Review: Yes ○   No ○

70. The sympathetic system of the autonomic nervous system is responsible for:
   A. constriction of the pupil of the eye.
   B. decrease in rate of heartbeat.
   C. dilation of bronchi of the lungs.
   D. constriction of blood vessels to skeletal muscles.
   E. slowing the pulse.

Answer: **C**
Why: The sympathetic system is responsible for stimulating the body's fight-or-flight response (stress). This response includes dilation of the bronchi. The parasympathetic system returns the body to normal activity by constricting the pupil and the blood vessels and by decreasing the heart rate or slowing the pulse.
Review: Yes ○   No ○

71. The portion of the brain that aids in the coordination of voluntary muscle action is the:
A. cerebellum.
B. thalamus.
C. medulla oblongata.
D. midbrain.

Answer: **A**
Why: The thalamus is responsible for relaying sensory impulses to the cerebral cortex of the brain. The medulla oblongata contains the respiratory center, which controls the muscles of respiration; the cardiac center, which helps regulate the rate and force of the heartbeat; and the vasomotor center, which regulates the contraction of smooth muscle in the blood vessel walls. The midbrain contains a relay center for certain eye and ear reflexes.
Review: Yes ○   No ○

72. Strabismus is a condition of the eye causing:
A. nearsightedness.
B. farsightedness.
C. drooping eyelids.
D. cross-eyed appearance.
E. redness of the sclera.

Answer: **D**
Why: Myopia is nearsightedness, and hyperopia is farsightedness. The term for drooping eyelids is blepharoptosis (blephar/o = eyelid, optosis = drooping, falling). The sclera is the visible white portion of the eye that can become red from inflammation and irritation.
Review: Yes ○   No ○

73. A structure found in the inner ear is the:
A. pinna.
B. tympanic membrane.
C. malleus.
D. cochlea.

Answer: **D**
Why: The earlobe is the pinna. The tympanic membrane, or eardrum, separates the external and middle ear. The malleus is one of the three small bones of the middle ear. The other bones are the stapes and incus.
Review: Yes ○   No ○

74. The clusters of cells called the islets of Langerhans are located in the:
A. adrenal glands.
B. anterior pituitary gland.
C. pancreas.
D. pituitary gland.
E. parathyroid glands.

Answer: **C**
Why: The islets of Langerhans, located in the pancreas, secrete insulin, which aids in the transport of glucose into cells, decreasing the blood sugar level.
Review: Yes ○   No ○

75. A goiter is associated with abnormal function of the:
A. thyroid gland.
B. parathyroid glands.
C. spleen.
D. pituitary gland.

Answer: **A**
Why: A goiter is a swelling in the neck region surrounding the thyroid gland. It is caused by hypertrophy, or chronic enlargement, of the thyroid gland.
Review: Yes ○   No ○

76. The Rh factor in blood is:
A. an antigen that affects a person's blood type.
B. responsible for protecting against infection.
C. used to transport oxygen.
D. one of the clotting factors.
E. an enzyme that breaks down cholesterol.

Answer: **A**
Why: Rh is a red cell antigen (protein) that contributes to a person's blood type. A person is Rh-positive if the antigen is present in the blood and Rh-negative if it is absent from the blood. This antigen can cause incompatibility problems in pregnancies and blood transfusions.
Review: Yes ○   No ○

77. The area of the heart that initiates a heartbeat is the:
- A. atrioventricular node.
- B. sinoatrial node.
- C. right bundle branches.
- D. Purkinje fibers.

Answer: **B**

Why: The SA node (sinoatrial node) initiates the heart contractions. Impulses travel next to the AV node (atrioventricular node), then to the bundle of His, to the right and left bundle branches, and, last, to the Purkinje fibers.

Review: Yes ○   No ○

---

78. A heart disease that is present at birth is:
- A. atherosclerosis.
- B. rheumatic heart disease.
- C. congenital heart disease.
- D. angina pectoris.
- E. maternal.

Answer: **C**

Why: The term **congenital** means "born with" or "at birth." Atherosclerosis is a degeneration of the inside of the blood vessels that causes a narrowing of the opening as the walls become thicker. Angina pectoris is caused by inadequate blood flow to the heart muscle and results in chest pain. Rheumatic heart disease is caused by an attack of rheumatic fever, usually in childhood. **Maternal** is a term meaning "to the mother" or "from the mother."

Review: Yes ○   No ○

---

79. Which of the following blood vessels is proximal to the heart?
- A. Iliac artery
- B. Carotid artery
- C. Ascending aorta
- D. Renal artery

Answer: **C**

Why: The term **proximal** means closest to a body part. The ascending aorta is an extension of the aorta and is the largest vessel in the body. It is the first blood vessel to exit the heart with oxygenated blood. The iliac artery is located in the hip area. The carotid arteries, right and left, are found in the neck, and the renal artery supplies blood to the kidneys.

Review: Yes ○   No ○

---

80. Acquired, natural, active immunity is achieved by:
- A. injection of immune serum.
- B. nursing babies with mother's milk.
- C. contracting the disease.
- D. injection of a vaccine.
- E. immunizing with antibodies of a disease.

Answer: **C**

Why: Injection of any serum or vaccine is an artificial means of acquiring immunity. Nursing a baby is a method of passing on antibodies from the mother to the baby, which is passive. If someone comes in contact with a disease and naturally manufactures antibodies, this is an active method of acquiring immunity.

Review: Yes ○   No ○

---

81. The human immunodeficiency virus is the cause of which disease?
- A. Hodgkin disease
- B. Leukemia
- C. Acquired immunodeficiency syndrome
- D. Sarcoma

Answer: **C**

Why: Acquired immunodeficiency syndrome (AIDS) is caused by the human immunodeficiency virus (HIV). Hodgkin disease, leukemia, and sarcoma are all forms of malignancy (cancer).

Review: Yes ○   No ○

82. Which of the following statements is accurate about the lungs?
  A. The bronchioles branch to form smaller structures called bronchi.
  B. The right and left lungs both have three lobes.
  C. The sac covering the lungs is the pleural sac.
  D. The least amount of gas exchange takes place in the alveoli.
  E. External respiration is the exchange of oxygen and carbon dioxide in the lungs.

Answer: **C**
Why: The bronchi are larger structures than the bronchioles. The right lung has three lobes, and the left has only two lobes. The most gas exchange takes place in the millions of tiny alveolar sacs. External respiration is the exchange of oxygen and carbon dioxide in the lungs. Internal respiration is the exchange of these gases in the capillaries and tissue cells.
Review: Yes ◯   No ◯

83. A communicable, infectious disease of the lungs is:
  A. emphysema.
  B. chronic obstructive pulmonary disease.
  C. asthma.
  D. tuberculosis.

Answer: **D**
Why: Emphysema, chronic obstructive pulmonary disease (COPD), and asthma are not infectious or communicable. COPD is a condition in which there is an obstruction of normal airflow. Air is trapped in the lung spaces, and there is no proper exchange of oxygen and carbon dioxide. Emphysema is one type of lung disorder classified as a COPD. Asthma is a condition that creates spasms of the involuntary muscles of the bronchial tube walls and causes labored breathing. Asthma may be caused by allergens such as dust, pollen, or foods.
Review: Yes ◯   No ◯

84. An example of an inflammatory bowel disease is:
  A. gastritis.
  B. pyloric stenosis.
  C. Crohn disease.
  D. Vincent disease.
  E. Hodgkin disease.

Answer: **C**
Why: Gastritis is inflammation of the stomach. Pyloric stenosis is a constriction of the pyloric sphincter, the ring of muscle between the stomach and small intestine. Vincent disease is a form of gum disease of the mouth. Hodgkin disease is a chronic malignant disease characterized by enlargement of the lymph nodes and spleen.
Review: Yes ◯   No ◯

85. A function of the liver is to:
  A. detoxify harmful substances, such as alcohol and certain drugs.
  B. produce insulin to metabolize glucose.
  C. absorb nutrients into the bloodstream.
  D. assist in digestion by producing hydrochloric acid.

Answer: **A**
Why: Insulin is a product of the pancreas. The small intestine is where most nutrients are absorbed into the bloodstream. Hydrochloric acid is produced in the stomach and is used to start the digestive process.
Review: Yes ◯   No ◯

86. The fluid contained within the body cells is called:
  A. lymph.
  B. plasma.
  C. interstitial fluid.
  D. isotonic.
  E. intracellular fluid.

Answer: **E**
Why: Lymph is the fluid that drains from the tissues into the lymphatic system. Plasma is the liquid part of blood, and interstitial fluid is tissue fluid found in the spaces between cells. Isotonic means the same concentration of fluid inside and outside a cell.
Review: Yes ◯   No ◯

87. Two important electrolytes found in the body are:
    A. zinc and magnesium.
    B. sodium and potassium.
    C. protein and carbohydrates.
    D. nitrogen and carbon dioxide.

Answer: **B**
Why: Zinc and magnesium are minerals, protein and carbohydrates are nutrients, and nitrogen and carbon dioxide are gases.
Review: Yes ○   No ○

88. A condition resulting from renal failure and causing high levels of blood urea nitrogen is:
    A. uremia.
    B. anemia.
    C. edema.
    D. hematuria.
    E. dehydration.

Answer: **A**
Why: Dehydration is an excessive loss of body fluid. Anemia is a condition of decreased amount of hemoglobin, or red blood cells, in the blood. Edema is an accumulation of fluid in tissue spaces. Hematuria is a condition of blood in the urine.
Review: Yes ○   No ○

89. The period of pregnancy is called:
    A. gestation.
    B. menarche.
    C. fertilization.
    D. ovulation.

Answer: **A**
Why: The term **menarche** refers to the first time a female has a menstrual cycle, usually occurring between ages 9 and 15. Fertilization is the impregnation of the female egg with the male sperm; the release of an egg from the ovary is ovulation.
Review: Yes ○   No ○

90. The hormone that causes contraction of uterine muscle during labor is:
    A. oxytocin.
    B. progesterone.
    C. follicle-stimulating hormone.
    D. testosterone.
    E. estrogen.

Answer: **A**
Why: Estrogen and progesterone are produced by the ovaries. Estrogen is important in the growth and development of sexual organs, and progesterone helps in development of mammary glands and preparation of the uterus lining for implantation of a fertilized ovum. Follicle-stimulating hormone is produced by the anterior pituitary and stimulates the growth of ovarian follicles. In the male, it promotes the development of sperm cells and growth of the testes. Testosterone is male hormone.
Review: Yes ○   No ○

91. The region located directly below the umbilical region is the:
    A. right iliac region.
    B. hypogastric region.
    C. hypochondriac region.
    D. epigastric region.

Answer: **B**
Why: The hypogastric region is the region below the umbilicus (navel), in the middle of the lower abdomen. The hypochondriac regions are on the right and left at the base of the ribs. The epigastric region is above the umbilicus and is located over the stomach area.
Review: Yes ○   No ○

92. An example of exocrine glands are:
    A. sebaceous glands.
    B. parathyroid glands.
    C. adrenal glands.
    D. ovaries.
    E. testes.

Answer: **A**
Why: The parathyroid, adrenal glands, ovaries, and testes are examples of endocrine glands that secrete their hormones directly into the bloodstream and do not require ducts or tubes to transport the hormones.
Review: Yes ○   No ○

93. The order of the vertebral column from top to bottom is:
A. cervical, thoracic, sacral, lumbar, coccyx.
B. thoracic, lumbar, sacral, coccyx, cervical.
C. coccyx, sacral, lumbar, thoracic, cervical.
D. cervical, thoracic, lumbar, sacral, coccyx.

Answer: **D**
Why: The spine starts at the top with the cervical area in the neck region and ends with the coccyx, or the tailbone.
Review: Yes ◯   No ◯

94. The muscle located on the anterior thigh and that functions to extend the leg is the:
A. tibialis anterior.
B. quadriceps femoris.
C. sternocleidomastoid.
D. sacrospinalis.
E. gluteus maximus.

Answer: **B**
Why: Muscles frequently are named for the bone or area located in proximity to the muscle. The tibialis anterior lies in front, or anterior to, the tibia, the lower leg bone. The sternocleidomastoid connects the sternum, the mastoid process, and the clavicle. The sacrospinalis is located in the region of the sacrum, ilium (hip), and lumbar vertebrae of the spine. The gluteus maximus is the largest muscle in the posterior hip area.
Review: Yes ◯   No ◯

95. The artery located in the upper arm is the:
A. brachial artery.
B. carotid artery.
C. radial artery.
D. subclavian artery.

Answer: **A**
Why: The brachial artery is located in the upper arm and subdivides near the elbow to form the radial and ulnar arteries, which lie over the radius and ulna bones of the forearm. The carotid arteries are located in the neck. The subclavian arteries are located in the armpit (axillary) area.
Review: Yes ◯   No ◯

96. Any foreign substance that enters the body and induces an immune response is a(n):
A. antibody.
B. antigen.
C. enzyme.
D. immunoglobulin.
E. globulin.

Answer: **B**
Why: An immunoglobulin, also known as an antibody, is a substance produced in response to an antigen. An enzyme is a protein produced in the body that causes a breakdown of food. A globulin is a protein in the blood associated with antibodies.
Review: Yes ◯   No ◯

97. The smaller leg bone, lateral to the tibia, is the:
A. femur.
B. tarsal.
C. patella.
D. fibula.

Answer: **D**
Why: The femur, the largest bone in the body, is the thigh bone. The patella is the kneecap. Tarsal refers to any one of the seven ankle bones.
Review: Yes ◯   No ◯

98. The small pouch that is the first part of the large intestine is the:
A. pylorus.
B. duodenum.
C. cecum.
D. ileum.
E. jejunum.

Answer: **C**
Why: The jejunum, duodenum, and ileum are parts of the small intestine; the pylorus is the region between the stomach and small intestine.
Review: Yes ◯   No ◯

99. The hormone that regulates the amount of water that is eliminated with urine is:
A. ADH.
B. ACTH.
C. FSH.
D. TSH.

Answer: A

Why: ADH, antidiuretic hormone, aids in regulating water retention or expulsion from the body. ACTH, adrenocorticotropic hormone, stimulates the adrenal cortex to produce cortical hormones that aid in protecting the body in stress and injury. FSH, follicle-stimulating hormone, stimulates the growth and activity of the ovarian follicle. TSH, thyroid-stimulating hormone, stimulates the thyroid gland to produce thyroid hormones.
Review: Yes ◯   No ◯

100. An excessive curvature in the thoracic portion of the spinal column, also known as hunchback, is:
A. kyphosis.
B. arthritis.
C. lordosis.
D. spina bifida.
E. spondylitis.

Answer: A

Why: Arthritis is inflammation of the joints. Lordosis is an excessive curvature of the lumbar spine, also known as swayback. Spina bifida is a congenital deformity exposing the spinal column. Spondylitis is inflammation of the joints of the spine.
Review: Yes ◯   No ◯

101. Diabetic retinopathy is a result of damage to the:
A. heart.
B. lungs.
C. eyes.
D. brain.

Answer: C

Why: Diabetic retinopathy causes damage to the retina of the eye from hemorrhage of vessels; it is usually progressive and related to the control of the diabetes.
Review: Yes ◯   No ◯

102. Which of the following statements is *true*?
A. Diabetes mellitus is an uncommon endocrine disorder.
B. Insulin dependent diabetic patients do not need to restrict their diets.
C. Diabetes mellitus results from an overproduction of insulin.
D. Type 2 diabetes is non–insulin-dependent diabetes.
E. Insulin assists glucose into the cells.

Answer: D

Why: Diabetes mellitus results from a low production of insulin. Diabetic persons who are diagnosed with type 1 diabetes require insulin as part of their treatment of this disease. Persons with type 2 diabetes do not require insulin. Insulin does not assist glucose into the cells but promotes the synthesis of carbohydrates. All diabetic patients need counseling regarding exercise and diet
Review: Yes ◯   No ◯

103. Which of the following is a protein found in the epidermis that makes the skin waterproof?
A. Melanin
B. Keratin
C. Collagen
D. Cilia

Answer: B

Why: Melanin is a substance that provides pigment for the skin. Collagen is a protein found in the dermis that provides strength and flexibility. Cilia are hairlike processes that trap and move foreign particles.
Review: Yes ◯   No ◯

104. What is the most common condition of the eye associated with aging?
A. Astigmatism
B. Strabismus
C. Macular degeneration
D. Hyperopia
E. Presbyopia

Answer: **E**
Why: Astigmatism is a condition causing impaired vision from an irregular curve of the cornea. Strabismus is an inability of both eyes to simultaneously focus on a subject. Macular degeneration is a progressive, abnormal growth of blood vessels or other materials in the retina. Hyperopia is a condition of farsightedness in which distant objects can be seen more clearly than closer objects.
Review: Yes ○   No ○

105. What structure is at the neck of the bladder and surrounds the urethra?
A. Prostate
B. Epididymis
C. Prepuce
D. Vas deferens

Answer: **A**
Why: The epididymis consists of two coiled tubules on the posterior of the testes that store and carry sperm. The prepuce is known as the foreskin. The vas deferens is a tubule that carries sperm from the epididymis to the seminal vesicles.
Review: Yes ○   No ○

106. The epigastric anatomical region of the abdomen is located:
A. posterior to the kidneys.
B. inferior to the colon.
C. anterior to the pelvis.
D. distal to the sternum.

Answer: **D**
Why: The epigastric anatomical region of the abdomen is located below the sternum and above the umbilical region.
Review: Yes ○   No ○

107. Collagen, a substance found in the dermis, is a/an:
A. neurotransmitter.
B. fibrous protein.
C. catecholamine.
D. enzyme.
E. genetic material.

Answer: **B**
Why: Collagen is a fibrous protein found in the dermis, connective tissues, tendons, and ligaments. It is sometimes referred to as the body's glue, providing strength and flexibility.
Review: Yes ○   No ○

108. Which of the following glands are located on the sides of the vaginal opening and produce mucus?
A. Prostate
B. Cowper
C. Bartholin
D. Endocrine

Answer: **C**
Why: Bartholin glands are located on the sides of the vaginal opening and produce mucus. The prostate and Cowper glands are glands associated with the male reproductive system. Endocrine glands have no ducts and secrete hormones directly into the bloodstream.
Review: Yes ○   No ○

109. The organ located in the right upper abdominal quadrant beneath the diaphragm is the:
A. spleen
B. stomach.
C. liver.
D. pancreas.
E. kidney.

Answer: **C**
Why: The spleen and stomach are located on the left side, and the pancreas is behind the stomach with only it's head on the right side. The kidneys are located retroperitoneal on both the right and left sides.
Review: Yes ○   No ○

110. The master gland of the body is the:
A. adrenal.
B. pituitary.
C. pineal.
D. thyroid.

Answer: **B**
Why: The pituitary gland is an endocrine gland located at the base of the brain in the cavity. It is called the "master gland" because of the number of hormones it secretes and the functions it serves.
Review: Yes ⃝   No ⃝

---

111. A fracture of the radius characterized by bending of the bone with the skin left intact is referred to as:
A. greenstick.
B. transverse.
C. comminuted.
D. radial.
E. Colles.

Answer: **A**
Why: A greenstick fracture is an incomplete break or bending of the bone with the skin left intact and unbroken. This type of fracture frequently involves the radius bone and is common in children.
Review: Yes ⃝   No ⃝

---

112. Spermatozoa normally fertilize the female ovum in the:
A. ovary.
B. cervix.
C. uterus.
D. fallopian tube.

Answer: **D**
Why: Fertilization of the female ovum normally occurs in the fallopian tube after the ovum, the egg, has been released from the ovary where it is produced. The cervix is the neck of the uterus, the structure that houses and nourishes the growing fetus and placenta.
Review: Yes ⃝   No ⃝

---

113. The glomerulus is a cluster of blood capillaries found in the:
A. renal pelvis.
B. calyx.
C. loop of Henle.
D. bladder.
E. nephron.

Answer: **E**
Why: The renal pelvis is a cavity in the kidney where urine collects. A calyx is one of the points forming the renal pelvis. The loop of Henle is the bottom of the paperclip-shaped segment of the nephron.
Review: Yes ⃝   No ⃝

---

114. The disorder characterized by uncontrollable episodes of falling asleep is:
A. narcolepsy.
B. epilepsy.
C. Bell palsy.
D. Parkinson.

Answer: **A**
Why: Epilepsy is an abnormal electrical activity of the brain resulting in seizure. Bell palsy is a condition of unilateral facial muscle paralysis. Parkinson disease is a chronic progressive neurologic condition characterized by fine tremors and muscle weakness and rigidity.
Review: Yes ⃝   No ⃝

---

115. The regulation of body temperature is controlled by the:
A. pancreas.
B. thalamus.
C. pituitary.
D. medulla oblongata.
E. hypothalamus.

Answer: **E**
Why: The pancreas produces juices that metabolize sugar, the thalamus serves as relay for sensory input, the pituitary is the master gland, and the medulla oblongata controls heart rate, respiration, and blood pressure.
Review: Yes ⃝   No ⃝

116. Which of the following substances is *not a* neurotransmitter?

A. Acetylcholine
B. Norepinephrine
C. Epinephrine
D. Aldosterone

Answer: **D**
Why: Acetylcholine, norepinephrine, and epinephrine are neurotransmitters. Aldosterone is a hormone that regulates sodium and potassium levels.
Review: Yes ○   No ○

117. Cranial nerve I, the olfactory nerve, is related to the sense of:

A. sight.
B. smell.
C. sound.
D. taste.
E. touch.

Answer: **B**
Why: The olfactory nerve transmits smells from the nasal mucosa to the brain. The sense of sight, sound, taste, and touch are controlled by other cranial nerves. See Box 6-4.
Review: Yes ○   No ○

118. A blood cell that carries oxygen and has no nucleus is a/an:

A. leukocyte.
B. platelet.
C. erythrocyte.
D. thrombocyte.

Answer: **C**
Why: The erythrocyte is a red blood cell that contains hemoglobin that carries oxygen. The RBC has no nucleus. Platelets and thrombocytes are responsible for clotting. Leukocytes are white blood cells that do not carry oxygen and do have a nucleus.
Review: Yes ○   No ○

119. During respiration, exhaled air contains primarily:

A. oxygen.
B. nitrogen.
C. carbon dioxide.
D. carbon monoxide.
E. nitrous oxide.

Answer: **C**
Why: During the respiratory cycle, primarily oxygen is inhaled, or breathed in, and carbon dioxide is exhaled, or breathed out. Carbon dioxide is the waste product of respiration.
Review: Yes ○   No ○

120. A condition causing a backflow of stomach acid through an incompetent esophageal sphincter is called:

A. GERD.
B. SAD.
C. CVA.
D. IDDM

Answer: **A**
Why: GERD stands for gastroesophageal reflux disease.
Review: Yes ○   No ○

CRITICAL THINKING CASE REVIEW

The medical assistant is reading the medical record of Robert, an 18-year-old male patient coming in for a follow-up visit. He was in a high-speed motorcycle accident while wearing a helmet. At the scene, his upper left thigh was covered with bright red blood and bleeding profusely. A bone was penetrating through his slacks at the sight of the wound, and he was disoriented to time and place.

1. The bleeding was probably coming from the:

A. inferior aorta.
B. femoral artery.
C. femoral vein.
D. iliac artery.
E. iliac vein.

Answer: **B**
Why: An artery pumps bright red blood, and the femoral artery is located in the upper thigh.
Review: Yes ○   No ○

2. The type of fracture is:
   A. comminuted.
   B. Colles.
   C. compound.
   D. complex.

Answer: **C**
Why: Also known as an open fracture; the bone was penetrating through his skin.
Review: Yes ○   No ○

3. Robert also most likely suffered a:
   A. MTBI.
   B. MI.
   C. TIA.
   D. IM.
   E. ROM.

Answer: **A**
Why: MTBI is the mild traumatic brain injury or concussion that would account for his disorientation at the scene of the accident.
Review: Yes ○   No ○

4. The involved bone is the:
   A. tibia.
   B. fibula.
   C. patella.
   D. femur.

Answer: **D**
Why: The femur is the bone located in the upper thigh.
Review: Yes ○   No ○

5. The medical assistant reading the medical record is:
   A. in violation of HIPAA.
   B. not part of the job.
   C. appropriate.
   D. difficult to do with an EHR.
   E. the only staff member who should have access to the record at that time.

Answer: **C**
Why: Knowing why a patient is presenting to the medical office and the type and location of injuries is necessary to prepare for the visit and considered continuity of care.
Review: Yes ○   No ○

CHAPTER 7

Human Behavior and Professional Communication

Review Tip:

Take this time to evaluate your review process and progress. Is your environment comfortable and conducive to studying? Are you spending the time as you initially planned? Are you staying focused and motivated (especially after the "killer" "Anatomy and Physiology" chapter)? Is your study group (if you have one) productive? Are you asking family, friends, and employers for assistance and encouragement? Revise your plan if necessary, but DO NOT PROCRASTINATE. Remember why you are taking the exam!

Communication is the process of forming and transmitting a message (**encoding**) to a receiver who interprets that message (**decoding**) and, in most cases, transmits a message back to the original sender, repeating the process (Fig. 7-1).

Every phase of health care requires communication, whether it involves patients, their families and friends, physicians, coworkers, other members of the health-care team (such as hospital personnel), vendors, attorneys, governmental agencies, or other entities.

Many of the serious errors that result in patient harm are associated with faulty communication. Other consequences of miscommunication include malpractice suits, anger, distrust, and stress. Communicating in a professional, culturally sensitive manner helps ensure that messages are properly sent and correctly perceived by the recipient, and that the recipient responds appropriately to the sender. A leading principle of communication in health care is *confidentiality*. The majority of information in this chapter addresses communication between the patient and the health-care provider and appropriate aspects of psychology.

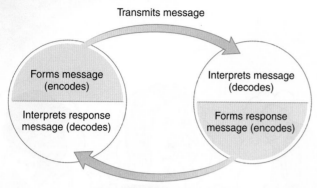

FIGURE 7-1 The communication process.

PSYCHOLOGICAL STAGES OF DEVELOPMENT

Although there are several theories on what is called behavioral development, the stages are generally divided into specific age groups. There are distinct processes that normally should occur in each of these stages of development. When communicating with people of various ages, keep in mind the behavior pertinent to each group. Familiar psychologists, Piaget and Erickson, described general stages of development, which are listed in Figure 7-2, and developmental milestones are found in Table 7-1.

COMMUNICATION GOALS

All communication has goals, either conscious or subconscious, that a person must understand to correctly formulate a message. Sometimes, there is more than one goal per message. Some examples of communication goals are to

- Obtain information
- Provide information
- Develop trust
- Demonstrate caring
- Relieve stress

TYPES OF COMMUNICATION

- Formal—a style associated with decorum, etiquette, and a person's recognized role
- Informal—a style associated with an easygoing, open role, and relationship
- Verbal—word-of-mouth communication; may be formal or informal
  - Face to face
  - Telephone
  - Television
  - Audio technology (compact disks, tapes)

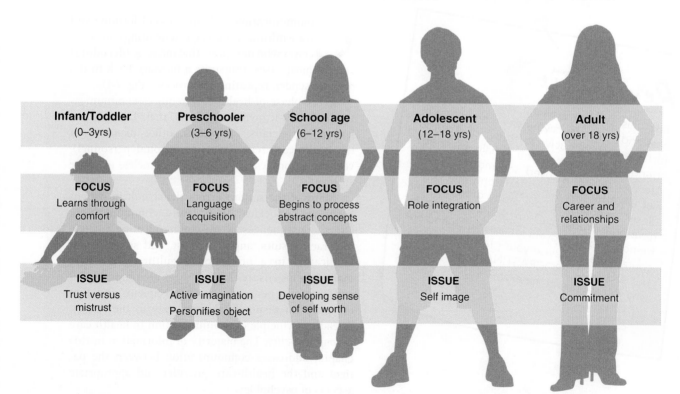

FIGURE 7-2 General stages of development.

TABLE 7-1 ▶ Developmental milestones: Ages 2 months to 4 years

Age	Social/Emotional	Language/Communication	Cognitive	Physical Development
2 mo	Begins to smile at people	Coos, makes gurgling sounds	Pays attention to faces	Can hold head up
4 mo	Copies some movements and facial expressions	Begins to babble	Recognizes familiar faces	Head is steady unsupported
6 mo	Likes to play with others	Responds to own name	Brings things to mouth	Rolls over in both directions
9 mo	May be afraid of strangers	Understands "No"	Plays peek-a-boo	Crawls
1 y	Cries when mom or dad leaves	Responds to simple spoken requests	Finds hidden things easily	Walks or stands holding on
2 y	Copies others	Knows names of body parts	Begins to sort shapes and colors	Kicks a ball, runs
4 y	Is more creative with make–believe	Tells stories, knows first and last name	Names colors and counting	Hops, pours, cuts (with supervision)

- Written—communication using the printed word; may be formal or informal
  - Medical records
  - Letters
  - Memorandums
  - E-mail
  - Books
  - Reports
  - Posters
  - Faxes
  - Bulletin boards
- Nonverbal—communication using body language and other nonwritten or nonoral methods
  - Open—receptive, positive appearance (e.g., the recipient leaning forward to listen)
  - Closed—nonreceptive, negative appearance (e.g., the recipient standing with frown on face and folded arms)
  - Indicators—signs that imply open or closed communication
    - Facial expressions, such as a smile or frown
    - Voice tone (e.g., soft or shrill)
    - Gestures, including sign language (e.g., extending hand for handshake or shaking a finger at a person, indicating anger or disapproval)
    - Body stance and posture, such as standing straight with arms at side or slouching with arms folded

COMMUNICATION BARRIERS

- Noise
- Inadequate listening
- Withdrawal or lack of attention
- Lack of privacy
- Embarrassment
- Cultural differences
  - Concepts of health and illness (e.g., only visiting the physician in the case of illness; not seeking preventive care)
  - Folk beliefs and practices (e.g., the belief that burying the umbilical cord when it falls off will help the child develop normally)
  - Child-rearing traditions (e.g., "a fat baby is a healthy baby")
  - Religion (e.g., Jehovah's Witnesses prohibit blood transfusions)
  - Politeness (e.g., in some Native American cultures, it is taboo to make eye contact with another person)
  - Who speaks for whom (e.g., in some cultures, the husband speaks for his wife at the health-care facility)
  - Family ties (e.g., all members of family and extended family expected to stay with ill person)
  - Death and dying traditions (e.g., required rites, blessings, or ceremonies)

- Educational differences
- Language barriers
- Physical and developmental impairments
- Pain or discomfort (including hunger, thirst, uncomfortable room temperature)
- Prejudice (holding a negative or positive opinion or bias concerning an individual because of his or her affiliation with a specific group; this includes gender bias)
- Stereotyping (believing that all members of a culture, subculture, or group are the same)
- Emotions
- Judgmental or critical behavior
- Substance abuse

PSYCHOLOGICAL DEFENSE MECHANISMS

People commonly react to injury and illness with anxiety and, often, defensive behavior. **Defense mechanisms** are psychological behaviors that protect a person from guilt and shame. Some uses of the mechanisms are considered normal. Overuse or exaggerated use may become pathologic. Recognizing defense mechanisms assists in understanding and managing the behavior and the circumstance.

- Compensation—overemphasizing certain behaviors to accommodate for real or imagined weaknesses (e.g., giving a child expensive gifts to make up for not spending time with him or her)
- Denial—refusal to accept unwanted information or unpleasant circumstances (e.g., the parent who will not consider that his or her child is using drugs despite very clear indications to the contrary)
- Displacement—transferring negative feelings, sometimes hostility, to something or someone unrelated to a negative situation (e.g., being rude to the medical office receptionist because your insurance company does not have you listed on the physician's roster)
- Introjection—identifying and assuming characteristics or feelings of another (e.g., the expectant father who has food cravings similar to his pregnant partner)
- Projection—placing blame or accusing another for actions or feelings committed by the person himself or herself (e.g., the patient blaming the health-care provider for continued illness when the patient was noncompliant with the care plan)
- Rationalization—justifying thoughts or actions whether right or wrong (e.g., spending money on a luxury item because you've had a bad day)

- Regression—escaping an unpleasantness by returning to an earlier stage or behavior in life (e.g., a child who reverts to baby talk when scolded to distract the parent's anger)
- Repression—dealing with a difficult situation by true temporary amnesia (e.g., a witness to a crime who cannot remember the crime or who he or she is)
- Sublimation—redirecting unacceptable thoughts or behaviors to acceptable ones (e.g., the alcoholic who goes from drinking every night to attending Alcoholics Anonymous meetings every night)
- Suppression—purposefully forgetting an unpleasant situation or avoiding it (e.g., victims of childhood sexual abuse who do not remember the molestation until, perhaps, an incident in adulthood triggers the memory)

HEALTH-CARE IMPLICATIONS

Every communication within the health-care setting has the potential for affecting a patient's outcome, physically and emotionally, positively or negatively. The relationship, good or bad, between the patient and the health-care provider is predominately the result of their interactions. Other considerations when communicating with patients are as follows:

- Are the patient's expectations of the health-care providers realistic?
- What feelings and emotions are involved?
- Does the patient have personal challenges (financial, home situation, etc.)?
- Are you maintaining professionalism at all times?
- Are both parties interpreting and understanding each other while accurately exchanging information?
- Are both parties accepting differences?
- Are both parties making reasonable accommodations?

THERAPEUTIC COMMUNICATION

The health-care team should strive to make every interaction with the patient and with all persons one of understanding and caring. The encounter should promote healing or acknowledgment in cases of serious disease or disability and provide some level of comfort. It is always

- Confidential
- Respectful and courteous
- Professional (friendly and capable but not too informal)
- Without bias regarding race, religion, age, gender, sexual orientation, or socioeconomic status
- Empathetic (sympathetic but not enabling)

- Nonjudgmental
- Tolerant and supportive
- Accepting
- Reassuring
- Mindful of the patient's individuality
- Honest and open
- Diplomatic and tactful
- Positive in attitude and body language

ENHANCING COMMUNICATION

The health-care provider should continually strive to develop and practice better communication techniques. To promote positive and effective communication, especially in the health-care setting:

- Provide a quiet, private, safe, and comfortable environment
- Listen carefully with no interruptions
- Provide feedback (paraphrasing, mirroring, repeating, restating to ensure understanding)
- Ask exploratory or open-ended questions (such as "Tell me about your pain"), not questions that can be answered with yes or no or one word
- Seek clarification (who, what, how, how much)
- Use silence to allow patients to add more information
- Demonstrate open body language
- Exhibit a confident demeanor
- Focus (stay on important topics)
- Observe boundaries (e.g., remaining at a friendly but professional distance, not discussing intimate parts of patient's life or health-care provider's life that do not pertain to the pertinent health-care issue; not allowing rambling; not giving advice outside of one's scope of practice)

RESPONDING TO CRITICISM

Criticism may come from a patient, employer, or other team member. The manner in which you deal with criticism, whether valid or not, could mean the difference between a therapeutic or detrimental encounter with a patient or a positive or negative outcome with your employer or other team member. Methods of dealing with criticism include the following:

- Listen and avoid being defensive
- Consider the validity by using introspection
- Take into account the situation of the person delivering the criticism (refer to previous-chapter topics)
- Think before you speak
- Respond in a professional, objective but caring manner
- Close on a warm positive note

SPECIAL COMMUNICATION NEEDS AND STRATEGIES

- Sight-impaired patients
  - Speak in a normal tone of voice
  - Describe surroundings and locations of structures
  - Explain what you are going to do and what you are doing
  - Alert patient before touching him or her
  - Explain unusual noises associated with a procedure
  - Notify patient of anyone who is entering the room or if you are leaving the room
  - Allow touching of instruments and use models when appropriate
  - Facilitate return demonstrations as needed
  - Obtain feedback
  - Encourage questions
- Hearing-impaired patients
  - Touch the patient gently on an arm or shoulder to get his or her attention
  - Address the patient directly
  - Determine level of hearing loss and what assistive devices are used by patient
  - Increase voice volume, if appropriate, but do not shout
  - Speak distinctly and more slowly, using short sentences with slight pauses
  - Eliminate as much background noise as possible
  - Offer notepads or other non–hearing communication devices
  - Use pictures and captioned videos as appropriate
  - Facilitate return demonstrations as appropriate
  - Obtain feedback
  - Encourage questions

Box 7-1 addresses one of the telecommunication devices for the deaf, which allows office personnel to communicate with hearing-impaired patients over the telephone.

- Diverse populations and no or limited English-language patients
  - Attempt to acquire some knowledge of culture to avoid negative communication (refer to "Cultural differences" in the section "Communications Barriers")
  - Provide an interpreter if possible (some insurance companies will arrange or cover the cost; some social agencies dealing with refugees and immigrants provide help; some offices contract with an interpreting service)

Telecommunication device for the deaf

Many of the larger medical practices maintain a telecommunication device for the deaf (TDD). This equipment allows the office to call a hearing-impaired patient and to type a message that is electronically transmitted to the receiver's TDD and vice versa. If the office does not have a TDD, the office's telephone carrier may be contacted to send a TDD-facilitated message to the patient. E-mail and texting are other effective communication technology for contacting hearing-impaired patients.

- Research the culture to determine if there are any restrictions regarding who may act as an interpreter (e.g., in some cultures, interpreter must be of the same sex as patient)
- Determine whether the patient is bringing an interpreter (children and young adolescents should not be used)
- Speak directly to the patient even when using an interpreter
- Speak in a normal tone but at a slightly slower pace
- Use simple, short sentences
- Avoid slang or idioms
- Observe patient's body language as questions are asked and answered
- Use visual aids, such as pictures, hand gestures, or demonstrations
- Provide forms, educational materials, and office signs in various languages, if possible
- Use dual dictionaries of English and the patient's language

■ Pediatric patients and patients with age-related developmental disabilities
- Always state the truth
- Position yourself at the same height as the patient
- Talk to the patient even if a caregiver is present
- Use vocabulary appropriate to the patient's developmental age
- Incorporate dolls, pictures, and other toys to enhance communication or obtain cooperation
- Allow patient to handle safe medical equipment
- Expect patient to regress emotionally during illness
- Maintain a calm voice and demeanor, even if the patient is "acting out"
- Utilize previously stated techniques to determine understanding and compliance

■ Adolescent patients
- Treat the adolescent with respect
- Avoid being judgmental
- Always state the truth
- Expect adolescents to demonstrate resentment in illness, especially in chronic illness
- Allow privacy from parents during assessment and treatment, if desired by the patient
- Maintain a calm voice and demeanor even if the adolescent is "acting out"
- Do not assume, regardless of the patient's age, that he or she possesses the correct terminology and knowledge related to body functions, especially those related to the reproductive system
- Consider typical teenage preferences and behaviors when providing self-care instructions
- Obtain feedback
- Encourage questions

■ Geriatric patients
- Accommodate for hearing, sight, or other impairments
- Ensure patient's comfort and privacy
- Maintain an unrushed environment
- Use feedback strategies often
- Facilitate staying focused on pertinent topics
- Include the patient in the conversation even if a caregiver is providing the information

■ Illiterate patients (illiteracy is not a reflection of intelligence)
- Use simple, short sentences
- Avoid slang or idioms
- Offer to assist with completing forms if patient is struggling
- Encourage questions
- Observe patient's body language for cues as questions are asked and answered
- Use visual aids, such as pictures or demonstrations rather than written material
- Provide educational materials and instructions that are understandable to the patient

■ Anxious or angry patient
- Consider why the patient is feeling as he is (for example, fear of a diagnosis; the physician was running late)
- Avoid becoming defensive
- Maintain professionalism
- Prevent stereotyping or bias
- Speak using a calm normal voice
- Acknowledge the patient's feeling ("you appear upset")

- Provide a neutral apology ("I can understand why you are feeling that way and I am sorry") and assure that you will try to help or will notify the appropriate person to help
- Report the situation to the physician or appropriate staff member
- End on a positive note if you are the person dismissing the patient

MASLOW'S HIERARCHY

Abraham Maslow, an American psychiatrist, theorized that people are motivated by their needs and that those needs are a progression from basic survival to reaching one's pinnacle, or self-actualization. Dr. Maslow ordered these needs in a hierarchy and listed them in a pyramid formation (Fig. 7-3). Generally, a person cannot progress from one level to the next until all needs are met in the lower levels.

The implications of **Maslow's hierarchy** or **pyramid** for health-care providers are substantial. Your communication with the patient will be more effective if you determine where that person is on Maslow's hierarchy. For example, a patient who does not have the money and other resources (e.g., transportation, child care) to visit a physician when he or she is sick will not be motivated to listen to advice regarding preventive health care or nutritional diets that are more expensive than a low-cost fast food, high-fat, high-carbohydrate diet. Effective therapeutic communication recognizes the stage on the Maslow hierarchy pyramid, provides empathy and understanding, and then strives to discover a motivating factor within that level. The health-care provider in

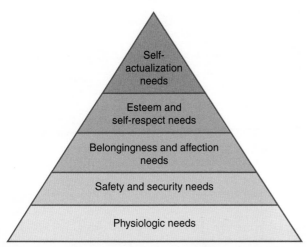

FIGURE 7-3 Maslow's hierarchy of human needs. (Reprinted with permission from Molle EA, Durham LS. *Lippincott Williams & Wilkins' Administrative Medical Assisting*. Philadelphia: Lippincott Williams & Wilkins, 2004.)

this example can explain that if the patient ignores the treatment plan, the potential for a life-threatening illness increases, which may result in leaving his or her children without support.

STAGES OF DEATH AND DYING

Another progression in human life involves the **stages of death and dying**. Elizabeth Kübler-Ross is credited as being the first to formally outline these stages. The patient and the patient's family and close friends all experience the continuum. Communication is more effective when the stage is recognized and appropriate accommodations are made.

- Denial—refusing to accept that death will soon occur or has occurred
- Anger—lashing out at a deity, family and friends, and health-care providers
- Bargaining—attempting to gain time through negotiating, pleading with a deity, with health-care providers to do more, and with self
- Depression—withdrawing, feeling low in spirits
- Acceptance—resigning to the situation, preparing (if time permits), and feeling tranquil

Sudden death is thought to be more difficult. The involved parties do not have the time for a distinct progression through the stages and are unprepared; their reactions are often chaotic.

In all cases of death or terminal illness,

- Be truthful while staying within your role (if the patient asks your opinion about a new "cure," say that you are not qualified to weigh it and he would have to speak to the doctor)
- Listen allowing people to vent their thoughts and feelings
- Provide an opportunity for questions
- Offer appropriate resources such as support groups

TERMS

COMMUNICATION REVIEW

The following list reviews the terms discussed in this chapter and **other important terms that you may see on the exam.**

communication the process of forming and transmitting a message to a receiver who interprets that message and, in most cases, transmits a message back to the original sender, repeating the process

compensation a defense mechanism in which a person overemphasizes certain behaviors to accommodate for real or imagined weaknesses

culture customary beliefs, traits, social forms, and behaviors associated with a religious, ethnic, or other group

decoding receiving and interpreting a message

defense mechanisms psychological behaviors that protect a person from guilt and shame

denial a defense mechanism in which a person refuses to accept unwanted information or unpleasant circumstances

diplomacy the art of handling people with tact and genuine concern

displacement a defense mechanism in which a person transfers negative feelings, sometimes hostility, to something or someone unrelated to a negative situation

encoding forming and sending a message

feedback paraphrasing, mirroring, repeating, or restating to ensure understanding

introjection a defense mechanism in which a person identifies and assumes characteristics or feelings of another

Maslow's hierarchy a progression of a person's needs from basic survival to reaching one's pinnacle, or self-actualization, identified by Abraham Maslow

nonverbal communication using body language and other nonwritten or nonoral methods; nonverbal communication may be formal or informal, open or closed

paraphrasing using different words to assure understanding of what the speaker said

prejudice holding a negative or positive opinion or bias regarding an individual because of his or her affiliation with a specific group

projection a defense mechanism in which a person places blame or accuses another for actions or feelings committed by himself or herself

rationalization justifying thoughts or actions whether right or wrong

regression a defense mechanism in which a person escapes an unpleasantness by returning to an earlier stage or behavior in life

repression a defense mechanism in which a person deals with a difficult situation by true temporary amnesia

stages of death and dying articulated by Elizabeth Kübler-Ross, a progression of feelings and behaviors that patients, families, and close friends experience when death is imminent or has occurred; these behaviors include denial, anger, bargaining, depression, and acceptance

stereotyping believing that all members of a culture, subculture, or group are the same

sublimation a defense mechanism in which a person redirects unacceptable thoughts or behaviors to acceptable ones

suppression a defense mechanism in which a person purposefully forgets an unpleasant situation or avoids dealing with it

REVIEW QUESTIONS

All questions are relevant for all medical assisting and medical administrative certification exams.

1. Which of the following is the best example of nonverbal communication?
   A. Clarification
   B. Feedback
   C. Body language
   D. Messages

   Answer: **C**
   Why: Nonverbal communication refers to a way of exchanging messages without using words. Body language uses types of behavior or gestures and facial expressions to send a message without saying anything.
   Review: Yes ○   No ○

2. When a person generalizes the behavior or characteristics of all members of a particular culture, race, or religion, it is referred to as:
   A. empathizing.
   B. stereotyping.
   C. discriminating.
   D. bias.
   E. Rationalizing.

   Answer: **B**
   Why: Bias occurs when personal values or opinions affect the way you treat others. Discriminating is the act of treating certain people unfairly or without respect because of their cultural, social, or personal values or beliefs. Empathizing means that you emotionally identify with what another person is feeling or experiencing. Rationalizing is the process of explaining on the basis of reason or logic.
   Review: Yes ○   No ○

3. Three elements necessary for basic communication include:
   A. message, sender, receiver.
   B. message, feedback, body language.
   C. clarification, sender, feedback.
   D. sender, receiver, body language.

   Answer: **A**
   Why: The message is the information that is to be relayed either verbally or nonverbally. There must be someone sending and someone else receiving the message. Clarification is the process of making a message clearer or more understandable to the receiver. Feedback refers to the responses returned from either the sender or the receiver about the message.
   Review: Yes ○   No ○

4. To have proper verbal communication with a patient, you should use:
   A. a monotone voice so the patient will listen better.
   B. elaborate medical terminology to impress the patient.
   C. negative body language to get the patient's attention.
   D. sarcastic remarks to get the patient's attention.
   E. conversation at the patient's educational level.

   Answer: **E**
   Why: A monotone voice occurs when a person is speaking without changing the pitch or key of the voice and is likely to cause the listener to lose interest in the conversation. Medical terminology is confusing for most laypersons; using such terminology will not lead to a patient understanding your message. Negative body language can make others uncomfortable and may cause them to ignore, turn away, or walk away from a conversation. Sarcastic remarks are rude and disrespectful and should not be part of any professional conversation.
   Review: Yes ○   No ○

5. Communicating with someone who is grieving the loss of a loved one is difficult when the person refuses to acknowledge the loss. This type of behavior is referred to as:
   A. sympathy.
   B. mourning.
   C. denial.
   D. depression.

Answer: **C**

Why: Sympathy is sharing someone else's feeling, especially during a difficult situation, such as the death of a loved one. When a person is experiencing the loss of a loved one, he or she is in a period of mourning. Depression is a feeling of low spirits and being withdrawn. Denial is the inability or refusal to accept reality—in this case, the loss of a loved one.

Review: Yes ○   No ○

6. To communicate with a sight-impaired patient, it is important to:
   A. transport the patient in a wheelchair to avoid an accident.
   B. use positive body language.
   C. raise your voice to make your conversation louder.
   D. tell the patient each time before you touch him or her.
   E. give directions in writing to ensure understanding.

Answer: **D**

Why: Always talk to the patient and explain procedures before touching or performing any procedures on him or her. If a patient is sight-impaired, it does not necessarily mean that the person is totally blind. The patient may be capable of walking safely without a wheelchair, but transporting the patient does not facilitate communication. It may be difficult for the patient to see you clearly, so body language is not going to be easily seen by the patient. The patient may not be deaf or hard of hearing, so raising your voice is not necessary. Written instructions are difficult for a sight-impaired patient to read and will not be an effective method of communication.

Review: Yes ○   No ○

7. To communicate with a hearing-impaired patient, it would be advisable to:
   A. not call the patient at home, because of the hearing impairment.
   B. keep at a normal distance from the patient, but talk much louder and shout if necessary to be heard.
   C. write everything down instead of talking to the patient.
   D. speak slowly and distinctly to the patient.

Answer: **D**

Why: If a patient is hearing-impaired, it does not necessarily mean that he or she is completely deaf. It is appropriate to call this patient at home to confirm appointments. It is impolite to shout at a patient; therefore, it is appropriate to get closer to a hearing-impaired patient when having a conversation. It would not be necessary to write everything down, but you may want to write down the most important things you want the patient to remember. The key to communicating with a hearing-impaired individual is to speak slowly and clearly.

Review: Yes ○   No ○

8. Which of the following is an example of an open-ended question you would ask a patient?
   A. Did you follow the doctor's instructions?
   B. What time did you take your medication?
   C. Which insurance plan are you covered by?
   D. Will you tell me about your pain?
   E. What day can you come in for a follow-up appointment?

Answer: **D**

Why: An open-ended question is one that requires more than a single-word answer or a yes-or-no answer. This is a way to get patients to open up and talk or express their thoughts. All of the choices require only a single-word answer, except for choice D, which requires the patient to describe the pain he or she is experiencing.

Review: Yes ○   No ○

9. When communicating with a difficult, challenging patient, you should:
   A. exhibit a diplomatic attitude.
   B. display an attitude of authority.
   C. make sure the patient knows the office is correct.
   D. always ask the patient to put any complaints in writing.

Answer: **A**
Why: Diplomacy is the art of handling people with tact and genuine concern. Do not display an attitude of authority, because this may make a patient or client angry. Patients have rights in the physician's office, and the office may not always be correct. It is not appropriate to ask any patient to put his or her complaint in writing. Suggesting a patient "put it in writing" may be an invitation to a lawsuit. It is best to discuss concerns as they surface at the office.
Review: Yes ◯   No ◯

10. Which of the following is an example of behavior that demonstrates open nonverbal communication?
    A. Frowning eyes and mouth
    B. Folded arms across chest
    C. Leaning forward to listen
    D. Staring at the floor
    E. Sighing frequently during conversation

Answer: **C**
Why: Body language is a form of nonverbal communication. Open nonverbal communication is a positive, receptive way of communicating. The recipient usually leans forward to listen and makes direct eye contact with the person who is sending the message. Closed nonverbal communication is expressed through negative expressions such as frowning, folding arms, not making direct eye contact, and sighing during the conversation. These expressions reveal that an individual is not receptive to the communication.
Review: Yes ◯   No ◯

11. When an individual is overemphasizing certain behaviors to accommodate for real or imagined weaknesses, he or she is:
    A. regressing.
    B. compensating.
    C. projecting.
    D. rationalizing.

Answer: **B**
Why: To regress, or to go backward, is to escape an unpleasant event or situation and to return to an earlier stage or behavior in life. Projecting is placing blame or accusing someone else for something you have done. Rationalizing means reasoning or justifying one's behavior.
Review: Yes ◯   No ◯

12. Maslow's hierarchy of human needs is based on the concept that:
    A. affection is the most important basic need for all people.
    B. a safe environment is placed above all other needs as the number one requirement of all persons.
    C. physiologic needs are the most basic but are necessary for a person to progress any further toward reaching self-actualization.
    D. esteem must always come from those around us.
    E. security is the most basic and important need.

Answer: **C**
Why: The physiologic needs are air, food, water, rest, and comfort. Without these basic foundational needs being met, a person cannot reach any higher levels on Maslow's hierarchy of human needs. Affection is important but not a basic need for all persons. A safe and secure environment is only achieved after the basic needs are met. Esteem needs are needs to feel self-worth. Esteem can be self-generated or can come from others who admire a person.
Review: Yes ◯   No ◯

13. When communicating with pediatric patients, you should:
   A. not allow children to handle safe medical equipment.
   B. use medical terminology so the child does not understand the procedure.
   C. not lie to a child but state the truth.
   D. talk louder and make sure the child understands that you are the adult.

Answer: **C**
Why: Children are capable of understanding many things, and the truth should always be told to them. If you lie to a child that a procedure will not hurt and then it does, the child may not trust health-care workers in the future. It is proper to allow children to handle safe equipment to help them feel comfortable. You should not use language the child does not understand and should not display an attitude of being an adult disciplinarian.
Review: Yes ○   No ○

14. The receiving and interpreting of a message is known as:
   A. decoding.
   B. feedback.
   C. encoding.
   D. acceptance.
   E. sending.

Answer: **A**
Why: Feedback is repeating or restating a message to ensure understanding. Encoding is the forming and sending of a message and does not involve receiving and interpreting. Acceptance means to resolve or be resigned to a situation, to accept the outcome. Sending is the process of carrying or transmitting a message.
Review: Yes ○   No ○

15. Psychological behaviors that protect a person from guilt and shame are:
   A. therapeutic techniques.
   B. defense mechanisms.
   C. cultural differences.
   D. language barriers.

Answer: **B**
Why: Therapeutic techniques include any activity that aids in a patient's recovery. Cultural differences are those traits specific to an ethnic culture or race. A language barrier is caused when people cannot communicate because they speak different languages.
Review: Yes ○   No ○

16. When communicating with a non–English-speaking patient, it is appropriate to:
   A. ignore the customs or taboos of the patient's culture.
   B. only communicate with the patient if accompanied by someone who speaks fluent English.
   C. raise your voice to increase understanding.
   D. use culturally acceptable gestures to demonstrate information.
   E. use negative body language.

Answer: **D**
Why: You should always take into consideration the customs of the patient's culture so that you do not unintentionally offend him or her. If an interpreter is available, this person may be able to better communicate the information to the patient. The interpreter may be a family member who is not fluent in English but who knows enough to relate the messages to the patient. It is not appropriate to raise your voice just because the patient does not speak English. Using appropriate descriptive gestures will help demonstrate what you are trying to convey to a non–English-speaking patient. Using negative body language is inappropriate and rude.
Review: Yes ○   No ○

17. Prejudice is a term that means:
   A. your personal values are not the same as others.
   B. you hold an opinion or bias concerning an individual because of his or her affiliation with a specific group.
   C. you recognize the fear and discomfort that a patient is feeling.
   D. you refuse to acknowledge something.

Answer: **B**
Why: All people are free to have their own personal values, which may not be the same as those of others, but when you hold an opinion or bias concerning an individual because of his or her affiliation with a specific group of people, this constitutes prejudice, which is also a form of stereotyping. Empathy means that you recognize the fear and discomfort a patient is feeling; denial is refusing to acknowledge something.
Review: Yes ○   No ○

18. To encourage further comments from a patient, the interviewer can repeat what the patient has said using open-ended statements that require the patient to respond. This technique is called:
   A. summarizing.
   B. reflecting.
   C. listening.
   D. focusing.
   E. encoding.

Answer: **B**
Why: Summarizing is restating information in a condensed format. Listening is the act of giving attention to the person who is talking and understanding what is being said. Focusing is the technique of staying on the same topic or subject during a conversation and not deviating onto other topics. Encoding is the forming and sending of a message.
Review: Yes ○   No ○

19. A patient who is withdrawn, weeping, and isolated from others may be experiencing:
   A. anger.
   B. denial.
   C. depression.
   D. empathy.

Answer: **C**
Why: Anger is lashing out at others. Denial is the refusal to accept a situation, and empathy is feeling the same as another feels in a situation.
Review: Yes ○   No ○

20. Maintaining a professional relationship with the patient means that you should:
   A. become personally involved with the patient.
   B. become socially interactive with the patient.
   C. disclose private, personal information about the physician.
   D. give the patient your private phone number in case of emergency.
   E. deliver patient care that allows you to continue to provide objective medical care.

Answer: **E**
Why: It is appropriate to be friendly with patients, but you should not become personally or socially involved with patients. Private or personal information about the physician should never be disclosed to patients. It is also inappropriate to disclose your private phone number or address to a patient.
Review: Yes ○   No ○

21. Proper flow of communication occurs in the following order:
   A. Message, response, clarification, feedback
   B. Response, clarification, feedback, message
   C. Feedback, message, clarification, response
   D. Clarification, message, response, feedback

Answer: **A**
Why: To ensure proper communication, there must first be a message or information to send. Clarification and feedback come after the message has been sent. A response cannot be given to something not yet received.
Review: Yes ○   No ○

22. The progression of a person's needs from basic survival to reaching one's pinnacle or self-actualization is known as Maslow's:
  A. rationalization.
  B. self-realization.
  C. hierarchy.
  D. mechanism.
  E. triangle.

Answer: **C**
Why: A hierarchy is a system of ranking or grading things from least to greatest or small to large. Maslow's hierarchy ranks a person's needs from basic needs for survival to a rank of fulfillment of oneself or one's capabilities.
Review: Yes ◯   No ◯

23. To avoid breaching confidentiality, you should:
  A. use the office intercom to notify another coworker of the name of a caller on the phone.
  B. only discuss patient problems during the office lunch hour.
  C. communicate in writing, not verbally, to coworkers about patients.
  D. avoid discussing patient problems in the office hallway.

Answer: **D**
Why: Patients' names should not be announced over an intercom. Patient information should never be discussed outside the office, such as in a restaurant during lunch. At the office, patients should only be discussed in a private area, not in the hallway. Written messages are not appropriate for all communication in the office. The written message is not efficient; paper still needs to be either discarded properly or stored in a confidential area.
Review: Yes ◯   No ◯

24. Communication techniques that are used when interviewing a patient include:
  A. reflecting and summarizing.
  B. language barriers.
  C. stereotyping.
  D. bargaining and acceptance.
  E. criticizing.

Answer: **A**
Why: Reflecting and summarizing are communication techniques that allow the interviewer to encourage more conversation from the patient and clarify information for accuracy. Language barriers exist when the people who need to communicate do not speak or understand the same language. Stereotyping is the belief that all members of a culture or group are the same. Bargaining and acceptance are stages of dealing with grief. Criticizing is the act of judging and analyzing to find fault with something.
Review: Yes ◯   No ◯

25. To set the stage for successful communication, you should:
  A. ask closed-ended questions instead of open-ended questions because they are less time-consuming and more efficient.
  B. sit at the patient's level, eye to eye, and maintain eye contact with the patient if culturally appropriate.
  C. avoid using any body language such as appropriate facial expressions.
  D. discourage any additional comments from the patient because the physician will question the patient again during the examination.

Answer: **B**
Why: You should sit at the level of the patient and maintain good eye contact during the interview. This creates an atmosphere of focus on the patient. The use of facial expression and open body language will also add to a positive communication environment. Asking closed-ended questions and not encouraging additional comments will cause the patient to shut down and not express what is actually going on with his or her health. It may be more difficult for the patient to talk to or discuss anything further with the physician.
Review: Yes ◯   No ◯

26. Which of the following is an issue that becomes predominant during the adolescent stage of development?
    A. Commitment
    B. Self-worth
    C. Mistrust
    D. Imagination
    E. Self-image

Answer: **E**
Why: According to noted behavioral psychologists, the predominant issue for the adolescent group is self-image. Commitment is an adult issue. Mistrust is an infant or toddler issue. School-age children have issues with developing a sense of self-worth, and preschoolers develop imagination as a form of communication.
Review: Yes ○   No ○

CRITICAL THINKING CASE REVIEW

Sara Mariano is a 13-year-old patient of Dr. Patel who is scheduled for a sports physical. Sara is usually outgoing and jovial. Today she is very quiet and seems tense. Her mother is with her. The medical assistant asked the customary screening questions and the responses were normal, but the medical assistant senses something is amiss.

1. An appropriate action might be to:
    A. consider where Sara may be on Maslow's hierarchy.
    B. note in the medical record that she is regressing.
    C. inform the physician of your observation.
    D. ask her mother to wait in the reception area.
    E. not get involved with any issues.

Answer: **C**
Why: Although "A" is always appropriate, it is not the best answer. Being quiet and tense are not signs of regression, and unless it is office policy for that age group to have parents wait outside of the exam room this is not a good approach. In this situation, it is best to inform the physician of your observations and do as instructed.
Review: Yes ○   No ○

2. According to the stages of development, a normal issue of a 13-year-old would be:
    A. commitment.
    B. self-image.
    C. developing a sense of worth.
    D. trust versus mistrust.

Answer: **B**
Why: Commitment is usually related to adulthood; developing a sense of worth during early school age and trust versus mistrust in the infancy/toddler stage. Self-image is associated with adolescence.
Review: Yes ○   No ○

3. Dr. Patel informed Mrs. Mariano that at Sara's age he likes to spend some time talking to the patient without the parent present. The physician is:
    A. being culturally sensitive.
    B. removing a communication barrier.
    C. encouraging feedback.
    D. decoding the message in the communication process.
    E. bargaining.

Answer: **B**
Why: During the teenage years, when it comes to personal and many health-related issues such as sexual or other age-appropriate concerns, teens are often reluctant to speak openly in front of parents. Therefore, the presence of a parent would be considered a communication barrier.
Review: Yes ○   No ○

4. Sara discusses with the physician that she has attended a class at school that discusses sexual education topics but she has many questions and is not comfortable asking her mother. She has also gone online and is finding contradictory information which is confusing her further. The doctor schedules a time for her to return, and the medical assistant will meet with her to go over information and assure all her questions are answered. The sexual orientation is important in Sara's stage of development related to:

A. role integration.
B. commitment.
C. trust versus mistrust.
D. processing abstract concepts.

Answer: **A**

Why: Prior to adolescence, the human is learning how to satisfy basic needs such as hunger, how to acquire language and abstract concepts such as thinking. At adolescence, one begins to realize and integrate the various roles inevitably assigned to us, often by place in the family, level at school, and our gender, including sexual orientation and processes.

Review: Yes ○   No ○

5. If Sara begins a discussion with the medical assistant, in order to promote positive and effective communication, the medical assistant should engage in a discussion with her that:

A. includes asking only closed-ended questions.
B. demonstrates good listening skills without being judgmental.
C. involves Sara's mother so that no legal action might be taken against the practice for treating a minor without parental consent.
D. provides frequent feedback to Sara in the form of paraphrasing everything she says.
E. shares the medical assistant's personal opinions based on when she was a teenager and went through the same things.

Answer: **B**

Why: Effective communication is necessary when working with patients. It involves listening to the patient and not judging their ideas or thoughts. Although it would be appropriate to provide feedback to the patient, as in answer D, it is not necessary to paraphrase everything that the patient says. It is also inappropriate to impose any personal opinions or ideas to a patient.

Review: Yes ○   No ○

CHAPTER

8

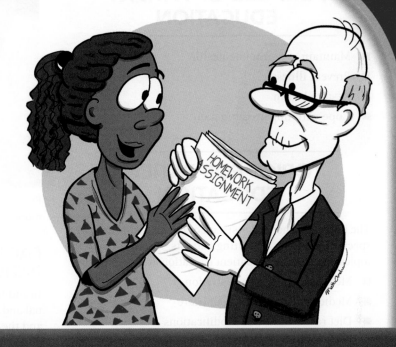

Patient Education

Review Tip:

Study the chapter on communication (Chapter 7) before you begin this chapter. The information supplied in that chapter also applies to patient education and should be integrated with the material presented here. Pick a topic pertinent to the medical office where you work or the field in which you are interested in working and develop a patient education plan. Ask your peers, supervisors, and physicians to critique it and provide input.

The emphasis on patient education in the health-care setting continues to grow. **The Joint Commission** (TJC) and the **National Committee for Quality Assurance** (NCQA), both of which accredit health-care organizations, have multiple patient education standards and requirements. The result is that more responsibility in this area is placed on the medical practice. Federal and state governments, health plans, insurance companies, hospitals, physician offices, other health-care agencies, and the public spend millions of dollars each year producing patient computer programs, online products, information pamphlets, videos, DVDs, and other instructional materials. Better-informed patients tend to be more compliant with care and more apt to participate in preventive services. The intended outcome is improved health. Patient education frequently contributes to quality improvement in health-care outcomes (see Chapter 4).

PURPOSE OF PATIENT EDUCATION

- Maintain and promote health
- Prevent illness
- Restore health
- Cope with impaired function

TOPICS FOR PATIENT EDUCATION

The role of the medical assistant or medical administrative specialist includes educating patients. A few of the many topics encountered in patient education are given below:

- Medication self-administration
- Medical equipment use and care
- Diet restrictions and modifications
- Prediagnostic test or procedure instructions
- Postdiagnostic test or procedure instructions
- Physical exercises
- Activity modification
- Preventive health schedules (e.g., immunizations, well-woman exams)
- Rehabilitative modalities
- Health warning signs
- Self-exams (e.g., for testicular and breast cancer such as Fig. 8-1)
- Health monitoring (e.g., blood pressure readings and glucose testing)

CONSIDERATIONS FOR PATIENT EDUCATION

Several areas must be considered when developing plans for patient education. These include the following.

DOMAINS OF LEARNING

Domains of learning are the areas of a person's being that affect his or her capacity to learn. The educator should be aware of the person's domains of learning when formulating the teaching plan. The domains are as follows:

- Cognitive (knowledge, comprehension)
- Affective (values, attitudes, opinions)
- Psychomotor (mental and physical abilities, sensory skills)

FIGURE 8-1 Instructing patient on self-breast exam using a model.

FACTORS INFLUENCING PATIENT EDUCATION

In addition to domains of learning, other factors, both internal and external to the patient, influence the teaching plan and the likelihood that the patient will comply or not comply with the plan. Some of these factors are given below:

- Motivation (refer to Maslow's hierarchy in Chapter 7)
- Goals
- Adaptation to illness
- Age
- Developmental age
- Impairments (e.g., hearing, sight)
- Pain
- Language
- Cultural or religious barriers
- Socioeconomic barriers
- Ability of the educator to convey information
- Learning style preference

LEARNING STYLES

Individuals learn in different ways. The three basic learning styles are as follows:

- Audio—learn by listening such as lectures
- Visual—learn by seeing such as videos and demonstrations
- Tactile or experiential—learn by performing or "hands on"

A combination using the follow steps is a good teaching model:

- explain the information and why;
- Use visual reinforcement such as pictures, videos or a demonstration if it is a procedure that requires a "hands on" activity

- request a return demonstration or other feedback from the patient such as asking to explain what they learned back to you
- Offer an opportunity to ask questions.

ENVIRONMENT CONDUCIVE TO LEARNING

After accounting for the domains of learning and other factors influencing patient education, the health-care provider must also consider the learning environment. A person is less likely to assimilate information in a chaotic setting than in one that is conducive to learning. Selecting and preparing the environment is part of the teaching plan. An environment conducive to learning is described as below:

- Quiet
- Comfortable
- Private
- Free from interruptions
- Trusting
- Appropriate for any needed equipment or materials

TEACHING AIDS AND MODALITIES

The tools and materials selected by the educator to provide patient instruction are important to the success of the teaching plan. As an example, you do not want to provide only written material to a person who has a low reading level. Many types of instructional tools and methods are available. They include:

- Pamphlets and other written material
- Internet sites such as YouTube and patient portals
- Braille materials
- Hearing devices
- Videos, compact disks, DVDs, audiotapes
- Oral presentations and discussions
- Demonstrations/return demonstrations
- Anatomic models, dolls
- Posters and other illustrations
- Record-keeping logs and journals
- Support groups
- Referral programs
- Family participation
- Feedback

COMMON SOURCES OF MATERIALS AND INFORMATION FOR PATIENT EDUCATION

Sources of patient educational materials are plentiful. Some sources will provide material at no cost; other sources may charge to cover their cost or to make a profit. In some cases, the insurance company will assume the cost. Use only credible sources, especially on the Internet, with medically known and professionally accepted sites, publications, and authors. All materials used or proposed should be approved by the physician or appropriate supervisory person in the medical office. Sources include:

- Professional organizations, such as the American Medical Association (AMA)
- Government agencies, such as Centers for Disease Control and Prevention (CDC)
- Nonprofit organizations, such as the American Diabetes Association (ADA)
- Commercial publishers of books and videos or DVDs
- Credible Internet Websites
- Computer programs designed to individualize information
- Libraries (public, private, and medical)
- Educational and medical supply companies for models, compact disks, videos, etc.
- Insurance and health-care companies (these frequently publish informational materials for members)

EDUCATIONAL PLAN

After arming yourself with the tools required for educating a patient, you are ready to begin creating the individual **patient educational plan**. TJC and NCQA standards recommend a **multidisciplinary**, or team, approach to developing the plan. Some plans are simple, such as explaining to the patient that he or she needs to reschedule an appointment, the importance of keeping that appointment, and, perhaps, escorting him or her to the scheduler, who will then arrange the required appointment. Educating a parent on how to obtain and use a small-volume nebulizer requires a more complex plan. This process could be multidisciplinary, involving the insurance company to approve rental or purchase of equipment and a medical supply company to provide the equipment. Teaching a patient about diabetes may include referring the patient to a diabetes educator. Even simple plans tend to be multidisciplinary, involving other members of the health-care team. The steps of the plan are as follows:

1. Identify the purpose and topic
2. Assess the patient's individual needs and abilities (domains of learning)
3. Develop the plan (Who will do the teaching? What will be taught and what materials for which learning style(s) are needed? Where will the teaching occur? How will it be done?)

- Review the plan with the physician or the supervisor as appropriate
- Include the appropriate patient support personnel and medical team members

4. Implement the plan

5. Evaluate the patient's understanding of your plan
   - Use feedback from the patient to evaluate the effectiveness of your teaching
   - Revise or repeat instruction if needed

6. Provide a form of written instruction for the patient to take home (frequently patients sign documents that confirm that they have received and understood information)

7. Document the education provided in the patient's medical record

8. Reevaluate effectiveness using follow-up visits, letters, e-mails, or telephone calls per office policy and procedure

OTHER CONSIDERATIONS

Some offices use computer programs with standardized or patient-specific information or compile information in packets that may contain videos, DVDs, calendars, compact disks, and even bound books. For instance, an obstetrics office may offer information on fetal development, diet and exercise during pregnancy, or what a pregnant woman can expect in each trimester. Your responsibility may be to discuss with a patient the information contained in a particular packet and to elicit and answer any questions that arise. Each patient should be considered individually, and emphasis should be placed on areas of need for that patient. If a patient is overweight, for example, more time should be spent discussing diet.

Accommodations must be made for special-needs patients and those with high-risk conditions. The medical record documentation should note what materials and information were given and explained and any areas of special emphasis. These entries should include the date, the time, and your signature. Some medical practices have forms with checkoff boxes, which are signed by you and by the patient. The medical record, in addition to providing information for the patient and members of the health-care team, is a legal document that can protect the health-care provider from liability if documentation is complete and accurate. Noncompliance by the patient could be reason for terminating that patient from a medical practice.

Accrediting bodies, governmental agencies, and contracted insurance plans also audit medical records to determine the extent and appropriateness of patient education. Failure to provide adequate patient education might be a reason for not obtaining full accreditation or for an insurance company not renewing a contract with a medical office.

EVOLVING RESPONSIBLITIES

Two major factors have contributed to the evolution of new roles and responsibilities:

1. The health-care system has become too complex and overwhelming for most nonmedical persons, especially those with major and chronic illnesses, to understand.

2. Economic-related needs (e.g. food, housing, employment; consider Maslow's hierarchy) prevent many people from being compliant with their health-care recommendations.

To help deal with these issues, informal and formal roles are evolving. The most common are called the patient advocate and the patient navigator. These terms are often used synonymously, but they are not the same.

PATIENT ADVOCATE

The **patient advocate** is a person, who through an informal or formal role, helps a patient to seek information and resources (e.g. low-cost health care, diagnostic test results, support groups) and to help to resolve issues with the health-care system (e.g. medication availability, billing problems). The patient advocate may be one of the following:

- A friend or neighbor (informal)
- A person with a specific advocacy agency such as the ADA (formal)
- An employee of a health-care organization designated for this role (formal)
- An employee of a health-care organization who includes patient advocacy issues in his or her every day patient care role such as providing patient education on community resources (formal)

PATIENT NAVIGATOR

The **patient navigator** is a formally designated role that guides patients through and around barriers to help ensure timely diagnosis, treatment, and follow-up to improve health outcomes. The navigator is usually associated with a specific disease or process such as cancer or diabetes or organ transplantation. Other titles are care coordinator, health coach, and case manager. These positions are growing rapidly with the initiation of the **Patient Centered Medical Home** (PCMH) certification, a primary care model designed to improve health by delivering services that are

- Comprehensive (address all modalities within and without the practice)
- Coordinated (facilitate all needed referrals and follow-ups)
- Oriented toward the whole person (address issues impeding health such as food availability and other needed community resources)
- Accessible around the clock (a member of the health care is readily available 24/7)
- Quality and safety-driven (outcomes are measured, addressed, and followed)

TERMS

PATIENT EDUCATION REVIEW

The following list reviews the terms discussed in this chapter and **other important terms that you may see on the exam.**

affective relating to a person's values, attitudes, opinions; a domain of learning

cognitive relating to knowledge and understanding; a domain of learning

domains of learning areas of a person's being that affect learning; the three domains are cognitive (knowledge, comprehension), affective (values, attitudes, opinions), and psychomotor (mental and physical abilities, sensory skills)

motivation a circumstance or a tangible item that drives a person into action

multidisciplinary a team approach involving different fields of knowledge and expertise

National Commission for Quality Assurance (NCQA) a national accrediting body for health-care organizations

noncompliant failure or refusal to comply or do something as asked

patient advocate a person who helps a patient to seek information and resources and to help to resolve issues with the health-care system

Patient Centered Medical Home (PCMH) a primary care model and certification delivering comprehensive, coordinated, always accessible quality care to the whole person

patient educational plan a design to provide education to a patient on a specific topic

patient navigator guides patients through and around barriers to help ensure timely diagnosis, treatment, and follow-up to improve health outcomes

psychomotor relating to a person's physical and mental capabilities and sensory skills; a domain of learning

The Joint Commission (TJC) formerly the Joint Commission on the Accreditation of Healthcare Organizations or JCAHO a national accrediting body for health-care organizations

REVIEW QUESTIONS

All questions are relevant for all medical assisting and medical administrative certification exams.

1. The process of acquiring information from a patient to determine health-care needs and abilities is called:
   A. assessment.
   B. evaluation.
   C. documentation.
   D. planning.

   Answer: **A**
   Why: Assessment is the gathering or acquiring of information. Evaluation is the process that indicates how well a patient is adapting or progressing. Documentation is the writing or recording of a patient's needs and progress and the physician's evaluation notes. Planning is the using of this information to fulfill the patient's needs.
   Review: Yes ○   No ○

2. Properly written patient educational materials should:
   A. include paragraphs rather than outlined information.
   B. always include charts or diagrams.
   C. include medical terms and phrases.
   D. focus on key points.
   E. be lengthy.

   Answer: **D**
   Why: Narrative paragraphs are usually not as easy to read or comprehend as outlined materials. Charts and diagrams are very valuable in the education process because they are visual but are not *always* appropriate. Medical terms and phrases usually confuse the layperson not familiar with medical language. Patient information materials should not be lengthy but should only include necessary information. Presenting information in the simplest way possible will help ensure the patient understands it.
   Review: Yes ○   No ○

3. The best way to reinforce verbal instructions for a patient is to:
   A. explain the directions using pronounced body language.
   B. provide the patient with written instructions.
   C. reassure the patient using constant therapeutic touch.
   D. ask the patient to call you in a couple of days to see if there are any questions.

   Answer: **B**
   Why: Before leaving the office, it is best if the patient has written instructions that will act as a reminder. This is the best way to reinforce what has been discussed with the patient.
   Review: Yes ○   No ○

4. As the best way to document that a patient received written instructions to take home, you should:
   A. have the receptionist file a note in the patient's chart.
   B. write an entry in the patient's chart stating that the patient received the materials.
   C. have the patient sign a document, to be placed in the patient's chart, verifying receipt of the materials.
   D. have the patient answer questions about the materials to see if he or she read the information.
   E. conduct a follow-up phone call to the patient.

   Answer: **C**
   Why: Placing a note or entry in a patient's chart or having a patient answer questions does not provide documented proof that the patient received educational materials. If the patient signs a document for the file verifying receipt of the materials, there is definite documentation that the event happened.
   Review: Yes ○   No ○

5. An environment conducive to learning is characterized by:
   A. privacy.
   B. music.
   C. noise.
   D. activity.

Answer: **A**

Why: An environment that is conducive to learning is quiet, free of interruptions, and private. A patient is more likely to concentrate on the information you are providing in this kind of place than in one that is noisy and full of activity.

Review: Yes ○   No ○

---

6. When evaluating a patient's progress in a patient educational program, if you discover noncompliance, this means that the patient is:
   A. following the instructions exactly as they were provided.
   B. not progressing as quickly as expected.
   C. not following prescribed orders.
   D. having a reaction to prescribed medication.
   E. progressing quickly and healing properly.

Answer: **C**

Why: Noncompliance means that the patient is not following prescribed orders. A compliant patient follows instructions exactly as they were provided. Not all patients progress at the same rate, even given the same treatment plan. Some have quick results, whereas in others, it may take longer to notice change or progress in their health. If a patient is having a reaction to a medication, this implies compliance. Because the drug does not agree with the patient, this is a case of incompatibility.

Review: Yes ○   No ○

---

7. When developing written patient educational materials, it is most important to consider:
   A. the patient's cognitive level of understanding.
   B. the patient's gender.
   C. incorporating more complex medical terminology in the information.
   D. including as many topics as possible in the same written brochure to avoid questions.

Answer: **A**

Why: The cognitive level of understanding means the level at which a person is knowledgeable or comprehends information. It is important to develop patient educational materials at a basic level the reader can understand. It is not necessarily important to consider the patient's gender when developing written patient educational materials. Using complex language or placing too many diverse topics in one document may be confusing for the patient.

Review: Yes ○   No ○

---

8. To provide patient education for a patient who is blind, which of the following formats of training materials would be most helpful?
   A. Posters
   B. DVDs
   C. Braille materials
   D. Pamphlets and brochures
   E. Internet websites

Answer: **C**

Why: Braille is a form of writing that blind people usually can understand. It is a writing system that uses raised dots to represent each letter of the alphabet. The other materials listed are not options for use in training someone who is blind.

Review: Yes ○   No ○

---

9. A team approach to patient education that includes different fields of knowledge and expertise is referred to as a(n):
   A. joint venture.
   B. multidisciplinary plan.
   C. quality assurance.
   D. accommodation.

Answer: **B**

Why: Multidisciplinary means that people from different areas of specialty or knowledge are involved together to assist patients in education. The front and back office personnel work together with other trained professionals to provide the specific information necessary to educate the patient.

Review: Yes ○   No ○

10. The first step in development of a patient educational program is to:
   A. document the educational plan in the patient's chart.
   B. identify the purpose and topic of the educational program.
   C. elicit patient feedback for documentation.
   D. evaluate effectiveness of the educational plan.
   E. decide the format for the materials to be developed.

Answer: **B**
Why: To design an appropriate patient educational program, you must first establish the reason or purpose of the educational program. This is the main objective of the education. You cannot gather feedback or document in the patient's chart unless you first know what the educational program is. Evaluating the effectiveness is also not possible until the program has been implemented. The format for the materials should be selected after the purpose has been established.
Review: Yes ○   No ○

11. When asked to provide dietary information for a patient, an organization that could provide the most valuable materials is the:
   A. Centers for Disease Control and Prevention.
   B. American Academy of Family Physicians.
   C. National Dairy Council.
   D. American Lung Association.

Answer: **C**
Why: The National Dairy Council is the organization that developed a nutritional guide that complements MyPyramid, the guide to basic nutrition and food group categories. The other organizations specialize in other areas of health.
Review: Yes ○   No ○

12. Patient educational materials are best implemented when the:
   A. patient is sent packets of materials in the mail.
   B. physician tells the patient to contact a professional organization to answer questions about the materials.
   C. patient is given the materials as he or she exits the office.
   D. patient's family is not involved.
   E. materials are discussed with the patient.

Answer: **E**
Why: If a patient is simply handed materials or is sent materials in the mail without any discussion or opportunity to ask questions, there is no assurance that the patient understands the information. Therefore, it is best to discuss the materials with the patient and answer any questions before the patient leaves the office.
Review: Yes ○   No ○

13. A national accrediting body for health-care organizations that has established standards and requirements for patient education is the:
   A. CDC.
   B. AMA.
   C. FDA.
   D. NCQA.

Answer: **D**
Why: The NCQA (National Committee for Quality Assurance) is a national organization that establishes standards for practice in health-care facilities. Among these standards are requirements for informing and educating patients on health-care issues. The CDC is the Centers for Disease Control and Prevention, the AMA is the American Medical Association, and the FDA is the Food and Drug Administration.
Review: Yes ○   No ○

14. The cognitive domain of learning refers to:
    A. attitude.
    B. physical abilities.
    C. sensory skills.
    D. opinions.
    E. comprehension.

Answer: **E**
Why: Cognitive refers to having knowledge or comprehending information. Mental and physical abilities and sensory skills are types of psychomotor learning. Attitudes and opinions are factors of affective learning.
Review: Yes ○   No ○

---

15. The process used to carry out the agreed teaching plan in patient education is called:
    A. assessment.
    B. evaluation.
    C. implementation.
    D. documentation.

Answer: **C**
Why: Implementation means carrying out or providing the means for accomplishing. Assessment, evaluation, and documentation are other processes necessary in the patient education process.
Review: Yes ○   No ○

---

16. The overall purpose of patient education is to:
    A. meet with patients one on one.
    B. improve patient health.
    C. provide excessive information.
    D. involve patients in community activities.
    E. comply with accrediting agencies.

Answer: **B**
Why: Patients who are better informed about their health are more likely to comply with the physician's treatment plan. This ultimately will help prevent disease and promote improvement in the patient's health.
Review: Yes ○   No ○

---

17. A patient who needs information about drug addiction could receive education and help from an organization that specializes in:
    A. prescription medications.
    B. preventive health.
    C. substance abuse.
    D. nutrition management.

Answer: **C**
Why: Substance abuse refers to excessive use of and dependency on legal or illegal drugs. This could include prescription drugs or illegal "street" drugs. Alcohol is also categorized as a substance that is frequently abused.
Review: Yes ○   No ○

---

18. If a diabetic patient is reluctant to learn how to give himself or herself insulin injections, the first thing you should do is:
    A. notify the patient's physician for further assistance.
    B. recommend that the patient see an endocrinologist.
    C. ask the patient to return to the office only when ready to comply with the instruction.
    D. refer the patient to a diabetic support group or a social worker who specializes in diabetes.
    E. volunteer to give the patient the injections.

Answer: **A**
Why: You must only perform duties under the direct supervision of the physician and should always inform the physician of the problem with the patient. It is the physician who is responsible for determining what the next step will be in this patient's care. The physician may actually refer the patient to another person who specializes in this type of problem. You should never go beyond the level of patient education approved by the physician.
Review: Yes ○   No ○

19. Of the following, which patient is the least likely to respond to learning objectives?

A. A patient who has reached the level of esteem and self-respect on Maslow's hierarchy of needs

B. A patient who perceives the information as important to his or her health

C. A patient who perceives the health-care team as condescending

D. A patient who has the same culture and ethnic background that you have

Answer: **C**

Why: The word **condescending** means "regarding another as being lower in status or knowledge than you." This attitude will discourage the patient from working with you. All the other answers are a positive indication that the patient will be receptive to the education or instruction. It is especially helpful if the medical assistant and the patient come from the same cultural and ethnic background. It gives them something in common.

Review: Yes ○   No ○

20. Of the following, which is very important for the person who is performing patient education?

A. Producing patient brochures

B. Using technical words when instructing

C. Documenting in the patient record whatever teaching is performed

D. Learning other languages to facilitate job performance

E. Assuring the patient considers you his or her friend.

Answer: **C**

Why: Although all of the answers might be helpful, if documentation does not occur, it is as if nothing happened. Documenting events is an important task to properly monitor and evaluate the progress of the patient. C is the best answer.

Review: Yes ○   No ○

21. One of the factors that is the most helpful in promoting patient learning is:

A. the height and weight of the patient.

B. the patient's gender.

C. a positive emotional outlook.

D. the patient's insurance company.

Answer: **C**

Why: The patient's height, weight, gender (sex), and insurance company usually have no effect on the patient's learning. If the patient has a positive emotional outlook, more than likely, he or she will also approach the patient education as a positive event.

Review: Yes ○   No ○

22. To ensure that a patient follows up with appointments for evaluation of the prescribed plan of treatment, you should:

A. assign a project or homework for the patient to complete between appointments.

B. ask the patient to call the office to schedule a follow-up appointment when it is convenient.

C. provide the patient with a written appointment slip with the date and time of his or her next session.

D. call the patient a week in advance to confirm the appointment.

E. have the physician contact the patient if the appointment is missed.

Answer: **C**

Why: It is always best to provide the patient with something in writing as a reminder. Asking the patient to call the office or even calling a couple of days in advance is not as effective as handing the patient a written appointment slip before he or she leaves the office. It may be considered a form of homework to ask the patient to keep a journal of progress to report on during return visits. It is not appropriate to have the physician contact a patient because of a missed appointment.

Review: Yes ○   No ○

23. A way to evaluate the patient's understanding of educational information is to:
   A. document in the patient's medical record that he or she received the materials.
   B. design a colorful brochure.
   C. ask for feedback from the patient.
   D. assess the patient's individual needs and abilities.

Answer: **C**

Why: To find out if the patient understands the information, ask for feedback. Documenting receipt of the materials does not ensure the patient understands them. Designing a brochure and assessing the patient's needs are done before the evaluation process.
Review: Yes ○   No ○

24. When providing patient education, you should:
   A. encourage questions from the patient.
   B. use only written materials for training.
   C. discuss training materials with the patient in the hallway so you do not occupy an exam room when the physician needs to use it.
   D. use the same method of training with all patients for consistency.
   E. present the materials at a level much higher than the patient's cognitive level.

Answer: **A**

Why: You should encourage the patient to ask any questions about the educational materials. Using only written materials may not be appropriate for all patients. You should always discuss training materials in a private exam room to maintain the patient's confidentiality. Varying the type of presentation is needed to accommodate different patients. It is important to understand the patient's level of comprehension so the training is meaningful for the patient.
Review: Yes ○   No ○

25. One factor that is a positive contribution to the patient's learning process is:
   A. just keeping quiet and only listening.
   B. maintaining noncompliance to directions or instructions.
   C. having family support.
   D. possessing a know-it-all attitude.

Answer: **C**

Why: A patient who has a good support system from his or her family will probably take the learning more seriously and have better progress with his or her health needs. If the patient is quiet and does not ask questions, learning may be hindered. Noncompliance means the patient does not do what is asked. A know-it-all attitude may cause the patient not to listen to instructions and then not know what he or she is to do later.
Review: Yes ○   No ○

26. The patient's mental and physical abilities are referred to as:
   A. psychosomatic.
   B. psychomotor.
   C. psychological.
   D. psychosocial.
   E. psychiatric.

Answer: **B**

Why: Psycho- refers to mind or mental capacity. *Motor* refers to a person's ability to perform physical functions such as body movement.
Review: Yes ○   No ○

27. The domain of learning that includes values, attitudes, and opinions is referred to as:
   A. cognitive.
   B. congenital.
   C. aberrant.
   D. affective.

Answer: **D**

Why: Cognitive refers to knowledge and comprehension. Congenital means born with, and aberrant means wandering from the norm.
Review: Yes ○   No ○

CRITICAL THINKING CASE REVIEW

Mr. Smith was diagnosed with type 1 diabetes. Dr. Chang's medical assistant, medical administrative assistant, and diabetic educator spent a great deal of time working with Mr. Smith on complications of diabetes, appropriate diet, how to test his blood sugar, administration of insulin, and the importance of keeping follow-up appointments that were scheduled.

1. The approach of using more than one team member for the patient education plan is known as:
   A. team approach.
   B. feedback.
   C. TJC compliant.
   D. multidisciplinary.
   E. domains of learning.

   Answer: **D**
   Why: Multidisciplinary refers to a team approach involving different fields of knowledge and expertise. Team approach is a correct answer but not the best answer. Feedback is a method of assuring the patient's understanding of the plan. TJC does require a multidisciplinary team, but that is not the best answer to the question; "domains of learning" refers to areas of a person's being that affect his or her capacity to learn.
   Review: Yes ○   No ○

2. Mr. Smith was shown how to administer insulin. To assure his understanding, the best strategy would be to ask:
   A. if he has any questions.
   B. for feedback.
   C. for a return demonstration.
   D. if a family member would also learn.

   Answer: **C**
   Why: While all other answers are correct; when it comes to performing a "hands on" procedure, a return demonstration is the most accurate method for assuring accurate knowledge.

3. Before leaving the office, the CMAS:
   A. advised Mr. Smith to call for a follow-up appointment.
   B. instructed Mr. Smith to call only for problems.
   C. told Mr. Smith the office would make a follow-up call.
   D. made a follow-up appointment for Mr. Smith.
   E. gave Mr. Smith a pamphlet on diabetes.

   Answer: **D**
   Why: With chronic illness to help maintain and restore health and to prevent further illness, follow-up care is essential. It is not appropriate or efficient to wait for the patient to make a follow-up appointment after he leaves the office or to call *only* for problems. While informing a patient of follow-up calls the follow-up appointment is the best answer. Giving Mr. Smith a pamphlet should have been done during the teaching to allow opportunities for questions or any clarification.

4. Mr. Smith would need a glucose monitor and reagent strips, syringes, and insulin; instructions on how to obtain these materials is:
   A. an important part of patient education.
   B. not included as part of patient education.
   C. the sole responsibility of the patient to work with his insurance company.
   D. to have the medical practice supply them.

   Answer: **A**
   Why: If the patient does not know how or where to obtain the materials prescribed by the doctor, the patient cannot be compliant. In many cases, the medical office must also work with the patient's insurance for approval and contracted vendors. The medical office is not responsible nor is it feasible to be a supplier.

5. After missing several scheduled appointments and many issues with care plan noncompliance by Mr. Smith, Dr. Chang instructed the medical assistant to terminate the patient from the practice. This requires:

A. an attorney.
B. notification ending the relationship and a period of time for the patient to obtain another care giver.
C. full HIPAA disclosure to the patient and his insurance carrier.
D. the office to locate another health-care provider for the patient.
E. Mr. Smith to agree to no longer being Dr. Chang's patient.

Answer: **B**

Why: The patient should be notified using a reliable method that the office will no longer see him after a certain date and advise him to find another health-care provider prior to that date. If this is not done, it may be considered patient abandonment (refer to Chapter 4, Law and Ethics). An attorney is not necessary; HIPAA disclosure should be done when the person first becomes a patient. It is not required for the current health-care provider to find the patient a new doctor or for the patient to agree to the termination.

Administrative Practice

Administrative Practice

Administrative Technologies

Review Tip:

Complete the chapters on communication (Chapter 7) and patient education (Chapter 8) before beginning this chapter. Many of the principles discussed in those chapters also apply to administrative techniques. This chapter lends itself to lunchtime reading and other "learning moments." Carry the review book with you and open it when you have a free moment.

Chapter 1 explained that this is a review book, not a text for primary learning. Many textbooks describe the telephone with its features (e.g., hold and transfer buttons), explain how to place long-distance calls, identify time zones, and discuss other operational functions. Although these areas are necessary for you to know in practice, they have a very low probability of appearing on the national exams. The information included in this chapter has "exam probability."

TELEPHONES

Despite the increasing use of advanced technology, the telephone remains the number one technologic method for patients and health-care providers to communicate with each other. The use of specific skills and guidelines helps ensure that telephone communication is effective.

TELEPHONE VOICE QUALITIES

- Enunciation—speak clearly
- Pronunciation—say words correctly

- Volume—use normal voice level
- Speed—use normal rate of conversation
- Inflection—change voice pitch to avoid a monotonous tone that implies boredom
- Facial expression—put a "smile" in your voice by having a pleasant look on your face while speaking, even though the caller cannot see you
- Courtesy—speak politely, without irritation or impatience
- Attention—focus on the caller and listen

MEDICAL OFFICE CALLS

- Attempt to answer by the third ring
- Use standard office greeting
  - Greet caller (e.g., "Good morning")
  - Provide name of facility
  - State your name
  - Inquire "How may I help you?"
- Use standard closing
  - Thank the patient for calling
  - Allow caller to hang up first
- Direct multiple incoming calls
  - Obtain permission of the first caller to be placed on hold. Explain that you have another incoming call. Allow time for the patient to respond before placing him or her on hold
  - Ask the second caller to wait; allow time for response before placing him or her on hold
  - Attempt to respond to callers within 30 seconds
  - Provide options if the hold will be longer
  - Thank the caller for waiting
- Screen calls
  - Know who and where to refer patients for appropriate assistance
  - Manage physician's time by referring necessary calls only and taking messages for other calls
- Route calls
  - Tell caller to whom you are forwarding the call
  - Provide the forwarding phone number to which you are transferring the call in case of disconnection
  - Inform the patient that if the party does not respond, the patient may leave a voice mail message (if available). Suggest the patient include a time when he or she is available for a return call
- Know the office policy regarding calls that should be directed to the physician
  - Forward calls from other physicians, hospital staff, and patients to whom the physician indicated

he or she would like to speak directly (e.g., close colleagues)
  - Provide the patient's medical record (chart or file) for the physician when transferring a call or leaving a message if he or she does not have access to the EMR
  - Assure a patient who insists on speaking only to the physician, when the physician is unavailable, that the physician will return the call; if possible, provide a time range during which the call will be returned
  - Inform callers who will not identify themselves that you need their name and number to have the physician return the call
- Record message
  - Use carbonized message pad, e-mail (more information later in chapter), or other methods that allow the message to be forwarded but saved
  - Maintain a copy of the message in the patient's medical record if that is office policy
  - Record the caller's name (confirm spelling), date, time, reason for call, phone number of caller, and convenient time to return call
  - Inform the caller who will return the call and give an approximate time the call will be returned
  - Initial and forward the message to the appropriate person with the patient's medical record, if needed
- Deal with emergencies
  - Notify the physician immediately
  - Activate the emergency medical system (EMS/911); if telephone system allows, keep the caller on one line while you notify 911
  - Instruct caller to hang up and activate EMS himself or herself, if the office phone system does not have at least two lines
  - Provide EMS or emergency facility with information, including advance directives and other important details
  - Follow up with the emergency facility
- Manage difficult callers
  - Keep your voice at a normal level and remain calm with angry callers
  - Determine the problem and notify appropriate staff to help the patient
  - Follow up to ensure the problem was addressed
  - Ensure that the physician or the administrator is aware of irate callers or callers with unresolved problems
  - Attempt to obtain identity of threatening callers and notify the physician or the administrator immediately

TEXTING

Texting or text messaging is an electronic communication sent from one cellular phone to another by typing words, often in a shortened form. Some practices use texting to

- Confirm appointments
- Remind patients of the need for preventive services
- Send simple messages such as confirming that a prescription has been sent
- Communicate with the hearing-impaired for select matters

The patient's consent should be obtained prior to using text messaging and abbreviations or shortened words should be avoided.

CALL CENTERS

Many large practices with multiple sites utilize *call centers* to screen and route calls and, in some cases, to make appointments. A call center is a centralized office used for the purpose of receiving or transmitting a large volume of requests by telephone. Some offices will use a call center for after-hours answering services.

SCOPE OF PRACTICE AND CALLS

All health-care providers *must* stay within the scope of practice for their role. The same principles apply to the phone as with other communication technologies. Remember, only the physician or mid-level provider diagnoses, provides medical advice, or says anything that may be construed as such. The following are telephone calls that a nonphysician may handle if he or she is the designated person in that office:

- Appointments (scheduling, rescheduling, canceling, reminding, recalling)
- Patient financial statements, insurance, fees, and service questions
- Prescription refills verified by the physician
- Diagnostic testing and other procedural preparations as written
- Satisfactory test results if reviewed and approved by physician following Health Insurance Portability and Accountability Act (HIPAA) guidelines
- Routine and satisfactory progress reports from patient if office policy allows
- Reinforcement of patient educational plan
- General information regarding office policies, locations, or appointment preparation
- Schedule procedures at other facilities

- Record diagnostic and other procedural results telephoned from health-care facilities (within the continuity of care or with patient consent)
- Activate answering service
- Retrieve messages from answering service or voice mail

Telephone Confidentiality

The HIPAA confidentiality standards, expected in all health-care activities, also apply to the telephone.

- Give information only to authorized persons (*Note:* Spouses, friends, parents of adults, or adult children of patients are not generally authorized unless specifically approved by the patient in writing.)
- Verify that you are giving information to an authorized person (e.g., the patient's insurance carrier)
- Ensure telephone conversations are not overheard or that messages are not seen by unauthorized persons
- Avoid discussing telephone conversations except in carrying out medical assisting duties with authorized persons
- Avoid leaving information on the patient's voice mail; only state the name of the office and the phone number. Ask the patient to return the call, and leave the name of the party he or she should request

OTHER TECHNOLOGIC DEVICES

In addition to the telephone, you will use other technologic devices. It is your responsibility to keep up with advances. At this book's press time, the national exams contained basic questions on the components of the computer and issues related to facsimiles (faxes) and the electronic health record (Chapter 11: Medical Records Management). The exams will continue to incorporate old and new technologies.

COMPUTERS

The *computer* is an electronic device programmed to take in, store, retrieve, and process data (Fig. 9-1).

- Hardware—the central processing unit (CPU), motherboard, hard drive, disk drive, keyboard, and monitor of the computer
  - Motherboard—the fiberglass plank of the computer that contains the CPU, memory, and other circuitry
    - Central processing unit (CPU)—circuit on a microchip that processes data; microprocessor

FIGURE 9-1 Basic components of a computer.

FIGURE 9-2 Compact discs and USB drives.

- ○ Random access memory (RAM)—main memory bank of a computer located on the motherboard; the more RAM the computer has, the more data and the faster the data manipulation; memory is measured in bytes (e.g., megabytes—one million bytes; gigabytes—one billion bytes)
  - Hard drive—a box containing the computer's programs and data files
  - Operating system (OS)—a collection of essential software that manages computer hardware providing instructions how to function; examples are Microsoft Windows and Apple (MAC)
  - Keyboard—a set of typewriter-like keys that plugs into the computer and allows input of data
  - Monitor—visual display terminal that allows data to be seen on a television-like screen
  - Disk drive—a device that allows information to be accessed from a compact disc (CD)
- ■ Accessories
  - Mouse—a device that plugs into the computer and allows the user to control the cursor (pointer) as viewed on the monitor
  - Modem—a device connecting the computer to a telephone line and allowing data to be transmitted over telephone wires
- ■ Software—computer programs that tell the computer what to do
- ■ Disks—magnetic disks that can be inserted in the disk drive; they allow for storage of data outside the computer and for transmission of data into and out of the computer

- ■ Compact disc (CD)—a disc that can be inserted into a CD-ROM (compact disc read-only memory) drive and read by a laser beam, allowing storage of data, including audio and visual programs, outside the computer and transmission of the data into and out of the computer (Fig. 9-2)
- ■ ZIP drive—a drive that allows several megabytes of data to be saved to a special disk; can be internal or external to the computer
- ■ Digital video disk (DVD)—a high-density optical disk, the contents of which can be displayed on a computer or television screen
- ■ USB (universal serial bus) drive—small, lightweight, removable data storage device; also called *USB stick*, *USB key*, *memory stick*, flash drive, or *thumb drive* (Fig. 9-2)

Common File Formats

A file format is a mechanism used by the computer to save and retrieve specific computer information, such as text or photographs.

- ■ DOC—document files (DOCX is a more current version, but the general recommendation is to save files in DOC for ease of opening from all senders)
- ■ GIF—graphics interchange format
- ■ JPEG—joint photographic experts group
- ■ RTF—rich text file
- ■ PDF—portable data format

Common Computer Networks

A computer network is the ability of two or more computers to communicate.

- ■ LAN (local area network)—a router is used to connect computers, generally of a single organization and all its sites

- WAN (wide area network)—using telephone systems, coaxial cables, or satellites, connects the computers of a geographic area; the Internet, which contains the World Wide Web (www), is the largest example of a WAN

Other Common Computer Terms

- **Blog**—a type of website, generally maintained by an individual who posts regular commentary or other material such as graphics or video
- **Social network**—a group of people interconnected by the Web for the purpose of interacting on a specific topic or multiple topics of common interest such as Facebook and Twitter
- **HTML** (hypertext markup language)—the language used to transfer documents on the Internet
- **HTTP** (hypertext transfer protocol)—how messages are formatted and sent over the Internet
- **Browser**—software that locates and displays Web pages on the computer; an example is Internet Explorer
- **Search engine**—an extensive program allowing searches for information and websites by using key words; examples are Yahoo and Google
- **Spreadsheet**—values arranged in columns and rows that may be electronically manipulated using formulas or other processes
- **URL** (uniform resource locator)—identifies the global address and domain to access Web pages
- **Website**—a collection of screens with text, images, videos, or other digital information with a common domain
- **Word processing**—one of the most common computer applications used to create, edit, and produce text documents

Common Computer Uses in the Medical Office

The uses of computers in the medical office continue to grow. The following are the more common applications.

- Appointment and procedure scheduling
- Patient statements
- Day sheets
- Financial ledgers
- Requisitions
- Payroll and other personnel functions
- Reports
- Correspondence
- Online patient registration
- Electronic medical records
- Insurance billing, coding, and claims
- Research using the Internet
- Digital imaging
- Patient educational materials
- Patient reminder and recall notifications
- Staff training
- Staff messaging (such as e-mail)
- Inventories
- Electronically operated patient tests and procedures
- Transmission of physician orders and prescriptions
- Transmission of diagnostic test results such as laboratory work and medical imaging
- Website information regarding the practice

Computers and Confidentiality

The health-care standards for confidentiality and release of patient information also apply to computers (Fig. 9-3). Computer-specific requirements and guidelines have come about through standard practice or HIPAA. One of the significant components of HIPAA is the filing of Medicare claims through a secure electronic database exchange. To ensure compliance

- Require authorized persons to use an exclusive "electronic signature" or password to view patient records
- Change passwords frequently
- Ensure computer screens are not in view of unauthorized persons
- Turn off computers when not in use
- Install privacy filters on monitors to prevent passersby from seeing the screen
- Protect computers from illegal access with appropriate security devices such as firewalls
- Shred confidential copied materials when no longer in use

MEDICAL TRANSCRIPTION AND EQUIPMENT

Transcription is basically a written copy of dictated or recorded information. With electronic health records, the use of transcription is decreasing. Although generally done by a person specifically trained in this field, medical transcription may be the duty of the medical assistant or the medical administrative specialist. Common information transcribed for the medical office is:

- Patient history and physicals
- Hospital admission and discharge notes
- Surgery and other procedural reports
- Consultations
- Correspondence

FIGURE 9-3 HIPAA standards also apply to computers.

The equipment used includes the following:

- Transcription machine with earpieces and foot pedals
- CDs or audiocassettes
- Computer and monitor
- Keyboard
- Specific software (e.g., medical terminology spell-check, pharmacology reference)

The important standard for medical transcription is if a word or phrase is not clear, *never* guess. Always go back to the person who dictated the information for clarification. Correct spelling is absolutely necessary to avoid incorrect information that can be harmful to the patient.

Other Common Electronic Devices

Many of the electronic devices allow remote communication and telecommuting with the medical office. HIPAA applies to all devices and communications. Extreme caution should be taken, especially in public places, not to inadvertently divulge information that might identify a patient.

- Facsimile machine (fax)—an electronic machine that sends copies of documents over telephone wires (fax confidential information only to secured areas; fax cover sheets should include a confidentiality statement)
- Scanner—software-required device that reads documents (text, graphics, photos) and transfers the image to the computer

- Automated routing unit (ARU)—programmable device that answers calls and plays prerecorded telephone messages to prompt a caller to choose options based on needs; the ARU automatically directs the caller to the chosen option; some ARUs are programmed to telephone patients and leave appointment reminders or other messages (these messages should not be left without patient consent)
- Electronic mail (e-mail)—a system of communicating messages, images, and sounds via a computer-type device through the Internet; e-mails should not be sent to patients without their consent. Since e-mails may be accessed from remote sites on unsecured devices, many practices have criteria what may be included related to patient identification and confidentiality.
- Cellular telephones (cell phones)—portable, wireless telephones; any type of personal cell phones should be in the silent mode and not used during working hours
- Smart phones—cellular phones that perform many of the functions of a computer, having an OS capable of running general-purpose applications that include medical resource e-books, access to e-mail, a search engine, and more
- Personal digital assistant (PDA)—a palm-sized, handheld, wireless computer that may be synchronized with other computers; an example is a PalmPilot; most have been replaced by the smart phone

- Electronic tablet (tablet)—a mobile computer with self-contained circuitry components and battery in a single unit, including cameras, microphone, and touchscreen or stylus that replace the mouse and keyboard. Differs from the *laptop computer* in that it usually does not have full document- and presentation-preparation capabilities.

- Pagers—battery-operated devices that alert a person to a message left through a telephone or wireless source; pagers may also display other information, such as news bulletins

- Digital camera—a camera that uses a memory card instead of film, allowing pictures to be viewed, altered, or printed through a computer

TERMS

ADMINISTRATIVE TECHNOLOGIES REVIEW

The following list reviews the terms discussed in this chapter and other important terms that you may see on the exam.

automated routing unit (ARU) programmable device that answers calls and plays prerecorded telephone messages to prompt a caller to choose options based on needs; the ARU automatically directs the caller to the chosen option

blog a type of website, generally maintained by an individual who posts regular commentary or other material such as graphics or video

browser software that locates and displays Web pages on the computer; examples are Internet Explorer or Google Chrome

Byte the unit of measure for the memory in a computer

call center a centralized office used for the purpose of receiving or transmitting a large volume of requests by telephone

cellular telephones (cell phones) portable wireless telephones

central processing unit (CPU) a circuit on a microchip that processes data; a microprocessor

compact disc (CD) a disk that can be inserted into a CD-ROM drive and read by a laser beam, allowing storage of data, including audio and visual programs, outside the computer, and transmission of data into and out of the computer

compact disc read-only memory (CD-ROM) a computer drive that reads CDs using a laser beam

computer an electronic device that is programmed to take in, store, retrieve, and process data

diction the style of speaking and enunciating words

digital camera a camera that uses a memory card instead of film, allowing pictures to be viewed, altered, or printed through a computer

digital video disk (DVD) a high-density optical disk, the contents of which can be displayed on a computer or television screen

disk drive a device allowing information to be accessed from a disk

disks diskettes; magnetic disks that can be inserted in the disk drive; they allow storage of data outside the computer and transmission of data into and from the computer

electronic mail (e-mail) a system of communicating electronic messages, images, and sounds via the computer through the Internet

electronic tablet (tablet) a limited mobile computer with self-contained circuitry components and battery in a single unit; including cameras, microphone, and touchscreen or stylus that replace the mouse and keyboard.

enunciation speaking clearly

facsimile machine (fax) an electronic machine that can send copies of documents over telephone wires

hard drive a box containing the computer's programs and data files

hardware the central processing unit, motherboard, hard drive, disk drive, keyboard, monitor, and mouse of the computer

HTML (hypertext markup language) the language used to transfer documents on the Internet

HTTP (hypertext transfer protocol) how messages are formatted and sent over the Internet

inflection changing voice pitch to avoid a monotonous tone implying boredom

keyboard a set of typewriter-like keys that plugs into a computer and allows input of data

LAN (local area network) uses a router to connect computers, generally of a single organization and all its sites

modem a device connecting the computer to a telephone line and allowing data to be transmitted

monitor visual display terminal (VDT) that allows data to be seen on a television-like screen

motherboard the fiberglass plank of the computer that contains the central processing unit, memory, and other circuitry

mouse a device that plugs into the computer and allows the user to control the cursor viewed on the monitor

operating system (OS) a collection of essential software that manages computer hardware providing instructions how to function

pagers battery-operated devices that alert a person to a message left through a telephone or wireless source;

pagers may also display other information, such as news bulletins

personal digital assistant (PDA) a palm-sized, hand-held wireless computer that may be synchronized with other computers; an example is a PalmPilot

photocopy a duplicate copy of a written document

pronunciation saying words correctly

random access memory (RAM) main memory bank of a computer located on the motherboard

scanner software-required device that reads documents (text, graphics, photos) and transfers the image to the computer

scanning a process of transferring a written document or image into an electronic version using computer hardware called a scanner

search engine an extensive program allowing searches for information and websites by using key words; examples are Yahoo and Google

smart phones cellular phones that perform many of the functions of a computer, having an operating system capable of running general-purpose applications

social network a group of people interconnected by the Web for the purpose of interacting on a specific topic or multiple topics of common interest

software computer programs that tell the computer what to do related to that topic (e.g., word processing)

spreadsheet values arranged in columns and rows that may be electronically manipulated using formulas or other processes

texting or text messaging an electronic message sent from one cellular phone to another by typing words, often in a shortened form

transcription a written copy of dictated or recorded information

URL (uniform resource locator) identifies the global address and domain to access Web pages

USB (universal serial bus) drive small, lightweight, removable data storage device; also called USB stick, USB key, memory stick, flash drive, or thumb drive

WAN (wide area network) using telephone systems, coaxial cables, or satellites, connects the computers of a geographic area; the largest example of a WAN is the Internet

website a collection of screens with text, images, videos, or other digital information with a common domain

word processing one of the most common computer applications used to create, edit, and produce text documents

www (world wide web) the Internet

ZIP drive a drive that allows several megabytes of data to be saved to a special disk; can be internal or external to the computer

REVIEW QUESTIONS

All questions are relevant for all medical assisting and medical administrative certification exams.

1. When assigned to answering the telephone in a physician's office:
   A. some callers are angry and it is acceptable to hang up.
   B. you should be able to determine which calls are routine, nonemergent, or emergent situations.
   C. it is routine to give family members who call normal results of laboratory findings.
   D. when many phone calls are coming into the office at one time, it is appropriate to immediately put all calls on hold and then return to each one in the order received.

Answer: **B**

Why: Hanging up on an angry patient will likely exacerbate the problem. You should try to address the caller's concern or find someone who can. All calls coming into a physician's office should be answered promptly and first determined whether they are an emergency. Only after it is known that the call is not an emergency should you place the caller on hold. HIPAA and standards prohibit giving out medical information over the telephone unless under the direction of the physician and only to authorized individuals.

Review: Yes ○   No ○

2. The style of speaking and enunciating words is referred to as:
   A. diction.
   B. pronunciation.
   C. expression.
   D. conversation.
   E. inflection.

Answer: **A**

Why: Diction is the act of articulating words distinctly as you speak so that you are clearly understood. Pronunciation is the manner of pronouncing or speaking words using phonics (speech sounds that make up a language). Expression is the use of feeling or character when speaking to help convey the spoken word. Conversation is an exchange of words, ideas, or thoughts. Inflection means to change voice pitch to avoid a monotonous tone.

Review: Yes ○   No ○

3. When answering phones during a busy time of day, it is only appropriate to place a caller on hold after you ask the following:
   A. May I have your phone number so I can call you back?
   B. Will you please hold?
   C. Are you a regular patient at this office?
   D. We are busy now; will you call back later?

Answer: **B**

Why: It is appropriate to place a caller on hold only after you have asked the caller's permission to be placed on hold. If it is an emergency, the caller will usually state that he or she cannot hold and needs immediate attention.

Review: Yes ○   No ○

4. Which of the following is a phone call that ordinarily does not require the party to speak directly to the physician?

A. A pharmacist calls to verify information written on a prescription form.

B. A patient calls complaining of shortness of breath, sweating, and heart pounding after taking new medication.

C. A referring physician calls to relate information of an abnormal electrocardiogram on a patient.

D. A nurse from the local hospital emergency room calls for orders on a patient just admitted.

E. One of the physician's family members calls to talk with the physician about an emergency.

Answer: **A**

Why: You would refer to the prescription information written by the physician in the patient's medical record and communicate the information to the pharmacist. All the other responses would require intervention by the physician.

Review: Yes ○   No ○

5. The transmission of a hard copy of a written document through a phone line is called a(n):

A. electronic mail.

B. facsimile.

C. photocopy.

D. scan.

Answer: **B**

Why: The facsimile (usually shortened to *fax*) is an electronic machine that sends written images over telephone wires. Electronic mail is used in conjunction with the Internet via the computer. A photocopy is a duplicate copy of a written document. Scanning is a process of transferring a written document or image into an electronic version using computer hardware called a scanner.

Review: Yes ○   No ○

6. The primary purpose of screening telephone calls is to:

A. manage the physician's time by referring only necessary calls.

B. place patients on hold as soon as they contact the office.

C. decrease the number of telemarketing calls to the office.

D. intercept personal calls.

E. increase the physician's patient load.

Answer: **A**

Why: You will screen phone calls to determine which calls must be forwarded to the physician and which can be handled by you.

Review: Yes ○   No ○

7. The physician has asked you to contact a patient to schedule a return office visit to discuss laboratory results. The patient is not available when you call. It is appropriate to:

A. leave a message with the person answering the phone indicating that the patient should contact the office for laboratory results.

B. contact the patient's workplace to leave a message for the patient to contact the physician's office to go over some blood test results.

C. try to reach the patient later but also send a letter with the information.

D. call the person who is listed as the emergency contact on the patient's information sheet.

Answer: **C**

Why: If a patient cannot be reached by phone, it is not appropriate to leave a message regarding test results with anyone other than the patient. Because this is not an emergency situation, a letter can be sent to the patient—but you should also try to reach the patient by telephone later.

Review: Yes ○   No ○

8. When assigned to work in the reception area of the office, you should attempt to answer all incoming telephone calls:
   A. after assisting all other calls on hold.
   B. by the third ring.
   C. by the fourth ring.
   D. by the fifth ring.
   E. in between rooming patients.

Answer: **B**
Why: It is usually impossible to answer all phone calls on the first or even second ring. All efforts should be made to answer calls by the third ring.
Review: Yes ◯   No ◯

9. Which of the following is an appropriate standard opening for an incoming call to the physician's office?
   A. Will you please hold?
   B. Who's calling please?
   C. Good morning, Dr. Smith's office.
   D. 555-2456, may I help you?

Answer: **C**
Why: The first thing a caller should hear is a pleasant greeting and the name of the facility.
Review: Yes ◯   No ◯

10. When transferring a patient call to the physician, you should:
    A. interrupt the physician in an exam room to forward the information about the caller.
    B. not forward the call, but ask the caller to call back later when the physician is finished with all patients for the day.
    C. inform the patient that the physician will be upset if interrupted.
    D. inform the patient that there will be an office visit charge for the call.
    E. have the patient's medical record available for the physician if no EMR access.

Answer: **E**
Why: The physician will want to have the patient's medical record available in the event questions arise during the conversation that require information from the medical record. It is inappropriate to tell the patient the physician will be upset with the call, and you should not interrupt a physician while in an exam room unless the call is an emergency. Offices typically do not charge patients for phone calls.
Review: Yes ◯   No ◯

11. After a caller has been placed on hold, you should make every attempt to respond to the caller within:
    A. 10 seconds.
    B. 30 seconds.
    C. 1 minute.
    D. 5 minutes.

Answer: **B**
Why: If a caller needs to be placed on hold, it is recommended that you check back with the caller at least every 30 seconds. Even if you are still busy with another patient, at least the caller will be encouraged to continue holding.
Review: Yes ◯   No ◯

12. When dealing with a difficult caller, you should:
    A. forward the call to the physician.
    B. forward the call to the office manager.
    C. tell the caller you will hang up if he or she continues to be difficult.
    D. determine the problem and the appropriate staff member who can help the caller.
    E. put the caller on hold until he or she hangs up.

Answer: **D**
Why: When a caller is difficult to deal with, it will further exacerbate the situation if you also become angry or difficult. Keep your voice at a normal level and remain calm while you try to determine what the problem is and who can best help the caller.
Review: Yes ◯   No ◯

13. When a patient calls with a list of symptoms, including fever, chills, and body aches, that have lasted for the past several days, you should:
   A. offer the patient an appointment to see the physician.
   B. tell the patient to stay home in bed and to take aspirin and fluids.
   C. inform the patient that there is a lot of flu going around.
   D. tell the patient that the physician does not see patients unless they have been ill for at least a week and that it is probably a flulike illness that will pass.

Answer: **A**
Why: A patient with those symptoms may actually have the flu, but it is not within your scope of practice or responsibility to diagnose. The patient should be offered an appointment to see the physician to make an appropriate diagnosis.
Review: Yes ◯   No ◯

14. When placing calls to patients to confirm appointments, the calls should be made:
   A. the morning of the day of the appointments.
   B. only to patients who were not given appointment cards.
   C. one week before the appointment.
   D. only to those patients who you know missed their last appointment.
   E. in an area where you cannot be overheard by other patients.

Answer: **E**
Why: All patients should be contacted the day before their appointment, and the calls should be made from a place where other patients cannot overhear the call. Even if patients are given appointment cards, a reminder call is usually made.
Review: Yes ◯   No ◯

15. An electronic device that takes in, stores, retrieves, and processes data is a:
   A. disk drive.
   B. monitor.
   C. computer.
   D. operating system.

Answer: **C**
Why: A disk drive is a device located on the computer that allows information to be accessed from a disk or CD-ROM. A monitor is used to visually display the data, and the operating system is software providing instructions to the computer. The computer is the entire electronic device that takes in, stores, retrieves, and processes the data.
Review: Yes ◯   No ◯

16. A computer program that tells the computer what to do is the:
   A. disk drive.
   B. modem.
   C. software.
   D. mouse.
   E. keyboard.

Answer: **C**
Why: The disk drive is located on the computer and allows information to be accessed from a DVD or CD-ROM. A modem connects a computer to a telephone line and transmits data via that line. The mouse is the device that plugs into the computer and controls the cursor as viewed on the monitor. A keyboard is a set of typewriter-type keys that allows for input of data.
Review: Yes ◯   No ◯

17. The federal government enacted a standard practice for confidentiality and release of patient information as it applies to computers. This information is found in the federal register under the abbreviation:
    A. HCFA.
    B. HIPAA.
    C. HHS.
    D. HRSA.

Answer: **B**
Why: HIPAA stands for Health Insurability and Accountability Act, which is the name of the federal guidelines for confidentiality and release of patient information in all forms, including electronically. HCFA is the Health Care Financing Administration; HHS is the Department of Health and Human Services. HRSA is the Health Resources and Services Administration.
Review: Yes ◯   No ◯

18. When you are focusing on the conversation of the telephone call and ignoring outside distractions, you are:
    A. expressing yourself.
    B. actively listening.
    C. practicing diction.
    D. demonstrating time management.
    E. maintaining confidentiality.

Answer: **B**
Why: To actively listen to a conversation, you must not interrupt the speaker and you must ignore what is going on around you so that you can concentrate on the conversation.
Review: Yes ◯   No ◯

19. When routing a caller to another person, you should:
    A. forward the call immediately, not wasting time to talk to the caller.
    B. tell the caller you do not forward calls and ask the caller to call back when the person is available.
    C. place the caller on hold for up to 5 minutes while you locate the person to whom you need to transfer the caller.
    D. provide the phone number or extension to which you are transferring the caller, in case the call is disconnected.

Answer: **D**
Why: Before forwarding a call, you should inform the caller that you are going to forward the call and provide the phone number or extension in case the call is disconnected. If the person you need to forward the call to is unavailable, you can give the caller the option of calling back or leaving a message, but you would not tell the caller that you do not forward calls. You should not place a caller on hold for more than 30 seconds without checking in to see whether he or she is still willing to hold.
Review: Yes ◯   No ◯

20. To comply with the HIPAA requirements when using a computer, you should remember to do the following *except*:
    A. change passwords frequently.
    B. protect computers from illegal access with appropriate security devices.
    C. ensure computer screens are not in view of unauthorized persons.
    D. keep the computer on at all times to save time turning it on.
    E. turn off the computer when not in use.

Answer: **D**
Why: When not in use, the computer should be turned off. This will help maintain security of the computer and prevent illegal use or its being viewed by unauthorized persons.
Review: Yes ◯   No ◯

21. Which of the following is a necessary quality for a good telephone voice?
    A. Maintaining a monotonous tone
    B. Using a rapid rate of conversation
    C. Focusing on surrounding activity in the office while on the phone with a caller
    D. Speaking clearly and saying words correctly

Answer: **D**
Why: Proper telephone voice qualities include changing the pitch to avoid a monotone voice. Use a normal rate of conversation and actively listen to the caller without allowing the activity around you to interfere with your ability to concentrate on the conversation.
Review: Yes ◯   No ◯

22. When an unidentified caller insists on speaking with the physician, the medical assistant should:
A. hang up.
B. tell the caller that the physician is with a patient and you need a name and a number so the call can be returned.
C. put the caller on hold until he or she hangs up.
D. transfer the call immediately to the physician.
E. transfer the call to a coworker.

Answer: **B**
Why: Explain that the physician is not available to take the call but that you will forward the name and number so that the physician can return the call later. Most people will be willing to give their name and number if they know the physician will call them back.
Review: Yes ○   No ○

23. The proper way to deal with an emergency call is to:
A. ask the caller to hold while you call the local emergency room for instructions.
B. ask the caller to come to the office immediately.
C. keep the caller on the line while contacting the emergency medical system on another line if the office has multiple phone lines.
D. give the caller the number of the physician who is on call when his or her physician is not available.

Answer: **C**
Why: You would not want to waste time having the patient come to the office or contact the physician on call. In a true emergency, the patient should be instructed to activate 911/EMS (emergency medical system), or the physician's office should contact EMS for the patient, if possible.
Review: Yes ○   No ○

24. Telephone calls that the medical assistant or medical administrative specialist may handle include the following *except*:
A. refilling prescriptions verified by the physician.
B. providing a patient with laboratory test results just received from a lab.
C. scheduling procedures at other medical facilities.
D. answering patient financial statement questions.
E. confirming the time of an appointment for a patient.

Answer: **B**
Why: If the laboratory results were just received from the lab and have not been reviewed and approved for release by the physician, the medical assistant must not release the test results.
Review: Yes ○   No ○

25. To maintain telephone confidentiality, the medical medical office staff must:
A. give information only to authorized persons.
B. discuss telephone conversations anywhere in the office.
C. give information to the patient's employer if he or she contacts the office to inquire about the patient's absence from work.
D. give information to family members with or without authorization because of their relationship to the patient.

Answer: **A**
Why: The medical assistant or medical administrative specialist should only give patient information to those who are authorized to receive the information. This does not include the patient's employer or relatives unless the patient has given permission to release the information. Always discuss information in the office in an area where patients or unauthorized persons cannot hear the conversation.
Review: Yes ○   No ○

26. Which of the following is not a device used to save computer data?
    A. HTTP
    B. USB drive
    C. DVD
    D. ZIP
    E. CD-ROM

Answer: **A**
Why: HTTP (hypertext transfer protocol) is how messages are formatted and sent over the Internet. All of the other devices listed are devices used to save data.
Review: Yes ○   No ○

27. Yahoo is an example of an Internet:
    A. browser.
    B. search engine.
    C. LAN.
    D. CPU.

Answer: **B**
Why: A search engine is an extensive program allowing searches for information and websites by using key words. Yahoo is an example of an Internet search engine. A browser is software that locates and displays Web pages on the computer. LAN means local area network; CPU is a central processing unit; and a scanner is a device that reads documents (text, graphics, photos) and transfers the image to the computer.
Review: Yes ○   No ○

28. A patient history processed on the computer would most likely be saved in what type of file?
    A. RTF
    B. JPEG
    C. GIF
    D. DOC
    E. spreadsheet

Answer: **D**
Why: Word documents such as patient histories are most frequently saved in document files (DOC). Graphic images are saved in GIF format; photographic images are commonly saved in JPEG files. RTF, rich text file, can be used to save written documents; however, it is not commonly used.
Review: Yes ○   No ○
Note: This question is an example in which two answers are correct but one answer is a "better" choice or is more common. Your clue is the phrase "most likely." The exams will contain questions of this nature.

29. Equipment needed for medical transcription is a:
    A. copy machine.
    B. facsimile machine.
    C. telephone.
    D. computer.
    E. mouse.

Answer: **D**
Why: Transcription is a written copy of dictated or recorded information. A copy machine, facsimile machine, or telephone cannot transform oral information into a written format. The computer is the only instrument listed that can do this. This process can take place without the use of a mouse, although a mouse may be used minimally. The computer is the *best* answer.
Review: Yes ○   No ○

30. The correct spelling of heavy, uncontrolled bleeding is:
    A. hemmorrhage.
    B. hemorrhage.
    C. hemmorage.
    D. hemorhage.

Answer: **B**
Why: A medical terminology spell-check in use while performing medical transcription would indicate that choice B (hemorrhage) is the correct spelling.
Review: Yes ○   No ○

CRITICAL THINKING CASE REVIEW

Dr. Gerard has a very busy internal medicine practice that includes adult patients of all ages and cultures. The office has an excellent reputation in the medical and academic communities and precepts many health-care students, also, of all ages and cultures. Dr. Gerard has three sites.

1. Due to the many students, the practice encourages them to use their own technology as resources during their preceptorships. Appropriate use of personal electronic devices in a medical office would be to:
   A. access medical records.
   B. post assignments on Facebook.
   C. allow the student's children to call in an emergency.
   D. research a drug using Wikipedia.
   E. spell check a word using a medical terminology application.

Answer: **E**
Why: It is a violation of HIPAA to access private medical information on a nonsecured site or to post information for anyone not involved in the patient's care or on a nonsecured site such as Facebook. A student's electronic devices should not be on during work hours except when using them as directed by the practice. Children should be instructed to call the main number and inform the answerer who they are and that it is an emergency. Wikipedia is not considered a credible source for medical information. Using a medical terminology application for spell-check is extremely appropriate.
Review: Yes ○   No ○

2. One of Dr. Gerard's patients speaks only Farsi; there is no one on site fluent in the language. A reasonable alternative is to use:
   A. an Internet translation application such as Google.
   B. an electronic Farsi dictionary.
   C. a translator contracted through the telephone service.
   D. a student who is studying Farsi.

Answer: **C**
Why: Internet translation applications are only semireliable with single words which may have many meanings and unreliable with phrases, syllables, or concepts. The same applies with an electronic dictionary. Most facilities do not let staff (or students) translate unless they have gone through a translation certification process. The most reliable option is to use a contracted translation service through the telephone company (refer to Chapter 7: Human Behavior and Professional Communications)
Review: Yes ○   No ○

3. Due to the high volume of calls, Dr. Gerard finds it effective to answer telephones using:
   A. an ARU.
   B. three students.
   C. a CMAS and a student.
   D. a call center.
   E. a landline and cell phones.

Answer: **A**
Why: Most busy offices use an automated routing unit or ARU to direct callers. Call centers may be used but are more frequently used in conjunction with an ARU or for after-hours calls. Three students by themselves on busy lines is not an option conducive to learning or efficiency. A CMAS and a student is an option but not the best one given the practice has three sites.
Review: Yes ○   No ○

4. When orienting students, the practice emphasizes:
   A. answering the phone on the second ring.
   B. focusing on the caller.
   C. memorizing the script used for answering the phone.
   D. using e-mail to provide all the details of a patient call to the physician.

Answer: **B**
Why: It is not an expectation to answer the phone on the second ring. Nor is it expected to memorize a telephone script when it can be read. Since e-mails are not generally considered secure, most offices have criteria to include only minimal patient information. Focusing on the patient should be emphasized during every call.
Review: Yes ○   No ○

5. When speaking with a patient on the phone and listening to his problem, the student said, "That sounds like the flu." This statement is:
   A. probably true since a lot of flu was going around.
   B. possibly not accurate since many illnesses are similar.
   C. outside of the student's scope of practice.
   D. a method for establishing trust with the patient.

Answer: **C**
Why: Since the statement can be considered diagnosing, it is clearly outside of the student's scope of practice.
Review: Yes ○   No ○

CHAPTER 10

Appointment Scheduling and Reception

The goal of appointment scheduling is to maintain a smooth efficient office flow while accommodating the needs of the medical practice and the patient. The type of scheduling used depends on the following:

- Nature of practice
- Patient population needs
- Doctor's preferences and habits
- Available facilities and staff

TYPES OF SCHEDULING

Many practices have multiple sites and utilize call centers (figure 10.1), centralized-computer-program-driven scheduling, and even *patient portals* for automated scheduling. However, the exams will probably require you to identify the different standard scheduling modalities:

- Open hours (tidal wave, open booking)—no appointments needed; first-come, first-served
  - Used primarily in urgent care centers
  - Eliminates broken appointments

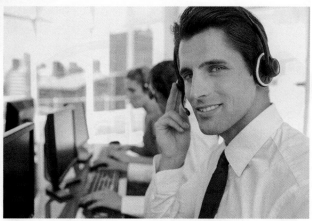

FIGURE 10-1 Appointments made through a call center.

- Limits medical records and procedures preparation
- Prohibits control of number of patients arriving at one time
- Requires triage system
■ Clustering (group procedures, categorizing)—similar procedures scheduled on predetermined days or in predetermined time blocks, such as new patient exams, sports physicals, and immunizations; they are designated when the appointment book **matrix** is developed
  - Increases efficiency and speed for procedures
  - Theoretically, allows better utilization of equipment and staff
■ Select scheduling (Box 10-1)
  - Double booking—two or more patients scheduled at the same time

- Used by practices with short visits or a high no-show rate
- Increases patient waiting time
- Reduces physician downtime
- Wave—a specific number of patients, usually four, scheduled at the beginning of the same hour
  - Allows specific procedures, such as a routine ECG, to be performed prior to the physician seeing the patient, reducing physician "downtime"
  - Intended to start and finish each hour on time allowing for up-to-date knowledge of patient flow
  - Increases waiting for patients seen later in the hour
  - Creates issues of who is seen first if more than one person arrives at the same time
- Modified wave—hour-long blocks broken down to smaller time increments (usually 10 or 15 minutes each) and individual patients scheduled within those increments
- Intended to start and finish each hour on time
  - Decreases patient waiting time compared with wave scheduling
  - Avoids issues of who should be seen first
- Time-specific (streaming)—patient given an appointment based on length of time needed and on available time; this is the most common scheduling method
■ Other scheduling considerations
  - Fasting patients—schedule their appointments as early in the morning as possible

---

BOX 10-1

Comparison of double booking, wave, modified wave, and time-specific schedules

Double Booking

9:00	Susan F. Garcia 602-1234 Ref
	John S. Habib 602-2345 S/R
9:15	Tony McCall 456-3456 CPE
	Jane P. Morgan 564-4567 CPE
9:30	Taylor Roberts 324-6789 Inj
	Michael Sanchez 324-7890 NP
9:45	Joseph Armat 567-1234 Ref
	Selena Green 765-7890 F/U

Wave

9:00	Susan F. Garcia 602-1234 Ref
	John S. Habib 602-2345 S/R
	Tony McCall 456-3456 CPE
	Jane P. Morgan 564-4567 CPE
10:00	Taylor Roberts 324-6789 Inj
	Michael Sanchez 324-7890 NP
	Joseph Armat 567-1234 Ref
	Selena Green 765-7890 F/U

Modified Wave

9:00	Susan F. Garcia 602-1234 Ref
9:15	John S. Habib 602-2345 S/R
9:30	Tony McCall 456-3456 CPE
9:45	Jane P. Morgan 564-4567 CPE
10:00	Taylor Roberts 324-6789 Inj
10:15	Michael Sanchez 324-7890 NP
10:30	Selena Green 765-7890 F/U

Time-Specific

9:00	Susan F. Garcia 602-1234 Ref.
9:15	John S. Habib 602-2345 S/R
9:30	Tony McCall 456-3456 CPE
9:45	⇓
10:00	Jane P. Morgan 564-4567 CPE
10:15	⇓
10:30	Taylor Roberts 324-6789 Inj

- Diabetic patients—determine what type of blood glucose testing will be done such as fasting or *postprandial* (after eating) and schedule accordingly; avoid scheduling close to a mealtime in case appointments are running late
- Physician or office delay—keep patients informed of waiting time; offer opportunity to reschedule or wait
- Time allotment for visits and procedures—established criteria indicate the time required for the common procedures and visits in a practice (e.g., a complete physical exam may be 45 minutes, suture removal may be 10 minutes); new patients are usually allotted more time than established patients
- Emergencies—office criteria and, often, algorithms for handling urgent medical situations in the office and on the telephone, including involvement of the emergency medical system and poison control centers
- "Walk-ins"—patients who come to the office without an appointment expecting to be seen; urgency and available appointment time should be considered
- Referrals—urgency of referrals should be communicated by the referring physician; appropriate medical records, including diagnostic results, should be sent to the consulting physician who will send a consultation report back to the referring physician
- Repeat appointments—schedule patients for a series of appointments (e.g., dressing changes, antibiotic administration) at the same time on the same day of the week, if possible; this reduces the incidence of missed appointments
- Flexible hours—varied hours on certain days; may include evenings and weekends
- Buffer zone—periods during the day with no appointments scheduled to accommodate emergencies and to allow the physician to catch up if running late
- Vendors—the norm has become to give vendors or sales representatives, such as with pharmaceutical companies, a designated appointment or to have a specific day or time of the day set aside for these visits
- Other visitors—attorneys and other nonmedical professionals may request to meet with the physician to function as expert witnesses or perform other consulting-type services; appointments are scheduled to accommodate the physician and the practice; these services are sometimes billed by time

EQUIPMENT AND MATERIALS

- ■ Appointment book—specially designed calendar-type book used to schedule appointments
  - Considered a legal document and can be subpoenaed
  - Remains open and conforms to desk or counter space size
  - Conforms to Health Insurance Portability and Accountability Act (HIPAA) privacy standards; not able to be seen by unauthorized people
  - Accommodates practice (e.g., it has an adequate number of lines for the number of physicians)
- ■ Daily log—separate from the appointment book; a ledger-type book listing the day's appointments and used for cross-referencing financial entries, data collection on types and number of procedures, and total patients seen
- ■ Worksheet—copy of daily patients by list or medical assistant assignment; used to prepare rooms and equipment; it is shredded at the end of the day in compliance with HIPAA privacy standards
- ■ Computer appointment scheduling—commercial or custom software that replaces the hard-copy appointment book (may also incorporate financial claims and procedures)
  - HIPAA (such as blocked computer screens), and other standard appointment guidelines must be met

PROCEDURE

- ■ Developing the matrix—preparing the appointment book or computer to show what times are available and unavailable for appointments
  - Block off times when appointments are not routinely scheduled, such as lunch, monthly staff meetings
  - Fill in physician's time away from the office, such as for hospital rounds, out-of-office procedures, meetings, vacations
  - If the cluster method of scheduling is used, mark days and times that are reserved for special procedures (e.g., if Mondays are reserved for sports physicals, the top of the day's matrix would be marked "sports physicals" and times would be blocked in the increments designated by the practice for each physical)
- ■ Scheduling
  - Begin with the first appointment available that has the time required for the specific visit

TABLE 10-1 ▶ Appointment abbreviations	
Abbreviation	**Definition**
Cons	Consultation
CPE	Complete physical exam
F/U	Follow-up
Inj	Injection
NP	New patient
NS	No-show
Ref	Referral
S/R	Suture removal
US	Ultrasound

- Consider patient and practice needs, such as fasting for blood work, preparation for procedures, or who does specific procedure
- Obtain patient's full name and telephone number
- Note reason for visit, using standard abbreviations (Table 10-1)
- Some offices will list the type of insurance

PATIENT PREPARATION

At the time the appointment is made,

- Verify that the office accepts the patient's insurance (the collection process begins when the appointment is made)
- Inform the patient of any co-pay and other office financial policies
- Instruct the patient to bring his or her insurance card, a picture identification and any necessary insurance forms, medical records, and immunization records
- Request that a new patient allow time before an appointment to complete registration material in the office or provide information for online registration
- Provide directions to office
- Mail preregistration material, which usually includes office policies and patient financial obligation if it is office policy to do so
- Obtain prior approval from the insurance company if required
- Explain any necessary preparations for procedures both verbally and in writing
- Confirm date and time of appointment at the end of conversation

PROCEDURES OUTSIDE OF THE PRACTICE

Depending on the type of practice, it may be necessary to schedule hospitalizations and procedures to be performed outside of the medical office. The following are guidelines:

- Inpatient scheduling for an illness or procedure that requires a hospital stay
  - Ensure insurance requirements, such as prior authorization, are met
  - Check patient's availability for expected length of stay (LOS)
  - Check physician's availability for procedure
  - Know appropriate diagnosis (*ICD-9* or *ICD-10* code) and procedure (*CPT* code)
  - If surgery or procedure, schedule with appropriate department within the hospital
  - Schedule the admission or reservation with the hospital Admissions Department (separate from scheduling the procedure to assure a bed is available on the appropriate unit afterward)
  - Provide patient preparation information and materials if appropriate
- Outpatient scheduling for a procedure that does not require a hospital stay
  - Ensure insurance requirements, such as prior authorization, are met
  - Check patient's availability
  - Check physician's availability for procedure
  - Know appropriate diagnosis (*ICD-9* or *ICD-10* code) and procedure (*CPT* code)
  - Schedule with appropriate facility
  - Provide patient preparation information and materials if appropriate

APPOINTMENT REMINDERS

Reminders are methods to alert the patient of upcoming appointments or the need for an upcoming preventive or follow-up service such as an annual well-woman check.

- Appointment cards—given at the time the appointment is established
- Tickler file—an index system with cards placed in chronologic order, usually by week or month; used as reminders for items that need attention in the future, such as immunizations
- Mailings—cards or computer-generated forms mailed to the patient informing him or her that an

appointment is coming up or to remind the patient to call and schedule an appointment if the patient is due for a procedure (e.g., annual well-woman check)

■ Telephone calls—made by the office the day before the appointment is scheduled; *leave messages only with prior patient permission* (usually obtained during initial registration)

■ E-mail—sent only with patient's permission

■ Text messages—sent only with patient's permission

■ Recall notices (not to be confused with reminder notices)—cards or computer-generated forms or the modalities as listed above sent to inform the patient that he or she *missed* a scheduled appointment or that he or she is overdue for a procedure (e.g., immunizations)

PATIENT FLOW ANALYSIS

Patient flow analysis is a periodic study conducted by the medical practice to assess the efficiency of scheduling and staff utilization. It may also be considered one of many tools in assessing patient satisfaction and generally measures the following times:

■ Sign in

■ Scheduled appointment

■ Placement in treatment room

■ Physician presentation

■ Discharge

The times are then evaluated and compared with established norms and benchmarks. Some insurance companies require or recommend a patient flow analysis at intervals or may conduct one as a follow-up to member complaints or other issues. In addition to participating in the process, the role of the medical assistant and the medical administrative specialist may be to report the findings and make recommendations. Changes should not be initiated without the approval of the physician or practice manager.

LEGAL ISSUES

■ Treat the appointment book and daily log, whether hardcopy or computer, as legal documents; as mentioned above, they can be subpoenaed

■ Maintain HIPAA standards by ensuring confidentiality with appointment information; if the system is computerized, screens should be protected from view, passwords changed frequently, and required firewalls in place if the system is part of a network

■ Document no-shows and cancelations that are not rescheduled in the patient's medical record and in the appointment book and log

RECEPTION

The expectation is that the reception area, formerly called the waiting room, adheres to all requirements involving asepsis, safety, confidentiality, and other issues under HIPAA, OSHA, and all regulating agencies.

■ **Confidentiality—** applies to all areas of reception as with the entire medical practice

• Block screens on computers

• Provide private areas for intake

• Use electronic sign-in sheet that records and sends patient's name and information prior to next patient or for hard copy, a method of blocking out names of patients as they sign in (marker, block-out tape)

• Be cautious of telephone and other conversations

■ **Accommodation and comfort—**ADA compliant; as with scheduling, the needs differ depending on the type of practice and patient population

• Avoid overcrowding

• Accommodate orthopedic, geriatric, and other physically impaired patients—space for wheelchairs and walkers to maneuver and rest, braille signs, handrails

• Pediatric offices—enough space to accommodate number of patients *and* parents; area for well-children and separate area for sick children; avoid toys that would allow spread of pathogens

• Consideration for service animals

■ **Safety—**observed as in all areas of medical office

• Practice an organized manner for opening and closing the office; a checklist is recommended

• Consider an alert system for unruly or potentially dangerous situations

• Assure a mechanism is in place for recognition and immediate reporting of patients in distress

• Avoid area carpets or other potential articles for tripping (risk management example)

• Observe and report any hazards or potential hazards such as frayed wire (risk management example)

■ **Asepsis or sanitation—**the general rules for asepsis apply (Chapter 17)

• Available PPE such as masks for coughing patients or staff, gloves for accepting specimens or other tasks involving body fluids, and emesis basins

• Appropriate method to dispose of contaminated material

• Alcohol-based hand sanitizer at counter and other areas

- Routine method and approved product for wiping down counters, furniture, toys, and other objects
- Appropriate postings and material for good health practices (cover your cough) and potential health hazards such as during flu season (patient education)

TERMS

APPOINTMENT SCHEDULING REVIEW

The following list reviews the terms discussed in this chapter and other important terms that you may see on the exam.

buffer zone period in the day with no scheduled appointments, intended to accommodate emergencies and allow the physician to catch up if running late

clustering (group procedures, categorizing) similar procedures are scheduled on predetermined days or in predetermined time blocks

daily scheduling log ledger-type book listing day's appointments; used for cross-referencing financial entries, data collection on types and number of procedures, and total patients seen

double booking scheduling two or more patients at the same time

length of stay (LOS) the time the patient is in or is expected to be in the hospital

matrix preparing the appointment book or computer to show what times are available and unavailable for appointments

modified wave scheduling method that uses hour blocks broken down into smaller time increments; individual patients are scheduled within those increments

open hours (tidal wave, open booking) scheduling method with no appointments needed; first-come, first-served

patient flow analysis a periodic study conducted by the medical practice to assess the efficiency of scheduling and staff

patient portal secure website giving patients 24-hour access to personal health information from an Internet connection and, in some cases, allow them to schedule their own appointments

postprandial after meals

recalls notices that inform the patient of a missed appointment and the need to reschedule

reminders cards or digital methods or sent to the patient informing him or her that an appointment is coming up or to remind the patient to call and schedule an appointment if the patient is due for a procedure

tickler file an index system with cards placed in chronologic order, usually by week or month; used as reminders for items that need attention in the future, such as immunizations

time-specific (streaming) patient is given an appointment time based both on length of time needed and on available appointments; this is the most common scheduling method

wave scheduling a specific number of patients, usually four, at the beginning of the same hour

worksheet a copy of daily patients by list or by medical assisting assignment, used to prepare rooms and equipment

REVIEW QUESTIONS

All questions are relevant for all medical assisting and medical administrative certification exams.

1. When setting up the appointment book by crossing off all times that will not be used for patient visits, this is known as setting up the:
   A. schedule.
   B. calendar.
   C. matrix.
   D. time frame.

   Answer: **C**

   Why: The matrix is the configuration of the appointment book after all the unavailable times are crossed out. These office times exclude vacations, meetings, lunch hour, and hospital visits.
   Review: Yes ○   No ○

2. Which of the following is a guideline that applies to using the appointment book?
   A. Erase any missed appointments from the book after it has been documented in the patient's chart.
   B. Discard all used appointment books.
   C. Always allow 1 hour per day for emergency appointments.
   D. Write or print clearly and make corrections neatly.
   E. Leave open one morning and one afternoon each week for any emergencies.

   Answer: **D**

   Why: The appointment book is considered a legal document and could be subject to subpoena. Always write or print clearly and make any corrections neatly. Missed appointments or canceled appointments are not erased from the book. Draw a single line through the entry and note the reason why the appointment was canceled or whether it was rescheduled. Used appointment books are not discarded but retained according to office policy, usually for the same period as patient records are retained. Most offices do not keep time available for emergency appointments; if an emergency arises, the office will try to prioritize the patient into the physician's schedule. In the event of a life-threatening emergency or serious injury, the patient may be referred to the local emergency room.
   Review: Yes ○   No ○

3. Of the following situations, which one constitutes a higher level of urgency and should be considered an emergency appointment?
   A. A patient needing an employment physical so that he or she can start a new job the next morning
   B. An 8-year-old child who sprained an ankle on the school playground that morning
   C. A 55-year-old man with difficulty breathing
   D. A patient who ran out of medication and needs her blood pressure checked so she can refill her medication

   Answer: **C**

   Why: Of the scenarios listed, none of them appears to be life-threatening *except* for someone who is experiencing difficulty breathing. Although all of these scenarios may seem like emergencies, especially to the patient, the only true emergency would involve a patient who is having difficulty breathing. The other cases can be handled as immediate status. Refer to Chapter 25 Emergency Preparedness.
   Review: Yes ○   No ○

4. The process of double booking in appointment scheduling means that:
    A. two or more patients are scheduled at the same time.
    B. one patient is scheduled but two appointment times are used.
    C. when two physicians are practicing in the same office, there are two appointment books used.
    D. at least four patients are scheduled for the same time at the beginning of the same hour.
    E. four patients are scheduled every 2 hours.

Answer: **A**
Why: Double booking schedules two patients at the same time and the patients are seen in the order in which they arrive at the office. This is used in practices in which physician visits are short.
Review: Yes ◯   No ◯

5. If the physician is delayed in arriving at the office for appointments, you should:
    A. immediately reschedule the patients.
    B. cancel the remaining appointments for the day.
    C. offer the waiting patients an opportunity to reschedule.
    D. offer to refer the patients to another physician's practice.

Answer: **C**
Why: When the physician is delayed, then you should keep patients informed of the approximate waiting time and offer to reschedule appointments.
Review: Yes ◯   No ◯

6. When making an appointment over the telephone for a new patient, it is important to secure the following information:
    A. Patient's place of employment
    B. Patient's date of birth
    C. Patient's co-pay amount
    D. Patient's home address
    E. Patient's insurance provider

Answer: **E**
Why: The patient's date of birth, place of employment, home address, and co-pay information can be obtained at the time of the appointment. It is important to know the patient's insurance company to ensure that the physician's office participates with the provider; if not, the patient can be informed of the payment procedures.
Review: Yes ◯   No ◯

7. When a specific number of patients, usually four, is scheduled at the beginning of the same hour, this is known as:
    A. modified wave scheduling.
    B. wave scheduling.
    C. cluster scheduling.
    D. group scheduling.

Answer: **B**
Why: In wave scheduling, the patients are seen in the order in which they arrive at the office. This reduces physician downtime but may increase waiting time for patients, who have to wait their turn if more than one patient arrives at the same time.
Review: Yes ◯   No ◯

8. When setting a series of repeat appointments for a patient, it is best to:
   A. have the patient call back no later than the end of the current week to schedule the return appointment.
   B. offer at least three alternative times for the return appointment.
   C. set the appointments at the same time on the same day of the week to enhance patient compliance.
   D. ask the patient to show up at a convenient time and you will work him or her into the schedule.
   E. vary the appointment times each week.

Answer: **C**
Why: Setting the return appointments at the same time and on the same day of the week will help the patient remember the appointments. It is easier to manage a schedule when there is consistency.
Review: Yes ◯   No ◯

9. The most critical aspect of the appointment book is that:
   A. the physician's personal time out of the office should not be reflected in the appointment book.
   B. when using the wave method of scheduling, always schedule one patient each hour regardless of the nature of the visit.
   C. allow at least 1 hour for lunch each day.
   D. the book is treated as a legal document, because it may be subpoenaed.

Answer: **D**
Why: The appointment book is a legal document and should be treated as any other legal document with regard to entries and corrections. It is important to build a matrix for scheduling that includes any time the physician will not be in the office. Multiple patients are scheduled per hour when using wave scheduling. The lunch break is determined by the practice and may actually be shorter or longer than 1 hour.
Review: Yes ◯   No ◯

10. The most common type of scheduling is:
    A. time-specific scheduling.
    B. wave scheduling.
    C. clustering.
    D. modified wave.
    E. tidal wave.

Answer: **A**
Why: Time-specific scheduling is the method of giving each patient an appointment time based on the length of time needed and what open time is available. Wave and modified wave scheduling are also used frequently but are not as common as time-specific scheduling. Clustering is the process of scheduling similar procedures on specified days or times. Tidal wave scheduling accommodates patients on a first-come, first-served basis.
Review: Yes ◯   No ◯

11. The abbreviation used in scheduling to designate a patient who has never been seen in the office before is:
    A. F/U.
    B. CPE.
    C. NS.
    D. NP.

Answer: **D**
Why: NP means new patient. F/U means follow-up, which would be used for a patient who is returning for an appointment. CPE means complete physical exam. NS is used to designate a patient who is a no-show.
Review: Yes ◯   No ◯

12. The reason for documenting a failed appointment in a patient's file is to:
   A. allow for scheduling another patient in that time slot.
   B. note all missed appointments in the event further action needs to take place.
   C. be able to erase the patient from the appointment book.
   D. allow the office to not schedule further appointments for that patient.
   E. notify the patient's insurance company.

Answer: **B**
Why: The physician may need to become involved to let a patient know that repeatedly missing appointments is disruptive to the office scheduling process. Occasionally, a patient's missing too many appointments may become of legal importance if the patient does not have a good medical outcome.
Review: Yes ◯ , No ◯

13. The type of scheduling used in a medical practice primarily depends on the:
   A. physician's preference.
   B. location of the practice.
   C. medical assistant's preference.
   D. size of the examination rooms.

Answer: **A**
Why: The physician always determines the type of scheduling used in the office practice. You may be asked for input on the decision, but ultimately, the physician makes the decision on scheduling preference. The location of the practice or size of the examination rooms has no impact on the type of scheduling the physician prefers.
Review: Yes ◯   No ◯

14. Which of the following is the least important concern when scheduling special procedures?
   A. The facilities available in the medical office at the time of the appointment
   B. The amount of time required for the procedure
   C. The patient preparation for the procedure
   D. The equipment required for the procedure
   E. The amount of the insurance co-pay

Answer: **E**
Why: When scheduling a patient for a special procedure, it is necessary to know what facilities are available, how much time the procedure will take, and what equipment is required for the procedure. You should also take into account any special patient preparation, especially if the procedure requires fasting. The first step in scheduling procedures is to assure the patient's insurance covers the procedure but the co-pay is the reponsibility of the facility where the procedure is to take place.
Review: Yes ◯   No ◯

15. A patient calls and requests an appointment immediately. What should be the first question you ask?
   A. The doctor is booked today. Can you come in tomorrow?
   B. Is it more convenient for you to come tomorrow morning or afternoon?
   C. When was the last time you were seen in this office?
   D. What are your symptoms and how long have you had them?

Answer: **D**
Why: You should always determine whether the call is an actual emergency or not. After this is determined, you can decide how soon the patient needs to be seen.
Review: Yes ◯   No ◯

16. When setting a return appointment for a patient, it is best to:
    A. have the patient call back from home after the patient checks his or her calendar.
    B. have preset appointment cards to distribute to patients with a set time and day when time is available in the appointment book.
    C. offer the patient a specific time and date.
    D. tell the patient you have only one available time and day that he or she will have to make work with his or her schedule.
    E. have the patient call the morning of the day he or she can come in for the appointment.

Answer: **C**
Why: The patient should be offered a time and day and see if they would be available to come in then. If that appointment is not acceptable, you can offer an alternative. It is too open to ask the patient to decide when to come in or to have the patient call the day of the desired appointment. They are not familiar with your scheduling procedures and may be indecisive.
Review: Yes ○ No ○

17. Scheduling duties include all the following EXCEPT:
    A. setting up the matrix of the appointment book.
    B. calling patients to remind them of their appointments.
    C. documenting any missed or rescheduled appointments in the patient's record.
    D. determining the time of day the office will accept appointments.

Answer: **D**
Why: The physician determines the appointment schedule for the office. This includes setting the time of the first and last appointments of the day and the break times throughout the day.
Review: Yes ○ No ○

18. When calling a hospital to schedule inpatient surgery, the information not necessary to have before the call is:
    A. patient's insurance co-payment.
    B. time and day requested by the physician.
    C. urgency for the procedure.
    D. type of sedation or anesthesia required.
    E. the physician's name.

Answer: **A**
Why: Inpatient surgery is scheduled with the hospital's operating room scheduler. Co-pays are the responsibility of the hospital.
Review: Yes ○ No ○

19. A tickler file is a(n):
    A. appointment card that is filed in the patient's chart.
    B. file used to hold laboratory reports if they cannot be filed right away.
    C. file of patient names who have missed appointments.
    D. filing system used as a reminder of things to do by a certain date or time.

Answer: **D**
Why: A tickler file may be a simple card file box with dividers placed in chronologic order by week or by month and containing items that will need attention in the future.
Review: Yes ○ No ○

20. A "walk-in" patient is one who:
   A. is able to ambulate without assistance.
   B. has arrived late for an appointment.
   C. arrives at the office without an appointment but wants to be seen.
   D. has an emergency.
   E. lives within walking distance of the office.

Answer: **C**
Why: A "walk-in" is a patient who shows up without an appointment but wants to see the physician. Unless it is an emergency, you should ask the patient to be seated in the waiting room and check with the physician to see whether the patient can be seen that day. If not, offer to schedule an appointment for the patient.
Review: Yes ◯   No ◯

21. When a patient needs a return appointment to discuss laboratory or X-ray findings with the physician, you should:
   A. call the lab and tell them to have the lab results available by the day of the appointment.
   B. call the lab to find out when the results will be available and make the return visit based on that date.
   C. ask the patient to contact the lab to determine when the results will be available.
   D. tell the lab that the results need to be back to the office by the next morning.

Answer: **B**
Why: The medical office is responsible for finding out when the lab results will be returned to the office so the return appointment can be scheduled accordingly. It is not appropriate to order tests by the next day unless the physician has made that request. The patient should not contact the lab.
Review: Yes ◯   No ◯

22. What type of scheduling is typical of an urgent care center?
   A. Tidal wave scheduling
   B. Wave scheduling
   C. Clustering
   D. Double booking
   E. Group scheduling

Answer: **A**
Why: Tidal wave scheduling means that there are no appointments set and patients are seen on a first-come, first-served basis. Wave scheduling is a type of scheduling in which several patients, usually four, are scheduled at the beginning of the same clock hour. Grouping and clustering are the same types of scheduling, in which patients having similar procedures are scheduled to come in on specified days or at specific times. Double booking means that two or more patients are scheduled at the same time.
Review: Yes ◯   No ◯

23. Types of patient appointment reminders used by offices include the following EXCEPT:
   A. postcards.
   B. appointment cards.
   C. telephone calls.
   D. facsimile.

Answer: **D**
Why: A facsimile, also called a fax, allows the medical office to send and receive printed material over a phone line. These machines are very popular in businesses but may not be found in homes. The fax machine is not used as a method to send appointment reminders.
Review: Yes ◯   No ◯

24. If the physician requests that the patient return for a fasting blood glucose and follow-up appointment, the best time of day to schedule this appointment would be:
    A. the first appointment after the lunch break.
    B. at the end of the day.
    C. the last morning appointment before the lunch break.
    D. the first appointment in the morning.
    E. any time 1 hour after the patient has eaten.

Answer: **D**
Why: This patient is having a fasting blood test performed, which requires the patient to have eaten nothing for several hours before the exam. By scheduling it as the first morning appointment, the patient can come to the office and have the blood drawn before eating breakfast.
Review: Yes ○   No ○

25. When a group of patients needs immunizations, the best type of scheduling for this is:
    A. tidal wave.
    B. clustering.
    C. modified wave.
    D. double booking.

Answer: **B**
Why: Clustering is a type of scheduling used when similar procedures are scheduled on specified days or at specific times. Tidal wave scheduling allows patients to walk in at any time to be seen. This type of scheduling is typically used in urgent care facilities. Modified wave scheduling is when hour-long blocks are broken down to smaller time increments (usually 10 or 15 minutes each) and individual patients are scheduled within those increments. Double booking means that two or more patients are scheduled at the same time.
Review: Yes ○   No ○

26. When conducting a patient flow analysis, it is determined that patients wait in the treatment room for approximately 15 minutes prior to the physician presenting. As a result, you would:
    A. schedule patients 15 minutes later.
    B. schedule fewer patients in each hour.
    C. report the findings to the insurance company.
    D. report the findings to the physician.
    E. direct the physician to spend less time with each patient.

Answer: **D**
Why: The role of the medical assistant or medical administrative specialist participating in the patient flow analysis is to report the findings. Recommendations may also be made, but it is up to the physician or practice manager to make changes and approve what should be sent to the insurance company.
Review: Yes ○   No ○

27. When scheduling an outpatient procedure, it is important to know all the following EXCEPT the:
    A. LOS.
    B. procedure.
    C. diagnosis.
    D. date.

Answer: **A**
Why: A patient will not be staying in the hospital following an outpatient procedure; therefore, the length of stay (LOS) is not necessary. All other information is required.
Review: Yes ○   No ○

28. The primary purpose of a patient flow analysis is to:
    A. identify patients who are late for appointments.
    B. demonstrate to insurance companies that the office does a good job.
    C. determine the efficiency of the practice.
    D. fire ineffective staff.
    E. encourage the physician to see more patients.

Answer: **C**
Why: The primary purpose of a patient flow analysis is to determine the efficiency of the practice. The other answer choices may result, but these would only be incidental to the primary reason for initially conducting the analysis.
Review: Yes ○   No ○

29. When scheduling an inpatient procedure, the reason for scheduling the admission separate from the actual procedure is to:
    A. provide billing information.
    B. reserve a hospital bed.
    C. assure the patient has meals ordered.
    D. notify the insurance company.

Answer: **B**
Why: A time for a surgery, for example, may be scheduled in the operating room, but that does not guarantee that a hospital bed will be available for the patient afterward. The Admissions Department is the only area that takes the reservations for the actual hospital bed. The department where the procedure is done is only aware of patients for that department, not for all admissions throughout the facility.
Review: Yes ○   No ○

30. Electronic appointment scheduling is:
    A. only for practices with multiple sites.
    B. less personal than a manual system.
    C. difficult to learn.
    D. unlikely to require a subpoena.
    E. held to HIPAA standards.

Answer: **E**
Why: Whether appointment scheduling is manual or electronic, both HIPAA and governmental requirements must be met. Electronic scheduling may be used in single-site practices as well as multiple-site practices. It is not impersonal because it requires a staff member to conduct the appointment process, and it is generally not more difficult to learn than a manual system. As mentioned earlier, the same requirements are enforced for manual or electronic systems.
Review: Yes ○   No ○

CRITICAL THINKING REVIEW QUESTIONS

Dr. Maloney is a pediatrician and uses a variety of scheduling methods dependent on the day of the week and the time of the year.

1. In the month before school starts, the office is opened on Thursday evenings until 8:00 PM for scheduling required school immunizations and sports physicals; this is called:
   A. clustering.
   B. open hours.
   C. wave.
   D. modified wave.
   E. double booking.

Answer: **A**
Why: Clustering is when similar procedures are scheduled on predetermined days in predetermined time blocks.

2. The office is opened one Saturday per month from 8:00 AM to noon and no appointment is required. This is called:
   A. clustering.
   B. open hours.
   C. wave.
   D. modified wave.

Answer: **B**
Why: Open hours or tidal wave or open booking does not require an appointment; patients are seen on a first-come first-served basis.

3. As a pediatrician, many of his patients have time with a medical assistant for height and weight, eye exams, sometimes audio testing, blood work, and other requirements of the well-child or EPSDT visit, including parent teaching (Chapter 18). He also has many asthmatic patients and routinely orders peak flow measurements. He has found that to best utilize his time and that of the patient and staff, the _____ scheduling works very well.
   A. clustering
   B. open hours
   C. wave
   D. modified wave
   E. double booking

Answer: **C**
Why: Wave scheduling is when a set number of patients are given the same appointment time at the beginning of each hour. A medical assistant may be doing multiple routine tests and procedures with one patient while the physician is seeing another. When the physician does see the patient, he usually has the test results available and does not have to wait or come back to the exam room before completing the visit. At the end of every hour, the physician and staff know if they are running late.

4. The scheduling method that does not easily accommodate for testing and procedures prior to the physician seeing the patient or for reviewing the medical records prior to the start of the day is:
   A. clustering.
   B. open hours.
   C. wave.
   D. double booking.

Answer: **B**
Why: Open hours or tidal wave or open booking does not require an appointment; patients are seen on a first-come first-served basis. This makes it difficult to preplan for the appointment, since the doctor does not know why the patient is there until he sees him or her.

5. During flu season, it is sometimes necessary to use this scheduling method to accommodate the increased number of sick patients:
   A. Clustering
   B. Open hours
   C. Wave
   D. Modified wave
   E. Double booking

Answer: **E**
Why: Double booking schedules two patients in the same time slot and is accommodated slot by slot. It differs from wave scheduling. For example, with wave scheduling, four patients may be scheduled for the same hour and come at the same time, which could mean that eight patients would arrive at the same time which makes for a hectic and unrealistic day. Putting more than one patient in the same time slot is contrary to the definition of modified wave scheduling. When using double booking to accommodate urgent needs, the patient should be informed that he or she may have to wait.

CHAPTER

11

Medical Records Management

Review Tip:

Congratulations! Believe it or not, you are nearly at the halfway point of the review chapters. The road to completion becomes easier from here. Don't give up on your goal to become a nationally certified health professional. Be sure to complete Chapter 4, "Law and Ethics," before beginning this one—some material involving medical records, such as Health Insurance Portability and Accountability Act (HIPAA) and confidentiality, is found in that chapter.

The term **medical record** is used synonymously with *patient chart* or *chart*; it contains all information related to a patient's medical care. For a century, medical records were kept in a hard-copy form (Fig. 11-1). In 2009, the *Health Information Technology for Economic and Clinical Health (HITECH) Act* was passed to promote the adoption and *meaningful use* of health information technology, including the electronic health record (EHR) or electronic medical record (EMR).

FIGURE 11-1 In the early 1900s, the physician dictated the patient information to a stenographer who recorded it in shorthand then used a typewriter to document it for the medical record.

MEANINGFUL USE AND THE EHR

The federal government defines meaningful use as follows (http://www.healthit.gov/providers-professionals/meaningful-use-definition-objectives):

Using certified EHR technology to

- *Improve quality, safety, efficiency, and reduce health disparities*
- *Engage patients and family*
- *Improve care coordination, and population and public health*
- *Maintain privacy and security of patient health information*

Meaningful use involves a series of objectives that eligible professionals (EPs) must achieve to qualify for Centers for Medicare & Medicaid Services (CMS) financial incentive programs. In the future, complying with meaningful use will effect reimbursement for care to these patients. Refer to Chapter 1 for meaningful use directly impacting medical assistants and medical administrative specialists.

MEDICAL RECORDS

It is expected that the majority of health-care providers have or will convert to the EHR or EMR by the 2014 date

set by CMS at the time of this writing. However, not all existing hard-copy medical records will be converted to an electronic version. Consequently, a duel system of hard-copy and EMR management will continue to be utilized for some years and both forms will be found in practice. Refer to Table 11-1 for a comparison of the two modalities.

The Medical Records Management chapter is divided into three sections:

- Medical records management
- The individual medical record
- Documentation guidelines

MEDICAL RECORDS MANAGEMENT

The medical assistant and medical administrative specialist are usually responsible for the management of the office's medical records. With the EMR, these functions are now shared with an informational technology specialist and involve the following:

- Assembling—place or utilize all the forms or screens used by the specific practice in the patient record in the prescribed sequence
- Filing—have active (see definition below) medical records in the secured designated area as assigned by the facility and system utilized (electronic or manual); sometimes referred to as indexing
- Maintenance—ensure all documentation is in the medical record in the proper order and that the record is in a secured area (this may be a locked cabinet or a secure electronic data storage system with backup)
- Retrieving—recover the medical record from the secured storage as needed and document when and where the record was taken (hard copy); a portion of a record may be in hard copy and a portion in an electronic format.
- Transferring—send the record to another health-care provider when the proper consent for release of medical records is obtained or for continuity of care such as a referral (if sending hard copies, do not send originals); e-mail is not considered a secure method of transfer, although it is frequently used.
- Protecting—ensure the medical record is in secure area and complete with all computer and hard-copy safeguards in place.
- Auditing—examine medical record files to ensure accuracy (a common mistake in the EHR is clicking a drop down screen too rapidly resulting in incorrect information), completeness, and sequence of the documents; may be an internal file audit performed

TABLE 11-1 ▸ **Comparison of the traditional and the electronic health records**

Traditional Health Record	Electronic Health Record
Relatively low cost for start-up and maintenance	High cost for start-up and ongoing maintenance
Can only be accessed by one person at a time	Can be accessed from multiple sites at the same time
Legibility can be an issue resulting in errors	No issue with legibility decreasing errors
Accessible during technical and power outages	Requires manual backup system during technical and power outages
Does not interface with labs, pharmacies, billing, and other services requiring duplication and increased chance for errors	Interfaces with lab, pharmacies, billing, and other services avoiding increasing efficiency
Staff training minimal	Staff training resource intensive
Upgrades and subsequent costs infrequent	Upgrades and costs significant
Utilizes multifunctional staff	Requires specific IT staff or contracts
Lost records or information placed in incorrect record	Virtually no lost records or misplaced information
Extensive filing and storage space required	Filing and storage space minimal
Simple security issues	Complicated cyberspace security issues
Transcription costs	Reduced or no transcription costs
Requires actual medical imaging to be filed in separate area	Actual medical imaging may be incorporated in medical record

by the office staff or an external file audit performed by professional auditors of an organization or agency who are not employees of the practice

- Retention—keep the medical record for a prescribed length of time or statute of limitations; the term **conditioning** is sometimes used to describe preparation of the chart for retention: secure all loose documents for hard copy and examine the record for completeness whether hard copy or EHR
- Purging—remove medical records that are beyond the time period of the statute of limitations
- Destroying—shred or otherwise destroy the medical record, ensuring no identifying factors are recognizable, when the prescribed statute of limitations is reached; maintain a file indicating when the record was destroyed; even though the electronic capacity for retaining medical records is greatly expanded for the EHR, the statute of limitations is usually honored

In addition to the functions associated with medical records, you must be aware of other factors:

- Types of files (hard copy and electronic)
  - Active—patient seen within 2 to 5 years (dependent on practice type)
  - Inactive—patient *not* seen within past 2 to 5 years (dependent on practice type)
  - Closed—patient not expected to return to practice, such as if the patient is deceased, has moved, or has reached age limit in pediatrics

- Record storage
  - Hard copy
    - Shelving units (active files)
    - Locked units or units locked in self-contained area
  - EHR—complex HIPAA security requirements
    - Firewalls should be in place if located on a network or electronically transferred
    - Cloud type storage must be specific for health care and meet HIPAA requirements
    - Passwords for access are changed frequently
    - **Encryption**, making information unreadable except for authorized persons
    - Screen blockers are in use when accessing
  - Other storage modalities
    - Floppy disk, CD-ROM
    - Microfiche (for closed or inactive records)
- Filing systems
  - Alphabetic—charts filed by the units of the patient's name: letter by letter beginning with the patient's last name; whether hard copy or electronic, accurate input is needed or the file is lost (Table 11-2)
    - Unit 1—last name, letter by letter
    - Unit 2—first name, letter by letter
    - Unit 3—middle initial or middle name, letter by letter
    - Unit 4—prefixes and suffixes (e.g., Dr., Mrs., Jr., Sr., I, II, III): numbers appear first (e.g., I, II, III); Jr. follows numbers and comes before Sr.

TABLE 11-2 ▶ Alphabetic filing by units

Example of Using units	Patient Name	Unit 1 (Last Name)	Unit 2 (First Name)	Unit 3 (Middle Name)	Unit 4 (Title)
	John E. Smith	Smith	John	E.	
	John William Jones	Jones	John	William	
Two-word last names	Susan B. Saint Nicolas	Saintnicolas	Susan	B.	
Period in last name	Harry F. St. James	Saintjames (ignore period and spell out name)	Harry	F.	
Hyphens or apostrophes (considered a single unit)	Jose Garcia-Lopez Jesse Peter O'Hara	Garcialopez Ohara	Jose Jesse	Peter	
Using titles	Dr. Jose Garcia-Lopez Mary T. El (Mrs. John)	Garcialopez El	Jose Mary	T.	Dr. Mrs. John
Jr. and Sr. (Jr. filed before Sr.)	Joseph C. Tan, Jr. Joseph C. Tan, Sr.	Tan Tan	Joseph Joseph	C. C.	Jr. Sr.
Birth order (filed in chronologic order)	Tomas Jacob Love, I Tomas Jacob Love, II Tomas Jacob Love, III	Love Love Love	Tomas Tomas Tomas	Jacob Jacob Jacob	I II III
Jr., Sr., and numbers (numbers first in chronologic order, Jr. next, Sr. last)	Roberto De Rosa, III Roberto De Rosa, IV Roberto De Rosa, Jr. Roberto De Rosa, Sr.	Derosa Derosa Derosa Derosa	Roberto Roberto Roberto Roberto		III IV Jr. Sr.
Businesses and associations	A-One Medical Supply The McMay Insurance Group	Aone Mcmay	Medical Insurance	Supply Group	The

- Numeric—each patient is assigned a medical record number through manual or computerized means; through a manual or computerized system, numbers are cross-referenced with the alphabetic file, sometimes referred to as a *master file* or *tickler file*
- Consecutive numeric order—patients are assigned numbers in the order of their first visit to the practice; charts are filed in this order; used by small practices
- Terminal digit order—patients are assigned a six-digit number; to file the charts, the numbers are divided into three groups of two digits each and read from right to left
- Alphanumeric—system using a combination of numbers and letters
  - Initial filing done alphabetically by first letter of last name or subject; then numbers are assigned
  - Seldom used for medical records; more frequently used for other office files
- Medical records retention (hard copy or electronic)— the length of time a medical record should be retained

- Guidelines from federal/state statute of limitations; retention for adults is usually 7 to 10 years
- Retention for minors is the age of majority plus the statute of limitations (7 to 10 years)
- Guidelines may also be issued by insurance companies and accrediting and legal organizations
- Functional storage and retrieval systems required

■ Medical records destruction
- After completion of statute of limitations and recommended guidelines
- Total eradication (shredding, burning, deleting and scrubbing); safe shredding and disposal of documents may be done by an outside company specializing in those services
- Notation of record number, name, means of destruction, and date must be kept

THE INDIVIDUAL MEDICAL RECORD

The individual medical record is all the information related to a patient's medical care. This information may be in the form of paper (e.g., progress notes or letters), medical imaging (such as X-rays, ultrasounds), DVDs (e.g., audio, visual), disks, electronic printouts (e.g., electrocardiogram tracings), photographs, and any other materials whether hard copy or electronic including online that tell the "story" of the patient's medical journey. The medical record *material* is the property of the health-care provider. The *information* in the medical record is the property of the patient or the patient's legal representative who always has the right to access, restrict access, and request any reasonable amendment to it.

■ Uses of the medical record
- Facilitates good medical care through continuity
- Provides legal protection for the health-care provider and the patient
- Functions as a quality of care monitor
- Facilitates research
- Provides resource for education

■ Determination of record forms information and sequence (Box 11-1)
- Type of practice
- Physician preference
- Software selection
- Frequency of access

■ Potentials for legal and ethical dilemmas
- Confidentiality breach (see "Confidentiality" in Chapter 4)

BOX 11-1

Example of medical record forms or screen sequencing

Medical record sequence of forms

1. Patient information/insurance
2. Consent for assignment of benefits
3. Problem list
4. Medical, social, and family histories
5. Physical findings, including graphs, tables, flow sheets (e.g., height and weight)
6. Progress notes
7. Immunization record
8. Medication/prescription
9. Diagnostic reports
10. Reports of procedures done outside the office such as surgeries, endoscopies
11. Consultation/referral reports
12. Medical records from other providers
13. Correspondence, telephone notes, e-mails
14. Termination summary

BOX 11-2

Release of medical records

■ A release of medical records to insurance companies, other recognized reimbursement agencies, and health-care providers within the same health-care network is generally included in a general consent form and is obtained at the first office visit.

■ Release of medical records to other health-care providers, attorneys, or others requires a Release of Medical Information form signed by the patient or the patient's legal representative, such as a court-appointed guardian.

■ Lawful mandatory reporting situations or subpoenas do not require consent forms (refer to Chapter 4).

- Improper release of information (Box 11-2)
- Withdrawal from care; discharge of patient
- Broken appointments
- Patient noncompliance with his or her care plan
- Questionable medical records
  ◦ Delayed filing of tests or notes
  ◦ Incomplete information
  ◦ Illegible entries
  ◦ Improperly corrected entries
  ◦ Missing information
  ◦ Lost record (misspelled names will result in a lost record whether hard copy or electronic)

DOCUMENTATION GUIDELINES

Documentation, also referred to as *charting*, makes up the medical record. A caveat, referred to as the "golden rule," is *If it is not documented, it was not done.*

- "Cs" of charting (a list of terms beginning with the letter "C" to help with proper documentation)
  - Client's words or chief complaint (cc) (recommend quotation marks or "patient states..")
  - Clear
  - Complete
  - Concise
  - Chronologic or reverse chronologic order
  - *Confidential*
- Documentation inclusions
  - Name of the patient, additional identifier (e.g., medical record number), and date on each page, front and back, or screen
  - Dated entry for each visit and procedure
  - Health-care provider signature (may be electronic) or initials and title for all entries
  - Dated entry for no-shows, cancelations, or phone calls
  - Dated entry for failure to follow treatment plan
  - Dated entry for prescription refills
  - Notations or copies of forms or electronic reports for outpatient and hospital visits and consultations
  - Dated entry with explanation for termination of care
  - Documentation of reported and reviewed diagnostic results
  - Documentation of follow-up for all tests and procedures
  - Acceptable error-correction method (Box 11-3)
- Charting methods
  - Source-oriented medical record (SOMR)—this file is divided into sections by guides, such as a section for progress notes or diagnostic reports; may be used in conjunction with other charting methods
  - Problem-oriented medical record (POMR)—the patient's problems are numbered and listed on a form or screen (problem list) that is placed in the front of the chart; each visit or treatment is associated with a problem number (for example, if asthma is the primary problem, it is listed as #1 and documented as #1 throughout the chart); may be used in conjunction with other charting methods. In addition to the problem list, POMR usually contains the following:
    - Database—patient profile and demographics; baseline and assessment information, including cc and test results

BOX 11-3
Error correction

Hard-copy medical record
Draw a single line through the error with black ink and write "error" or "err." above. Never white out or completely eliminate the error. Correct the error above the entry if it involves only a few words or below the entry if the error is longer. Record the date and time and sign or initial the entry with your health-care provider title.

Example:
09/10/20XX 0900 urine specimen collected. Mary Smith, MA
sputum/M.S., MA

Electronic medical record
Most programs have a built-in system to detect any changes made in the EHR; it is important to document in the system if an event is a late entry (performed on a previous date) or if an error was made that could affect the patient's outcome (incorrect medication given). Consult the supervisor when in doubt.

- Treatment plan—course of procedures, medications, and other instructions for the patient's care
- Progress notes—continuing description of the patient's improvement or lack of improvement
  - SOAP documentation—format for documenting each visit using subjective information, objective information, an assessment, and a plan, in that order; may be used in conjunction with other charting methods
    - S—subjective data (symptoms the patient states that cannot be seen, heard, or measured, such as a headache)
    - O—objective data (measurable and observable signs, such as swelling, vital signs)
    - A—assessment (exam and impressions)
    - P—plan (design for tests, treatments, education, follow-up)
  - Reverse chronologic order—format with the most recent records filed on top: visits in 2014 would be closer to the front of the chart than visits in 2013; may be used in conjunction with other charting methods

TERMS

MEDICAL RECORDS REVIEW

The following list reviews the terms discussed in this chapter and other important terms that you may see on the exam, especially those with an asterisk.

active medical record the chart of a patient seen within 2 to 5 years (dependent on practice type)

audit examine medical record files to ensure accuracy, completeness, and sequence of the documents

chart the patient's medical record

closed medical record the chart of a patient not expected to return to the practice, such as a patient who is deceased or has moved

conditioning preparation of the chart for retention: secure all loose documents, and examine the chart for completion and correct filing order of documents

electronic health record (EHR) patient health information maintained in an electronic format, computerized record

encryption process to make information unreadable except for authorized persons

Health Information Technology for Economic and Clinical Health (HITECH) Act passed in 2009 to promote the adoption and meaningful use of health information technology

Health Insurance Portability and Accountability Act (HIPAA) originally enacted in 1996, contains requirements for patient confidentiality

inactive medical record the chart of a patient *not* seen at the specific medical office within the past 2 to 5 years (dependent on practice type)

medical record all patient information related to the medical care; may be in the form of paper, medical imaging, tapes, disks, electronic printouts, photographs, and any other material telling the "story" of the patient's medical history

medical records management processes of assembling, filing, maintaining, retrieving, transferring, protecting, retaining, and destroying medical records

out guides folders inserted on file shelf when file is in use; they designate who took it, when, and where it is (may be computerized instead of hard-copy folder)

problem-oriented medical record (POMR) the patient's problems are numbered and listed on a form (problem list) placed in front of chart; each visit or treatment is associated with the number of the corresponding problem (e.g., if asthma is #1, it is documented as #1 throughout chart)

reverse chronologic order format with the most recent documentation filed on top of the past documentation

SOAP documentation format for documenting each medical visit using subjective information, objective information, an assessment, and a plan, in that order

source-oriented medical record (SOMR) the patient file is divided into sections by guides, such as a section for progress notes or diagnostic reports

REVIEW QUESTIONS

All questions are relevant for all medical assisting and medical administrative certification exams.

1. When adding a laboratory report to a patient's chart, you should:
   A. file all materials in the front of the chart regardless of the type of record it is.
   B. photocopy all records and retain in a separate file.
   C. ensure that the physician has initialed all reports before they are inserted into the chart.
   D. sign all documents with the medical assistant title and file in the patient's chart.

Answer: **C**

Why: Whenever a new laboratory report or other clinically related document is generated for a patient's medical record, the physician must review the record before it is filed in the chart for storage. If there is abnormal medical information, the physician will want to act on the information to ensure proper medical care for the patient.
Review: Yes ○   No ○

2. The most common method of documentation for a patient medical record is:
   A. POMR.
   B. SOMR.
   C. SOAP.
   D. SOB.
   E. DOB.

Answer: **C**

Why: The abbreviation SOAP stands for subjective, objective, assessment, plan. This is the most common method of documenting used by physicians. In the EHR, all of these elements may not be on the same screen. POMR (problem-oriented medical records) and SOMR (source-oriented medical records) are methods used in organizing the patient's chart either by the patient's problem categories or by sources of information, respectively. SOB stands for shortness of breath and is associated with a condition a patient has, not a documentation method. DOB stands for date of birth, which is a charting abbreviation.
Review: Yes ○   No ○

3. Which of the following is a true statement regarding guidelines for alphabetic filing?
   A. When two male family members have the suffixes Junior and Senior, Senior is filed before Junior.
   B. The chart for a patient with the last name of Saint James would be filed in the J (James) section of the files.
   C. The name McMurray is filed before MacIntosh.
   D. John William Smith is filed before John Will Smith.
   E. When a last name has a hyphen, it is filed as if the hyphen were not there.

Answer: **E**

Why: Alphabetic filing guidelines dictate that Junior is filed before Senior. These guidelines also state that the name Saint James becomes one word and is filed in the S section under Saint. The John Smith names are the same except for the middle name; Will is filed before William. A name starting with Mc is filed in alphabetic order, after Mac.
Review: Yes ○   No ○

4. When a paper medical record is in use, a folder inserted on the shelf in place of the medical record file is a(n):
   A. closed file.
   B. inactive file.
   C. file label.
   D. out guide.

Answer: **D**

Why: A closed or inactive file indicates the status of the file, and a file label is affixed to a file to indicate its name. An out guide is a folder inserted on a file shelf to replace a medical record file that is in use. The out guide folder designates who took the medical file, when it was removed, and where it is.
Review: Yes ○   No ○

5. One of the "Cs" of charting includes:
   A. clear.
   B. closed.
   C. computerized.
   D. complex.
   E. conditional.

Answer: **A**
Why: The six "Cs" of charting include client's words, clear, complete, concise, chronologic, and confidentiality. These are essential guidelines of documentation.
Review: Yes ○   No ○

6. The "P" in the SOAP method of charting includes:
   A. measurable signs.
   B. physician's exam.
   C. symptoms the patient states.
   D. plan for tests and treatments.

Answer: **D**
Why: The "P" stands for the plan and includes the plan for the patient's tests, treatment, and follow-up. Measurable signs are objective (O), the physician's exam is assessment (A), and symptoms the patient states are subjective data (S).
Review: Yes ○   No ○

7. If filing using reverse chronologic order, which of the following is in the correct sequence?
   A. Laboratory test results from June 2007 would be in front of those from December 2010.
   B. Office visit entries from December 2014 would be in front of visits from June 2014.
   C. X-ray exam reports from November 15, 2013, would be in front of those from December 30 of the same year.
   D. A surgical report from an operation in 2001 would be in front of a report of a procedure performed in 2009.
   E. A physician's referral report from May 15, 2009, would be in front of a report from the same physician dated May 30, 2009.

Answer: **B**
Why: Reverse chronologic order means that the most recent records are filed in front of or on top of the past record. The only example of this is item B. All the other examples would place the older reports or events first.
Review: Yes ○   No ○

8. The proper procedure to correct an error in a patient's hard-copy chart is to:
   A. date and sign the correction.
   B. white out the error before writing in the correction.
   C. draw a single line through the error with red ink.
   D. always start a new line in the chart for corrections.

Answer: **A**
Why: A correction should always be dated and signed by the person making the correction. Corrections should not be covered with white out or lined out with red ink. If it is only a word or two to correct, the correction is written above the error after the error is crossed out with a single line in black ink.
Review: Yes ○   No ○

9. A system of filing made of combinations of numbers and letters is:
   A. direct filing.
   B. numeric filing.
   C. subject filing.
   D. demographic filing.
   E. alphanumeric filing.

Answer: **E**
Why: Alphanumeric filing uses letters ("alpha") and numbers ("numeric") for filing.
Review: Yes ○   No ○

10. Of the following patient names, which would come first in alphabetic filing?
A. Fisher, Bill
B. Fischer, William
C. Fishar, Bob
D. Fishare, Bill

Answer: **B**
Why: Alphabetic filing requires that each letter be considered as a unit. All these names start with the same first three letters, *F I S*. The next letter determines which name comes first in filing. *C* comes before *H*, so the name Fischer is first in filing.
Review: Yes ○   No ○

11. The "golden rule" in documentation is the following:
A. Always sign your complete name and title.
B. Always document in ink.
C. If it is not documented, it was not done.
D. Always date and time all entries.
E. The physician must initial all chart entries.

Answer: **C**
Why: All of the answers are part of proper documentation, but the "golden rule" of documentation is if it is not documented, it was not done.
Review: Yes ○   No ○

12. Determining the organization of the medical record and sequence of filing is dependent on the following factors EXCEPT:
A. type of practice.
B. location of practice.
C. physician preference.
D. frequency of access.

Answer: **B**
Why: The location of the medical practice has no bearing on how medical records will be organized or filed. The other factors listed will determine the best way to manage the patients' medical records.
Review: Yes ○   No ○

13. The database component of problem-oriented medical records (POMR) includes what information?
A. Patient's past medical problems
B. Treatment plan for the patient
C. Progress notes
D. Patient's present illness
E. Laboratory findings from 5 years ago

Answer: **D**
Why: POMR has four components, including database, problem list, treatment plan, and progress notes. The problem list includes past medical problems, but the database includes chief complaint, present illness, patient profile, review of systems, physical examination, and laboratory reports.
Review: Yes ○   No ○

14. The term used to describe the legal length of time regarding storage of medical and business records is:
A. statute of limitations.
B. release of medical records.
C. microfiche.
D. closed records.

Answer: **A**
Why: The statute of limitations may vary from state to state. It is the legal time limit you must retain medical and business records before they can be destroyed. Most states require a minimum of 7 years from the date of the last entry. Many practices store records permanently because of the possibility of a malpractice suit.
Review: Yes ○   No ○

15. The method of filing used when documentation is placed in order based on the date of occurrence is:
A. demographic grouping.
B. statistical numbering.
C. chronologic order.
D. consecutive numeric order.
E. alphabetic filing.

Answer: **C**
Why: The word *chronologic* means "arranged in the order of occurrence." Most charting requires the most recent reports or records to be placed in front of or on top of older information.
Review: Yes ◯   No ◯

16. An important rule for releasing hard-copy medical records is:
A. release the original medical record when the patient asks for it.
B. there is no need to obtain the patient's signature on an Authorization for Release of Medical Record form as long as the patient has given verbal authorization.
C. limit the amount of medical information you release over the telephone when you are not talking directly to the patient.
D. release a copy of the medical record, not the original.

Answer: **D**
Why: A practice never releases the original medical record, only a copy. It is required that the patient sign a form to release medical records. A verbal consent is not official authorization. Information, no matter how limited, is never given over the telephone to anyone but the patient.
Review: Yes ◯   No ◯

17. If a patient is not expected to return to the practice because he or she has moved away, the patient's record would be classified as:
A. inactive.
B. active.
C. closed.
D. transferred.
E. released.

Answer: **C**
Why: An inactive file would be for a patient who has not been seen within the past 2 to 5 years. An active file is used for a patient who has been seen within the past 2 to 5 years. The number of years is established by each practice, with 2 to 5 being the most common range. A closed file is used for a patient who will not be expected back to the practice. This would include deceased patients and patients who have moved away. A transferred file has been sent to another practice; it is released when the file has been approved for transfer to another health-care provider.
Review: Yes ◯   No ◯

18. The pages or screens of the medical record contained within the patient's file are the property of the:
A. patient.
B. physician.
C. insurance carrier.
D. spouse or guardian.

Answer: **B**
Why: The health-care provider, the physician, owns the form of the medical record. The patient can request the information contained within the record, but the actual record belongs to the physician.
Review: Yes ◯   No ◯

19. Indexing rules for alphabetic filing include the following EXCEPT:
  A. file records according to last name, first name, and middle initial.
  B. file abbreviated names as if they were spelled out.
  C. disregard apostrophes.
  D. Junior is filed before Senior.
  E. treat hyphenated names as two units.

Answer: **E**

Why: A hyphenated name is treated as one unit (i.e., Jane Fisher-Smith is filed as Fisher-Smith, Jane, not as Smith, Jane Fisher).

Review: Yes ○   No ○

....

20. One method of backing up a file to a computer medical record is called the:
  A. file folder.
  B. out guide.
  C. disk.
  D. electronic copy.

Answer: **C**

Why: A disk of a computer record can be used as a backup to the electronic system. A file folder is the holder of the medical records. An out guide is used to temporarily replace a medical file while it is in use. An electronic copy refers to the computerized version of the record.

Review: Yes ○   No ○

....

21. The process of gathering all chart items together and preparing them for filing by removing loose pieces of tape or paper clips and replacing them with staples is known as:
  A. conditioning.
  B. sorting.
  C. destroying.
  D. indexing.
  E. retrieving.

Answer: **A**

Why: Conditioning is the process of making sure the chart records are presentable for filing. It is inappropriate to file records that have paper clips, because they become too bulky and take up file space. Sorting the files into groups makes it easier to file records. They can be sorted alphabetically or numerically first and then placed in the appropriate space on the file shelf. Destroying is the process of shredding the medical record to permanently remove it from storage. Indexing is the process of separating business records from the patient's medical records. Retrieving is the process of recovering the medical record from the secured storage location.

Review: Yes ○   No ○

....

22. The federal government policy that sets standards for electronic transmission of medical information is included in the act adopted in 1996 called:
  A. OSHA.
  B. CLIA.
  C. HIPAA.
  D. CDC.

Answer: **C**

Why: HIPAA, the Health Insurance Portability and Accountability Act, was passed by the federal government and mandates that health-care providers adopt policies in their medical practice that regulate the electronic transmission of patients' medical information. In addition, the act sets standards on the disclosure and release of medical records. OSHA stands for Occupational Safety and Health Administration. CLIA stands for Clinical Laboratory Improvement Amendments. CDC stands for the Centers for Disease Control and Prevention.

Review: Yes ○   No ○

23. To avoid legal and ethical issues, patients' medical records should be properly maintained, which includes all of the following EXCEPT:
    A. entry of any broken or missed appointments.
    B. letter sent to patient to notify of withdrawal of care.
    C. notation of patient's noncompliance with the treatment plan.
    D. delay in filing test results.
    E. initialing of all corrections made in a medical chart.

Answer: **D**

Why: The patient's medical record should always document missed appointments and noncompliance with the physician's treatment plan, in case of a malpractice suit brought against the physician for questionable patient care. When a physician notifies a patient of withdrawal of care, a copy of the letter sent to the patient is included in the medical record. The medical assistant or medical administrative specialist should always ensure timely filing of reports and lab results. There is a chance these records will be lost if not filed promptly. When making corrections to a chart, draw a single line through the error, write the correct information above the error, and initial the entry.

Review: Yes ○   No ○

24. When using the SOAP method of charting, which of the following belongs to the O section?
    A. Patient's complaint of headache
    B. Order for an electrocardiogram
    C. Blood pressure reading
    D. Physician's request to have patient return for follow-up appointment

Answer: **C**

Why: The "O" stands for "objective data." Objective data include things that are measurable and observable. A patient's blood pressure is a measurable, objective sign. The patient's complaint of headache is subjective data—something that cannot be seen or observed. The physician's request for an electrocardiogram and follow-up appointment are all part of the plan for the patient.

Review: Yes ○   No ○

25. SOMR refers to:
    A. subjective–objective medical record.
    B. safe objective medical radiology.
    C. State Office of Medical Records.
    D. Secure Office for Medical Records.
    E. source-oriented medical record.

Answer: **E**

Why: The SOMR, source-oriented medical record, is a type of filing within the medical record that sorts the information by sections such as progress notes, diagnostic reports, and correspondence.

Review: Yes ○   No ○

26. When a medical record or patient file is audited, it is:
    A. purged.
    B. examined.
    C. destroyed.
    D. shredded.

Answer: **B**

Why: When a file is examined for completeness, for accuracy, and to ensure the documents are in the proper order, it is being audited. Purging, destroying, and shredding are methods of cleaning out old files and appropriately discarding medical records that no longer need to be retained or maintained.

Review: Yes ○   No ○

CRITICAL THINKING CASE REVIEW QUESTIONS

Dr. Roder is a geriatric practitioner and has been in practice 20 years. Last year, he converted to an electronic health record.

1. While the system was expensive, part of the cost was covered through:
   A. HIPAA.
   B. patient billing.
   C. long-term monetary savings.
   D. meaningful use.
   E. increased patients.

   Answer: **D**
   Why: Meaningful use is associated with the federal act to provide reimbursement to health-care providers who met established criteria for certified electronic health records.
   Review: Yes ○   No ○

2. The act that this initiative is part of is the:
   A. HIPAA.
   B. HITECH.
   C. CMS.
   D. SOAP.

   Answer: **B**
   Why: B is the Health Information Technology for Economic and Clinical Health Act. The only other act listed in this answer is HIPAA, which is the Healthcare Insurance Portability and Accountability Act, which does not provide reimbursement incentives.
   Review: Yes ○   No ○

3. From a quality of care aspect, the most important feature of the EHR is:
   A. the need for more specialized staff.
   B. the reduction of errors due to illegibility.
   C. the interface with other services.
   D. decreased need for storage space.
   E. the opportunity for the medical office staff and IT staff to work together.

   Answer: **B**
   Why: While all the answers could be correct, the one that is related to clinical quality outcomes is the legibility of the chart which directly decreases medical errors.
   Review: Yes ○   No ○

4. While Dr. Roder has been in practice 20 years and has many hard-copy records in storage, of the records in storage he is only required to keep the records of patients who:
   A. are classified as inactive.
   B. are deceased.
   C. reached the age of majority.
   D. have been seen within 7 years.

   Answer: **D**
   Why: Be cautious of the word "only." Dr. Roder is not *only* to maintain records in *storage* of patients not seen in 2 years. It only means that these can be removed from the active files. Records of deceased patients must also meet the statute of limitations. Seven years is generally the statute of limitations for adults, and since Dr. Roder is a gerontologist, he does not treat minors which would involve storing records until 7 to 10 years after the age of majority.
   Review: Yes ○   No ○

5. HIPAA is involved with the:
   A. patient's confidentiality.
   B. insurance industry.
   C. secure electronic transmission of patient information.
   D. health-care insurance for the needy.
   E. Americans Disability Act.

   Answer: **C**
   Why: While A, B, and C are correct, C is the best answer (refer to Chapter 4). Patient confidentiality has been a standard in health care for many years prior to HIPAA and can be found in many organizations' credo or rights. HIPAA was the first major attempt to secure the electronic transmission of patient data.
   Review: Yes ○   No ○

12

Correspondence

Written communication in the medical office takes many forms. E-mail, patient instructions, faxes, and various computer applications have been discussed in previous chapters. This chapter concentrates on written correspondence involving mail and transcription. The topics are generally prescriptive, which means they follow a custom or rule.

The majority of letters generated in the medical office use a template, or form, which is recommended by the physician's attorney, insurance carrier, or professional organization. Purposes include but are not limited to patient reports, office policies, termination of services, and protection of the practice from medicolegal risk. The few original letters are usually those dictated by the physician and sent to other physicians regarding patient findings or treatment. The medical assistant or medical administrative specialist must know the correct format, materials, and process for outgoing and incoming mail.

Review Tip:

Become familiar with the various correspondence formats and materials discussed in this chapter. Look for examples in your workplace, among your own mail, or in other available sources.

CAUTION

All outgoing correspondence should be *proofread* (checking the document for errors). One of the most common errors when using spell-check software is a word that is spelled correctly, but has a different meaning than intended. An example is the word "for" when "four" was meant. Spell-check will not correct it, since it is an actual word, although the meanings of both words are very different. The exams contain questions regarding misspelling of words, usually associated with medical terminology. Formatting errors are also common; ensure that paragraphs are lined up properly and correct spacing used.

Electronic correspondence, especially e-mail, should be treated the same as hard copy correspondence. Always use formal and correct construction, never informal and casual construction or wording. E-mails are easily misunderstood and subject to subpoena. The patient's written permission should be obtained to send an e-mail.

BOX 12-1

Frequently misspelled words

abscess	ischium
aneurysm	larynx
arrhythmia	ophthalmology
bronchi (plural of bronchus*)	
cirrhosis	pharynx
curettage	pneumonia
hemorrhage	rheumatic
hemorrhoids	roentgenology
humerus	sphygmomanometer
ileum	*Staphylococcus*
ilium	tonsillitis
ischemia	

*Many Latin-based medical terms that end in "-us" for the singular form and in "-i" for the plural form. Fungus (plural fungi) is another example. Virus is *not* one (plural viruses).

MATERIALS

- Letterhead—quality bond stationery used for the first page of correspondence; contains the name of physician or group, address, telephone number, and e-mail address (if appropriate), usually at the top of the page; white, gray, or buff paper is most common

- Following pages—plain quality bond stationery that matches the letterhead

- Envelopes—no. 10 is the size most commonly used because it fits 8½ × 11 inch paper folded in thirds; should be made of quality bond paper that matches the letterhead used for letters; lower-quality envelopes with clear windows may be used for patient statements that are folded to exhibit patient's address through the window; no. 6 are commonly used for statements

- Resources—medical offices have various books and other sources, including the Internet, to ensure that the grammar, spelling, and format for correspondence are correct. Some helpful resources are given below:

  - Desk or electronic dictionary
  - Thesaurus (a book listing synonyms or words with like meanings for words)
  - Medical dictionary/encyclopedia (the exams usually have questions on misspelled words; see Box 12-1)
  - Writing style books
  - *Physicians' Desk Reference* (PDR)
  - Other medical reference books
  - Date stamp—used to imprint date received for all incoming mail

LETTERS

- Styles
  - Full block—all lines begin at left margin; this is the most common style (Fig. 12-1)
  - Modified block—subject and complimentary closing and signature begin at the middle of the paper; other lines begin at left margin
  - Semiblock (indented modified block)—subject and complimentary closing and signature begin in the center, and the first line of each paragraph is indented five spaces; all other lines begin at the left margin
  - Simplified—the greeting and complimentary closing are omitted; all lines begin at the left margin

- Components
  - Margins—the blank space or border around the text on a business letter; the standard margin is 1 inch
  - Date—placed 15 lines from top of page or 2 to 4 lines below letterhead; key in full date: January 1, 2015, not 01/01/2015
  - Inside addresses—the sender's address is located on the letterhead; the recipient's address referred to as the inside address, is keyed at the left margin; abbreviations in addresses should not be used except for the state
  - Salutation (greeting)—keyed at the left margin, two lines below the recipient's address, followed by a colon

Family Medical Practice Associates
7865 Union Avenue
Maintown, XY 12345

October 12, 2015

Mr. Henry O'Brien
9876 East 12th Street
Maintown, XY 12346

RE: Physician Changes

Dear Mr. O'Brien,

We wanted to inform you of some exciting physician changes at Family Medical Associates.
Dr. Henrique Ramirez, a graduate of Stanford Medical School, will be joining us. Dr. Ramirez
has been serving as a colonel in the United States Army Medical Corp for the past ten years with
duty in Irag, Germany and San Antonio. He recently completed special training in geriatric
medicine at Mount Sinai Medical Center in New York and has extensive experience in adult
medicine.

Sadly, in December, Dr. William Chen will be retiring. Dr. Chen is one of the founders of
Family Medical Associates; providing quality care, advice and love to thousands of children and
adults over the past 40 years.

Please join us for an open house to wish him well and celebrate this new phase in his life on
December 4, 2015 from 3:00 p.m. to 6:00 p.m. at the above address. Dr. Susan Watson and
Dr. Charles Patel will continue to serve you along with Dr. Ramirez and the dedicated staff at
Family Medical Associates. Our mission of excellence in health care remains firm.

Most Sincerely;

Jesse Smiley

Practice Administrator

JS/el

enclosure

FIGURE 12-1 Example of full block correspondence.

- Subject (optional)—topic of letter, keyed two lines below salutation, usually at the left margin; sometimes begins with "RE": ("regarding")
- Letter body—begins two lines below the salutation or the subject line; the position of the paragraph beginning depends on the style of the letter
- Complimentary closing—two lines below the last sentence of the letter body; if the closing contains more than one word, only the first word is capitalized
- Keyed signature—usually four lines below the complimentary closing; use titles before *or* after name, *not* both (e.g., Dr. James Jones or James Jones, MD, not Dr. James Jones, MD). This format is currently considered correct but as nurse practitioners and physical therapists with doctorates use the title "doctor," the suggested but not-yet-approved format, for example, is Dr. Amalia Drew, FNP (for Family Nurse Practitioner)
- Reference initials—two lines below keyed signature; the initials of the individual signing the letter in uppercase letters followed by a colon and the initials of the individual word processing the correspondence in lowercase letters
- Enclosures—two lines below the reference initials; indicates that other items are included with the letter; may simply state "enclosures," or it may be followed by a colon and the titles of the enclosed document(s)
- Copies—"cc": or "Cc": (computer software often automatically capitalizes the first "C") literally means *carbon copy*, but is still used to indicate that a copy of the document is being sent to the person whose name follows the "cc":; this notation is listed one or two lines below the reference initials; when more than one person is copied, the names are listed in alphabetic order
- Envelope addresses
  - Start address 14 lines down from top of envelope and 4 inches from left edge when using a no. 10 envelope
  - Do not use punctuation except the hyphen when using expanded zip codes
  - Use all uppercase letters

MAIL

- United States Postal Service (USPS) Classifications—different types of mailings require different postage and handling costs. Generally, the speedier the delivery is, the more expensive the postage. The following classifications are in order according to the cost (most expensive to least expensive) and the speed of delivery
- Certified Mail®—mail service with a verification from the postal service that the piece was mailed and arrived at the designated address; the sender, for an additional fee, may request a signature for the correspondence indicating who received it; the sender has the option to use the USPS's "NetPost" at www.usps.com or a USPS branch; a similar service is offered by private (FedEx, UPS, DHL) businesses
- Express Mail®—delivery guaranteed the following day
- Registered Mail™—first-class mail insured for a named value
- Priority Mail Express®—fastest USPS mail handling for items 70 pounds or less; usually takes 1 to 2 days to arrive, 365 days a year to most locations; prepackaging boxes and envelopes available
- Priority Mail®—mail handling for items 70 pounds or less; usually takes 2 to 3 days to arrive
- First-Class Mail®—postage generally used for office correspondence, including patient statements; weight must be 13 ounces or less
- Standard Mail (bulk)—postage used for advertisement, newsletters, flyers, and small parcels; requires a minimum of 200 pieces or 50 lbs of mail; formerly called second- and third-class mail
- Periodicals (formal postal authorization needed)—newspapers, magazines, and other periodic publications transmitting information to an established list of subscribers or requesters; lower rates are offered for nonprofits

- Mail payment methods
  - Stamps
  - Postage meter—purchased or leased printing machines or services that print postage directly onto mail pieces or labels; postage-metered envelopes do not need to be canceled and therefore save time; meter date is automatically or manually changed daily; postage meter services may be purchased online

- Private mail service options—often used for specimens and other time-sensitive items
  - Federal Express (FedEx)
  - United Parcel Services (UPS)
  - DHL especially for global delivery

- Incoming mail procedure
  - Check e-mail correspondence on a regular schedule
  - Acknowledge receipt of e-mails to the sender on the day they are opened and read; If the response must be researched, indicate that the email was received and you are looking into it
  - Stamp hard copy items with date received
  - Staple or paperclip original envelope to incoming mail piece
  - Stamp payment checks with endorsement

- Ensure all envelopes are empty before disposing of them
- Sort according to type (e.g., insurance payments, diagnostic reports)
- Check clinical mail for urgency
- Distribute mail, hard copy or e-mail, to appropriate staff
- Carry out any assigned functions related to the mail, such as posting payments

OTHER CORRESPONDENCE

Two other types of correspondence important to medical offices are memorandums and transcription. Questions on these topics may be on the national exam.

MEMORANDUMS

Interoffice correspondence is usually in the form of a *memorandum* (plural is *memorandums or memoranda*), or memo.

- Components
  - Date—the day the memo is written; placed 13 lines from top of the page, with a 1-inch side margin; left justified
  - To—the parties to whom the memo is directed; two lines below "Date" line
  - From—the name of the party sending the memo; two lines below "To" line
  - Subject—the topic of the memo; two lines below "From" line
  - Message—begins three lines below "Subject" line
- Distribution
  - Hard copy sent to individual staff members (less frequent)
  - Hard copy posted in office
  - Electronic mail

TRANSCRIPTION

Transcription is the conversion of the dictated word of the health-care provider to a word-processed form. Letters, reports, and patients' medical histories and treatments are the most common transcribed documents in the medical office. Transcribed documents involving the patient become part of the patient's medical record. The rules of confidentiality apply, including when these documents may be mailed to other entities.

The transcriber should always check with the health-care provider if in doubt about any portion of the document; never guess. The format used is based on the type of document and the facility preference.

The electronic medical record is replacing a significant amount of transcription.

TERMS

CORRESPONDENCE REVIEW

The following list reviews the terms discussed in this chapter and other important terms that you may see on the exam.

Certified Mail first-class mail with a verification from the postal service that the mail arrived at the designated address; the sender, for an additional fee, may request a receiver sign for the correspondence

Express Mail next-day delivery service

full block style of letter writing with all lines beginning at left margin; most common letter style

letterhead quality bond stationery used for the first page of correspondence; contains, usually at the top of the page, the name of the physician or group, address, telephone number, and e-mail address (if appropriate)

memorandum (plural *memorandums or memoranda*) memo; interoffice correspondence consisting of *date*, *to*, *from*, *subject*, and a message; may be hard copy or e-mail

modified block style of letter writing in which the subject, complimentary closing, and signature begin in the middle of the paper; all other lines begin at left margin

postage meter purchased or leased printing machines or services that print prepaid postage directly onto mail pieces or labels

Priority Mail faster delivery than first-class mail; usually takes 2 to 3 days

proofread checking the document for errors

Registered Mail first-class mail insured for a named value

semiblock (indented modified block) style of letter writing with the subject, complimentary closing, and signature beginning at the center; the first line of each paragraph is indented five spaces; all other lines begin at left margin

simplified style of letter writing with the greeting and complimentary closing omitted; all lines begin at left margin

Standard Mail (bulk) postage used for magazines, periodicals, newspapers, catalogs, and flyers; requires a minimum of 200 pieces; formerly called second- and third-class mail

transcription the conversion of the dictated word of the health-care provider into a word-processed form

REVIEW QUESTIONS

All questions are relevant for all medical assisting and medical administrative certification exams.

1. The most formal and professional style of letter format is:
   A. memorandum.
   B. semiblock.
   C. full block.
   D. indented block.

   Answer: **C**
   Why: The full block letter is written so that all the left margins are indented at 1 inch. This style has the most professional look.
   Review: Yes ○   No ○

2. The standard business envelope is a:
   A. no. 6.
   B. no. 9.
   C. no. 10.
   D. no. 12.
   E. no. 8.

   Answer: **C**
   Why: A no. 10 envelope is used for standard 8½ × 11 inch paper folded into thirds.
   Review: Yes ○   No ○

3. The punctuation mark following the salutation of a professional business letter is a:
   A. period.
   B. hyphen.
   C. comma.
   D. colon.

   Answer: **D**
   Why: The salutation is the opening of the letter, which is followed by a colon in a professional letter.
   Review: Yes ○   No ○

4. The standard margin used for a business letter is:
   A. ½ inch.
   B. 1 inch.
   C. 1½ inches.
   D. 2 inches.
   E. 2½ inches.

   Answer: **B**
   Why: One inch is used as the standard margin for all sides of a letter. The letter appears standardized and professional.
   Review: Yes ○   No ○

5. The component of a letter that indicates the purpose of the correspondence is the:
   A. subject line.
   B. enclosure.
   C. letterhead.
   D. salutation.

   Answer: **A**
   Why: The subject line introduces the main topic of the letter and begins with the abbreviation "RE" (short for "regarding") followed by a colon. The word "enclosure" is placed below the reference initials, indicating that there are other documents included with the letter. Letterhead is stationery with the sender's name and address at the top of the page.
   The salutation is the greeting of the letter.
   Review: Yes ○   No ○

6. Which of the following is true regarding the date on a business letter?
   A. The date includes the month and year only.
   B. The date is not necessary on a business letter.
   C. It is proper to abbreviate the date to save space.
   D. The date is placed on the same line as the inside address on the right of the paper.
   E. The date is placed two lines below the letterhead.

Answer: **E**
Why: The date the letter is written should be placed two lines below the letterhead.
Review: Yes ○   No ○

---

7. Certified Mail is also considered or classified as:
   A. First-Class Mail.
   B. Second-Class Mail.
   C. Third-Class Mail.
   D. Express Mail.

Answer: **A**
Why: Certified Mail is sent first class, and the sender can request verification that the mail piece was delivered to the recipient. Second-Class Mail was used to send items such as magazines, and Third-Class Mail was the same as bulk mail and was typically used to send promotional materials. (These types of mail are now called Standard Mail.) Express Mail is sent with a guarantee of next-day delivery.
Review: Yes ○   No ○

---

8. The mail classification used to send most medical office mail is:
   A. Priority Mail.
   B. Second-Class Mail.
   C. Express Mail.
   D. First-Class Mail.
   E. Standard Mail.

Answer: **D**
Why: First-Class Mail is used for most office correspondence, including letters and postcards. Priority Mail and Express Mail expedite the delivery. Second-Class Mail is now called Standard Mail, and it is primarily used for newsletters, bulletins, and advertisements.
Review: Yes ○   No ○

---

9. The style of letter in which all the lines begin at the left margin except the subject and complimentary closing is:
   A. modified block.
   B. semiblock.
   C. simplified.
   D. full block.

Answer: **A**
Why: The modified block is a style of letter that is less formal. The subject, complimentary closing, and signature lines begin at the center of the page, with all other lines beginning at the left margin.
Review: Yes ○   No ○

---

10. The proper style of writing the date in a professional letter is:
    A. 2015.
    B. Jan. 1, 2015.
    C. January 1, 2015.
    D. January 1, '15.
    E. January 01, '15.

Answer: **C**
Why: The proper date in a professional letter should be written out fully. The month is not abbreviated, and four digits are used for the year.
Review: Yes ○   No ○

11. How many lines below the salutation should the body of the letter start?
   A. One
   B. Two
   C. Three
   D. Four

Answer: **B**
Why: Two lines is the standard amount of space between the salutation and the body of the letter. This amount of space allows the salutation to be set apart from the body.
Review: Yes ○   No ○

12. An example of a properly keyed signature is:
   A. Dr. James Jones, MD.
   B. Dr. Jones, MD.
   C. James Jones, MD.
   D. Doctor Jones, MD.
   E. J. Jones, MD.

Answer: **C**
Why: It is not appropriate to use both the title "Dr." and the initials "MD" in the same title. You may use either one, but not both. The first name and the last name of the person signing the letter should be spelled out completely.
Review: Yes ○   No ○

13. The classification of mail that guarantees delivery the following day is:
   A. First-Class Mail.
   B. Certified Mail.
   C. Registered Mail.
   D. Express Priority Mail.

Answer: **D**
Why: Express Priority Mail will ensure that the delivery will arrive the next day. This service is more expensive than other types of mail classes, but offices rely on Express Mail for sending records and office correspondence that must arrive by the next day. Certified Mail and Registered Mail are used when the sender wants to have confirmation of delivery or have the mail delivered to a specific person. First-Class Mail is the most common type of delivery used for letters but has no guarantee of what day the mail will be delivered. Typically, it will take 2 to 3 days for most first-class mail to reach its destination.
Review: Yes ○   No ○

14. At the bottom of a professional letter, the reference initials represent:
   A. the individual processing the letter, in uppercase letters.
   B. the individual signing the letter, in uppercase letters.
   C. the individual signing the letter, in lowercase letters.
   D. only the individual processing the letter.
   E. the individual receiving the letter.

Answer: **B**
Why: The initials for both the individual signing the letter and the person who processed the letter are indicated. The uppercase initials belong to the individual signing the letter; the lowercase initials belong to the person who processed the letter.
Review: Yes ○   No ○

15. The abbreviation "cc": or "Cc":, when used at the end of a professional letter, means:
   A. there is an enclosure in the envelope with the letter.
   B. the letter was sent to another person.
   C. the physician requested a copy of the letter.
   D. there is a copy of another letter enclosed with this letter.

Answer: **B**
Why: The abbreviation "cc": means *carbon copy*. With computer processing, the abbreviation "cc": is also proper and means *correspondence copy*. This is used to indicate that a duplicate or copy of the letter has been sent. The abbreviation is placed at the bottom left margin of the letter. The name of the person follows the abbreviation (e.g., cc: James Jones, MD).
Review: Yes ○   No ○

16. When mail arrives at the office, the first step in processing the mail is to:
  A. record all insurance payments.
  B. distribute the mail to the appropriate staff members.
  C. review it with the physician.
  D. dispose of advertisements.
  E. date stamp each item of mail.

Answer: **E**
Why: Before anything else is done with the mail, the mail is opened and stamped with the current date. This records the date it was received by the office in case there is a question in the future about the arrival date of materials. After that, the medical assistant or medical administrative specialist can sort the mail and determine distribution of the remaining mail.
Review: Yes ○   No ○

17. The process of converting the dictated word of the health-care provider to a word-processed form is:
  A. dictation.
  B. recording.
  C. transcription.
  D. documentation.

Answer: **C**
Why: Transcription is the process of converting the health-care provider's dictated words to a word-processed form.
Review: Yes ○   No ○

18. The style of letter in which the first sentence of each paragraph is indented five spaces is:
  A. full block.
  B. modified block.
  C. semiblock.
  D. simplified.
  E. block.

Answer: **C**
Why: The semiblock style is similar to the modified block except the first sentence of each paragraph is indented five spaces. This style is less formal than the full block but more formal than a simplified letter. All of these types of letters use the block format.
Review: Yes ○   No ○

19. When a professional letter requires more than one page, the pages following the first page:
  A. are printed on embossed letterhead the same as the first page.
  B. are not numbered.
  C. do not include the date of the letter.
  D. are the same paper as the first page with no letterhead printing.

Answer: **D**
Why: A professional letter is processed on quality bond stationery with the first page containing the physician's name, address, and telephone number. All pages following the first page should contain the name of the person to whom the letter is addressed, the date of the letter, and the page number.
Review: Yes ○   No ○

20. The inside address of a professional letter is the:
  A. address of the sending group practice.
  B. recipient's address written with abbreviations to save space.
  C. physician's home address printed at the left margin.
  D. physician's office address.
  E. recipient's address written without abbreviations.

Answer: **E**
Why: The inside address is the address of the person or company to whom the letter is being sent. It should not contain any abbreviations.
Review: Yes ○   No ○

21. If there are materials included in the envelope with the letter, this should be noted:
   A. below the inside address.
   B. within the body of the letter only.
   C. two lines below the reference initials.
   D. four lines below the complimentary closing.

Answer: **C**

Why: If there are materials to be mailed with the letter, it should be noted by using the abbreviation "Enc." or the word "Enclosures" followed by the name of the document or the number if there is more than one.

Review: Yes ◯   No ◯

---

22. The classification of mail used for at least 200 pieces of promotional information is:
   A. Certified Mail.
   B. Second-Class Mail.
   C. Standard Mail.
   D. Registered Mail.
   E. Priority Mail.

Answer: **C**

Why: Standard Mail is also known as bulk mail. This is a classification used to mail promotional pieces such as flyers or brochures. There must be a minimum of 200 pieces to qualify for this class of mail.

Review: Yes ◯   No ◯

---

23. A postage meter is a:
   A. device used to weigh letters or packages.
   B. scale to determine the classification of mail for letters.
   C. machine that prints prepaid postage onto mail pieces or onto an approved label.
   D. machine used to scan zip codes.

Answer: **C**

Why: A postage meter is a postage-printing machine or system used in the home or office. Meters print postage directly onto mail pieces or onto an approved label that you affix to your mail piece.

Review: Yes ◯   No ◯

---

24. The keyed signature is typed:
   A. four lines below the complimentary closing.
   B. two lines before the return address.
   C. two lines after the reference line.
   D. four lines below the salutation.
   E. six lines below the salutation.

Answer: **A**

Why: The keyed signature is the typed full name of the person signing the letter. It is placed four lines below the complimentary closing to allow space for the handwritten signature.

Review: Yes ◯   No ◯

---

25. The letterhead on stationery should include the following *except* the:
   A. physician's name.
   B. office address and office telephone number.
   C. physician's home telephone number.
   D. medical group's name.

Answer: **C**

Why: The physician's personal information should not appear on professional business stationery used for office correspondence. The physician's home telephone number is private and usually unlisted.

Review: Yes ◯   No ◯

CRITICAL THINKING CASE REVIEW QUESTIONS

Jules, the medical administrative specialist in the Family Medical Associates practice, has been attempting to inform Ms. Rodriquez of an abnormal diagnostic test. After sending a letter by first-class mail and leaving phone messages, Jules decides to e-mail the patient.

1. Prior to e-mailing the patient, the CMAS should verify that:
   A. the patient has an e-mail.
   B. the physician approves the e-mail.
   C. the diagnostic test is available as an attachment.
   D. the patient's phone number and e-mail were correct.
   E. the patient's written consent for e-mail was obtained.

   Answer: **E**
   Why: A, B, and D are also correct, but E is the best answer. Written consent from the patient to send an e-mail should be obtained.
   Review: Yes ○   No ○

2. In addition to a brief message, Jules attaches a copy of the positive diagnostic report which indicates a serious illness. This attachment:
   A. is standard procedure.
   B. assures the patient understands the severity.
   C. is inappropriate.
   D. is in accordance with HIPAA.

   Answer: **C**
   Why: When diagnostic tests are abnormal, the common practice is for either the physician or midlevel provider to notify the patient or for the MA or CMAS to set up an appointment with the patient so the physician can explain the results and the recommendations; since the diagnostic test is also part of the medical record and most home e-mails do not have the firewalls for security required by HIPAA, it is a violation to send it in this manner.
   Review: Yes ○   No ○

3. When no response was received from the first-class letter or the phone calls, the next step should have been to send a letter by:
   A. Priority mail.
   B. Priority Express Mail.
   C. Registered mail.
   D. UPS.
   E. Federal Express.

   Answer: **C**
   Why: Registered mail verifies that the letter reached the intended address and indicates the name and signature of the person who actually received it. This assures the letter is not sitting in the back of a mailbox and that someone at the address has it. If the letter is returned or an unknown person signs for it, that is a strong indication that the person is no longer at that address. In this case, the next action might be to call the emergency contact which should be in the medical record or send an e-mail, if there is permission, asking the patient to call the office using the same language that would be in a letter if a diagnostic test was abnormal.
   Review: Yes ○   No ○

4. Ms. Rodriquez received the e-mail with the results of the diagnostic test attached; she assumed that the word "positive" in the results was a good thing and did not pursue further contact with the medical office until her disease was quite progressed. The practice:

A. is not libel since several attempts were made to contact the patient and documented in the medical record.

B. is libel based on the four "Ds" of malpractice.

C. is not libel since the patient signed an agreement to follow her care plan when she became a patient.

D. is libel since HIPAA was violated.

Answer: **B**

Why: D is also correct, but the better answer is B. The practice had a **duty** to assure that the patient was informed of and understood the results of the diagnostic test. The office was **derelict** in this duty by not following standard procedure. **Damage** was sustained by the patient with progression of the disease without treatment. The **direct cause** was the attachment of the diagnostic test which was misunderstood by the patient (Chapter 4: Law and Ethics).

Review: Yes ○   No ○

5. After this incident, it became clear that the practice was in need of a policy regarding the correct usages and content of e-mail; this comes under the category of:

A. Negligence.

B. Professional Communication.

C. Correspondence.

D. HIPAA.

E. Risk Management.

Answer: **E**

Why: To some extent, all the answers are correct, but the best answer is E, Risk Management, which is a process to routinely assess, identify, correct, and monitor any potential hazards or risks to prevent harm and loss (Chapter 4, Law and Ethics).

Review: Yes ○   No ○

13

Medical Insurance

The intent of medical insurance is to provide financial protection for costs associated with sickness or injury. Because of the complex American social and health systems, the types of medical insurance and payers are varied and dependent on eligibility criteria.

Health care is one of the few services paid for by a party other than the one receiving the actual service. The insurance company, responsible governmental agency or private entity is known as the *third-party payer*—the party that pays the second party (doctor, hospital, pharmacy, etc.) for the medical bills of the first party (patient or insured individual). The term *third-party administrator* is sometimes used.

This chapter is organized differently from previous chapters. The types and sources of insurance are described with information that has "exam probability." The "Terms" section contains the remaining materials and definitions for medical insurance. *Do not skip it.*

COMMON TYPES OF MEDICAL INSURANCE PLANS

An insurance company (carrier), whether private or governmental, may offer all common plan types or a hybrid of multiple types. The medical assistant and medical administrative specialist must know not only the insurance company but also the type of plan covering the patient. Each plan has different costs and benefits to the patient and different payments to the health-care provider.

- **Health maintenance organization (HMO)**—a form of managed care organization (MCO), an association that is designed to provide all care (specialty care or care not available within the MCO or HMO may be referred out) to the insured person for a fixed fee, usually paid for by the insured or employer through a monthly premium; a co-payment may or may not be required

- **Indemnity**—private plan through which the insured person or the insured's employer selects his or her own health-care plan; an established amount or percentage of care costs is paid by the insurance plan on a fee-for-service basis to the provider; usually has deductibles and limits

- **Preferred provider organization (PPO)**—a list of physicians, hospitals, and other health-care services approved by the insurance plan to provide these services at a discounted rate and usually without a referral to specialists within the PPO

- **Major medical**—type of insurance that does not cover primary care, but covers costs associated with significant illness or injury (e.g., hospitalization, surgeries); premiums are lower than full-coverage insurance

SOURCES OF MEDICAL INSURANCE

The two major sources of insurance in the United States are the private sector and governmental agencies. The 2012 census reported approximately 55% of Americans were covered by private insurance, the majority are employer-based; 33% are covered by a governmental insurance and the remainder uninsured (you do not need to know these numbers).

COMMERCIAL PLANS

Commercial plans are for-profit companies that provide health insurance for a fee to individuals or groups; Blue Cross and Blue Shield is perhaps the most widely known. The cost may be totally provided by an employer, jointly funded by the employer and the employee or totally funded by an individual.

- **Individual plan**—coverage provided for a person and eligible dependents when premiums are made and designated criteria are met

- **Group plan**—generally associated with employment; coverage provided for employee and usually dependents for an additional charge; premiums may be paid by employer or shared with the employee

  - Eligibility—dependent on company and plan

  - Benefits—covered services dependent on plan selection, premiums, and eligibility criteria

- **Medigap**—also called Medicare Supplement Insurance, but it is a *commercial medical insurance* intended to cover Medicare deductible, coinsurance, and other uncovered items

GOVERNMENTAL PLANS

A variety of governmental plans are offered dependent on the eligibility and funding source. Some plans are totally funded by the government such as Medicaid and others are funded through individual contributions through payroll taxes such as Medicare.

- **Medicare**—federal insurance program established in 1965 under the Social Security Act (Title 18) and administered by the Centers for Medicare and Medicaid Services (CMS), formerly called HCFA; primarily designed for eligible citizens aged 65 years and older

  - Eligibility

    - Persons and spouses of persons aged 65 years or older who are eligible for Social Security benefits by contributing to the plan directly or through a spouse or parent

    - Railroad workers who receive disability pensions and meet criteria

    - Persons receiving Social Security disability benefits for 24 months

    - Persons with end-stage kidney disease who have contributed to Social Security

  Note: eligibility through a disability is often an exam question.

  - Benefits

    - Part A—benefit is automatic when eligibility and deductible are met; covers hospital inpatient costs, hospice, limited nursing facility stays, and home health

    - Part B—optional benefit; requires premiums, deductibles, and coinsurance; covers physician costs, outpatient services, durable medical equipment, and medical supplies; the premium is determined by insured's income from previous tax year

    - Part C—formerly called Medicare 1 Choice, now referred to as Medicare Advantage; requires participants to be covered under both Medicare Part A and Medicare Part B; allows participant to choose a Medicare Advantage plan, which is HMO-type coverage

- Part D—optional benefit; covers approved pharmaceuticals
  - Advanced Beneficiary Notice of Noncoverage (ABN)—notification to the beneficiary (person insured by Medicare) of their potential liability for payment of services under certain conditions that are not covered or approved for payment by Medicare, frequency of coverage such as a maximum number of glucose tests that will be approved for payment within a specific time frame is an example.

- **Medicaid**—federal insurance program established in 1965 under the Social Security Act (Title 19) and administered by the CMS, formerly called HCFA; eligibility, benefits, and name differ from state to state (e.g., in California, it is called MediCal); provides health coverage for the categorically needy
  - Eligibility—low-income (calculated as a percentage of poverty level, which differs by state) families and individuals who are citizens or, in some cases, select refugees and immigrants
  - Benefits—minimum benefits are mandated by the federal government, and other benefits are defined by the states; minimum medically necessary benefits include the following:
    - Primary care
    - Early, periodic screening, diagnosis, and treatment (EPSDT) for children
    - Hospitalizations
    - Outpatient services
    - Family planning
    - Skilled nursing facilities (SNFs)
  - **Medi/Medi** (dual eligibility)—persons eligible for both Medicare and Medicaid; Medicaid is *always* the payer of last resort

- **CHIP** (Children's Health Insurance Program)—provides health insurance coverage for children under 19 years of age in families who are not eligible for Medicaid but cannot afford private coverage
  - Eligibility—for children above the federal minimums with family income at or below the Federal Poverty Level (FPL) which is updated annually
  - Benefits—minimum benefits are mandated by the federal government, and other benefits are defined by the states; minimum medically necessary benefits include the following:
    - Inpatient and outpatient hospital services
    - Physician's services
    - Surgical and medical services
    - Laboratory and X-ray services
    - Well-baby and well-child care, including immunizations

- **TRICARE**—formerly CHAMPUS; offers three health-care benefit plans sponsored by the federal government, primarily for spouses and dependents of servicemen and -women
  - TRICARE Standard—program under TRICARE that automatically enrolls all eligible beneficiaries
  - TRICARE Prime—PPO-type TRICARE option with an annual deductible
  - TRICARE Extra—HMO-type TRICARE option with an annual deductible and co-pays
  - Eligibility
    - Spouses and dependents of active military personnel
    - Military retirees, spouses, and dependents
    - Spouses and dependents of deceased active or retired military personnel
    - Former spouses of active or retired military personnel who meet requirements
    - Spouses, former spouses, and dependents of court-martialed active-duty service personnel
    - Spouses, former spouses, and dependents of retirement-eligible military personnel who lost eligibility as a result of child or spousal abuse
    - Other select individuals
  - Benefits
    - Hospitalization
    - Maternity care
    - Inpatient and outpatient treatment for mental illness
    - Physician services
    - Diagnostic testing
    - Emergency services, including ambulances
    - Family planning
    - Durable medical equipment
    - Home health care

Note: the name of the coverage for military retirees is often a question.

- **CHAMPVA** (Civilian Health and Medical Program of the Veterans Administration)—a service benefit program with no premiums for select family members of specific veterans
  - Eligibility
    - Spouses and dependents of military personnel with permanent, total, service-related disability
    - Spouses and dependents of military personnel who died from a service-related disability
  - Benefits—the same as TRICARE Standard

- **Workers' compensation**—medical and disability insurance that covers employees in the event of a work-related injury, illness, or death
  - Eligibility
    - Federal coverage—federal employees, coal miners, and maritime workers

○ State coverage—all workers not covered by federal statutes

- Benefits
  ○ Medical treatment related to work associated illness or disability, including prostheses
  ○ Temporary disability payments
  ○ Permanent disability payments
  ○ Death benefits to survivors

THE HEALTH INSURANCE PORTABILITY AND ACCOUNTABILITY ACT

In addition to the other components of the Health Insurance Portability and Accountability Act (HIPAA) covered in previous chapters, the United States Department of Labor cites the act

- Limits the ability of a new employer plan to exclude coverage for preexisting conditions

- Provides additional opportunities to enroll in a group health plan if you lose other coverage or experience certain life events

- Prohibits discrimination against employees and their dependent family members based on any health factors they may have, including prior medical conditions, previous claims experience, and genetic information

- Guarantees that certain individuals will have access to, and can renew, individual health insurance policies

THE PATIENT PROTECTION AND AFFORDABLE CARE ACT

Passed in 2010, the act's full name is the Patient Protection and Affordable Care Act, but it is commonly known as the Affordable Care Act (ACA). The intent was to reform the United States health-care system, and it encompasses 10 complex major areas called "titles." While some issues remain unresolved at the time of this writing (Fig. 13-1), the basic points of the act

- Require nearly everyone to obtain health insurance beginning 2014 or be subject to a fine

- Establish minimum standards for health insurance plans, including preventive care

- Prohibit health insurers from rejecting persons with preexisting conditions or charging different rates due to patients' medical histories or gender

- Expand Medicaid to increase Medicaid eligibility to 133% of the FPL

- Establish Web-based health insurance exchanges or "marketplaces" for the public to compare policies and rates

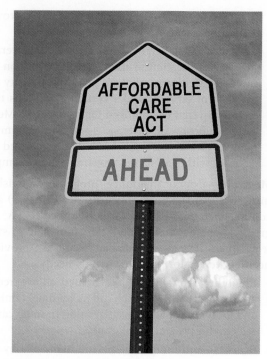

FIGURE 13-1 Affordable Care Act road sign.

- Impose an excise tax on medical devices

- Impose a limit on contributions to flexible spending accounts (FSAs)

- Impose on income tariff on persons in higher wage brackets

COMMON METHODS OF DETERMINING INSURANCE PAYMENT

- Fee schedule—list of a physician's customary charges; the basis for contracted discounts

- Resource-based relative value system or scale (RBRVS)—a method used to establish physician fees for specific medical services by assigning worth to a relative value unit (RVU); geographic-specific (Box 13-1)

  - RVU—a component (e.g., time) that is multiplied by a monetary conversion factor to establish physician payment; it includes the physician's
    ○ Service
    ○ Overhead
    ○ Cost of malpractice insurance
  - Relative value studies (RVS)—relative values listed by health-care procedure codes; allow comparison of reimbursement for different codes

- Usual, customary, and reasonable (UCR)—a method sometimes used by insurance carriers to establish

BOX 13-1

Breaking down relative value reimbursement

RBRVS = the **system** for reimbursement
(resource-based relative value system)

RVS = the list of **procedures** with the (relative) value for each
(relative value studies)

RVU = the **component** that is multiplied by a factor to determine the (relative) value ($)
(relative value unit)

provider payments based on a fee compendium of other like providers; in many cases replaced by the RBRVS

- Prevailing fee—the UCR fees of like providers in the same geographic area

■ **Co-payment**—a set amount owed by the insured at the time of service; routine waiving of co-payment by the medical office is against federal guidelines for Medicare and Medicaid; sometimes referred to as *co-insurance* which is not correct

■ **Coinsurance**—a percent of the covered insurance payment owed by the individual to the provider for the service

■ **Capitation**—payment made to a provider based on a fixed amount per enrollee assigned to that provider regardless of services provided

■ **Diagnostic-related groups (DRG)**—a classification of diagnoses used to determine hospital payment for Medicare inpatients; this method does not take into account length of stay (LOS)

■ **Preauthorization/Precertification**—under some health plans, individuals are required to receive advance authorization from the insurance provider for particular medical services; usually required for referral to a physician specialist

ELECTRONIC HEALTH-CARE CLAIMS

■ Claims are transmitted electronically from the provider's computer to the Medicare contractor's computer

■ When submitting electronic claims, the provider must use a computer with software that meets electronic filing requirements and national standards established under HIPAA

■ Claims are reviewed by the Medicare contractor for accuracy of submission, and the entire batch of submitted claims may be denied and returned for correction even if one claim is found with an area of noncompliance with submission standards (referred to as a dirty claim)

TERMS

MEDICAL INSURANCE REVIEW

The following list reviews the terms discussed in this chapter and other important terms that you may see on the exam.

Advanced Beneficiary Notice of Noncoverage (ABN) notification to the beneficiary (insured by Medicare) of their potential liability for payment of services under certain conditions that are not covered or approved for payment by Medicare

assignment of benefits authorization for the insurance company to send insurance payments directly to the health-care provider; also, an agreement with Medicare that the provider will accept the remittance as full payment

beneficiary a person eligible to receive insurance benefits

birthday rule a method used to determine the primary insurance carrier when children are covered under both parents' insurance plans; the parent whose birthday falls earliest in the calendar year becomes the primary carrier

capitation a health-care insurance payment made to a provider based on a fixed amount per enrollee assigned to that provider, regardless of services provided

carrier insurance company that provides the policy and benefits

CHAMPVA (Civilian Health and Medical Program of the Veterans Administration) a service benefit program with no premiums for select family members of specific, usually not retired, veterans

CHIP (Children's Health Insurance Program) provides health insurance coverage for children under 19 years of age in families who are not eligible for Medicaid but cannot afford private coverage

coinsurance a percentage of costs contractually assumed by the insured party; differs from co-payment

co-payment a set amount owed to the provider by the insured at the time of service; may be referred to as *coinsurance* which is not correct

deductible an established dollar amount of actual costs of medical services that must be paid by the insured party before the insurance carrier will cover costs; usually applies every year

dependent a person covered under the primary insured's policy

diagnostic-related groups (DRG) a classification of diagnoses used to determine hospital payment for Medicare inpatients

exclusion conditions or circumstances that are not covered under the insurance plan

explanation of benefits (EOB) a claim summary indicating what services were covered, what was not covered, and why; also referred to as *remittance advice*

fee for service a payment made to the health-care provider for each service rendered

fee schedule a list of a physician's customary charges; the basis for insurance companies to discount fees

health-care insurance exchange also called the "marketplace," Web-based organizations for persons to obtain information and sign up for health insurance plans under the ACA

health maintenance organization (HMO) an association that provides all care to the insured person for a fixed fee, usually paid for by the insured or employer through a monthly premium; a co-payment may or may not be required

indemnity a private plan through which the insured person or the insured's employer selects his or her own health plan; an established amount or percentage of care cost is paid by the insurance plan on a fee-for-service basis to the provider; usually has deductibles and limits

major medical a type of insurance that does not cover primary care but covers costs associated with significant illness or injury, such as hospitalization or surgeries; premiums are lower than full-coverage insurance

managed care organization (MCO) a system that requires the patient to go to specific health-care providers, including but not limited to doctors, hospitals, and diagnostic facilities

marketplace Web-based health insurance exchanges for the public to compare policies and rates

Medicaid provides health coverage for the categorically needy; a federal insurance program established in 1965 under the Social Security Act (Title 19) and administered by the Centers for Medicare and Medicaid Services (CMS), formerly called HCFA; eligibility, benefits, and name differ from state to state (e.g., in California, it is called MediCal)

Medicare primarily for people older than 65 and others eligible for Social Security; federal insurance program established in 1965 under the Social Security Act (Title 18) and administered by the Centers for Medicare and Medicaid Services (CMS), formerly called HCFA

Patient Protection and Affordable Care Act more commonly known as the Affordable Care Act (ACA) enacted 2010 with the intent of reforming the health-care system and requiring most citizens to carry health-care insurance or pay a fine

point of service facility where the health-care service took place (e.g., physician's office, emergency department)

preauthorization process of obtaining approval for a service through the individual's insurance company by establishing that it is a medical necessity

precertification process of determining whether a service is covered under the insured person's plan

predetermination a process of ascertaining the amount the insurance carrier will pay for a specific service

preexisting condition a diagnosed and treated health condition that the patient had before obtaining insurance

preferred provider organization (PPO) a plan allowing the insured person to select physicians, hospitals, and other health-care services from an approved list issued by the insurance plan to provide care at a discounted rate

premium a dollar amount the insured person pays for insurance coverage

prevailing fee the usual, customary, and reasonable fees of like providers in the same geographic area

primary care provider (PCP) physician contracted through a specific insurance plan to provide or to coordinate the care of all patients assigned through the insurance carrier

quality improvement organization (QIO) formerly called a peer review organization (PRO); group of professionals who monitor health-care treatments, length of hospital stays (LOS), outcomes, and other indicators for appropriateness and improvement opportunities

relative value studies (RVS) relative values listed by health-care procedure codes; allows comparison of reimbursement for different codes

relative value unit (RVU) the component (e.g., time) that is multiplied by a monetary conversion factor to establish physician payment for the resource-based relative value system or scale

resource-based relative value system/scale (RBRVS) a system that calculates physician reimbursement for services using relative value units (RVUs); geographic-specific

Temporary Assistance to Needy Families (TANF) formerly known as Assistance to Families with Dependent Children (AFDC); the federal welfare program

third-party payer the entity (usually the insurance company) that pays the second party (doctor, hospital, pharmacy, etc.) for the medical bills of the first party (patient or insured individual); also referred to as the *third-party administrator*

TRICARE formerly CHAMPUS; health-care benefit plans provided by the federal government, primarily for spouses and dependents of servicemen and women and retired military

usual, customary, and reasonable (UCR) a method used by insurance carriers to establish provider payments based on a compendium of other like provider fees

utilization review a process of reviewing and monitoring a provider's usage of health-care resources for appropriateness and comparison with peers

waiting period the time an individual is required to wait before being eligible for insurance benefits

waiver a special policy provision that forgoes a stipulation or requirement

workers' compensation medical and disability insurance to cover employees in the event of a work-related injury, illness, or death

REVIEW QUESTIONS

All questions are relevant for all medical assisting and medical administrative certification exams.

1. When a patient gives written authorization for reimbursement to the physician for billed charges, this is called:
   A. coordination of benefits.
   B. capitation.
   C. assignment of benefits.
   D. co-payment.

   Answer: **C**
   Why: Assignment of benefits is necessary if the physician agrees to wait for payment from the insurance company for billed charges.
   Review: Yes ○   No ○

2. Coordination of benefits means:
   A. the patient pays a specific amount of money for medical services before the insurance pays.
   B. one insurance plan will work with other insurance plans to determine how much each plan pays.
   C. there is a flat fee paid for each service.
   D. there is a deductible required by the patient before payment from the insurance is made.
   E. each insurance company will pay an equal amount of the patient's bill.

   Answer: **B**
   Why: Some patients have more than one benefit or insurance plan. Usually, there is a primary carrier, and the other becomes the secondary. The primary carrier determines an amount it will pay on a claim, and the secondary carrier will then determine the amount of the remaining balance that it will pay.
   Review: Yes ○   No ○

3. The person who is covered by a benefits plan is the:
   A. employee.
   B. carrier.
   C. administrator.
   D. insured.

   Answer: **D**
   Why: The insured is the person who is covered by the insurance benefits. This person could be an employee, but this would have to involve an employer-sponsored benefits plan. An administrator and a carrier are persons involved directly with the insurance provider.
   Review: Yes ○   No ○

4. A person's spouse or child who is covered under the benefits plan is called the:
   A. group member.
   B. coinsured.
   C. primary carrier.
   D. carrier.
   E. dependent.

   Answer: **E**
   Why: The dependent is related to the group member, the primary person covered, either as a family member or as an employee.
   Review: Yes ○   No ○

5. The amount that will be paid by the insurance plan for each procedure or service is based on the:

A. coinsurance.
B. capitation.
C. deductible.
D. fee schedule.

Answer: **D**

Why: A fee schedule is a list of a physician's customary charges, which are used to determine insurance plan–specific discounts. Coinsurance refers to the portion the patient is responsible for after the benefit plan pays a percentage of the eligible benefits and the member pays the deductible. Capitation is a system of payment used by managed care plans and refers to a fixed, per capita amount for each patient enrolled over a stated period. The deductible is the amount the insured must pay each calendar year before the plan begins to pay benefits.

Review: Yes ○   No ○

6. A government-sponsored program that provides health benefits to low-income or indigent persons is:

A. CHAMPUS.
B. CHAMPVA.
C. Medicare.
D. Medicaid.
E. Blue Cross and Blue Shield.

Answer: **D**

Why: Medicare, CHAMPUS, and CHAMPVA are all government-sponsored insurance programs, but only Medicaid determines eligibility based on income. States typically use the same criteria as their state welfare assistance programs. Blue Cross and Blue Shield is an independent health insurer.

Review: Yes ○   No ○

7. Expenses resulting from work-related illness or injury are usually covered by:

A. Medicare.
B. HMOs.
C. workers' compensation.
D. employee's health insurance.

Answer: **C**

Why: Employees in every state are covered by a workers' compensation program administered by the state. Medicare is a federal insurance program, primarily for people older than 65. A HMO is an association that provides all care to the insured person for a fixed fee. Employee's health insurance refers to an insurance program that an employee may voluntarily enroll in, but that does not usually cover illness or injury determined to be work-related.

Review: Yes ○   No ○

8. The statement issued to the provider and the patient that lists the details of a payment that has been made by the insurance plan is the:

A. fee schedule.
B. coordination of benefits.
C. assignment of benefits.
D. explanation of benefits.
E. deductible.

Answer: **D**

Why: The explanation of benefits (EOB), also known as remittance advice (RA), tells how the payment was made, including the deductible and coinsurance information. The EOB statement may show several claims that have processed during a particular period. A fee schedule is a list of a physician's customary charges. Coordination of benefits occurs when a person has insurance coverage from more than one company. The primary carrier will work with other insurance plans to determine how much each plan pays. Assignment of benefits occurs when a patient gives written authorization for reimbursement to the physician for billed charges. The deductible is an established dollar amount of actual costs of medical services that must be paid by the insured party before the insurance carrier will cover costs.

Review: Yes ○   No ○

9. If a patient is diagnosed with a disease before the effective date of the insurance plan, it is a(n):
    A. preexisting condition.
    B. crossover claim.
    C. exclusion.
    D. capitation.

Answer: **A**

Why: A preexisting condition is any illness or disease that was diagnosed before the effective date of the insurance plan. A typical illness that may be considered preexisting is cancer.

Review: Yes ◯   No ◯

10. The amount of eligible charges each patient must pay each calendar year before the plan begins to pay benefits is called:
    A. coinsurance.
    B. exclusion.
    C. eligibility.
    D. capitation.
    E. deductible.

Answer: **E**

Why: It is the patient's responsibility to pay the deductible amount before the insurance benefits will pay a percentage of the allowable charges. Most deductible amounts are between $1,500 and $2,500 per patient per year.

Review: Yes ◯   No ◯

11. Medicare is a federal health insurance program for:
    A. anyone over 62 years of age.
    B. disabled workers who are at least 65 years of age.
    C. blind individuals who are at least 50 years of age.
    D. individuals 65 years of age or older and are eligible for social security benefits.

Answer: **D**

Why: any individual who is 65 years of age or older who is retired and on Social Security or who retired from a railroad or civil service is eligible for Medicare. Blind and disabled individuals receiving Social Security benefits have no age restrictions.

Review: Yes ◯   No ◯

12. Medicare Part A provides coverage for:
    A. clinical laboratory services.
    B. physician's office services.
    C. hospitalization.
    D. physician's hospital services.
    E. outpatient referral fee for a specialist.

Answer: **C**

Why: Medicare Part A primarily covers the cost of inpatient hospitalization for the hospital room and board, general nursing, and hospital services and supplies. All of the physician's charges are covered under Part B.

Review: Yes ◯   No ◯

13. The process of determining whether a service or procedure is covered by the insurance provider is called:
    A. coordination of benefits.
    B. precertification.
    C. capitation.
    D. assignment of benefits.

Answer: **B**

Why: Contacting the insurance carrier for precertification determines whether the patient's insurance company will pay for a specific service or procedure. The patient may still be responsible for a portion of the charges after the insurance plan has paid a percentage of the charges. If the carrier does not precertify the service or procedure, the patient may be responsible for all the charges.

Review: Yes ◯   No ◯

14. The medical bills of spouses and children of veterans with total, permanent, service-connected disabilities are covered under:
   A. Blue Cross.
   B. HMO.
   C. workers' compensation.
   D. HCFA.
   E. CHAMPVA.

Answer: **E**
Why: The Civilian Health and Medical Program of the Veterans Administration (CHAMPVA) is a federal government–sponsored insurance that covers veterans' spouses and children. Blue Cross and Blue Shield is a private insurance company; a HMO is a type of insurance plan. Workers' compensation covers a patient who has a work-related illness or injury. HCFA is the Health Care Finance Administration (now called the Centers for Medicare and Medicaid Services, or CMS).
Review: Yes ○   No ○

15. The process of making a payment to a provider based on a fixed amount per enrollee assigned to that provider regardless of services provided is:
   A. exclusion.
   B. deductible.
   C. capitation.
   D. predetermination.

Answer: **C**
Why: Capitation is the process of paying a provider based on an established amount per person enrolled in the plan regardless of services rendered.
Review: Yes ○   No ○

16. A group of physicians who review cases for appropriateness of hospitalizations and discharges is called:
   A. relative value studies.
   B. preferred provider organization.
   C. quality improvement organization.
   D. third-party payer.
   E. state medical board.

Answer: **C**
Why: Physicians and specialists review cases from hospitalizations to determine whether the patient's care was provided in the most cost-effective setting. Many inpatient procedures are performed on an outpatient basis to save the patient excessive charges from an inpatient stay. The quality improvement organization (QIO), formerly referred to as the peer review organization (PRO), evaluates cases to ensure the procedures are necessary and cost-effective.
Review: Yes ○   No ○

17. A health maintenance organization is best described as:
   A. a group of physicians who have a contract to provide services to participating patients for a predetermined fee.
   B. independently practicing physicians providing services to patients covered under all types of insurance.
   C. a group of physicians who are partners in the same corporation.
   D. a group of physicians who specialize in wellness.

Answer: **A**
Why: A HMO (health maintenance organization) comprises physicians who work under contract to provide services to the subscribers of the plan. The plan is set up on a contracted fee-for-service basis, also known as capitation.
Review: Yes ○   No ○

18. A calculation of charges for each procedure indicating the charge of the majority of physicians in a geographic area is referred to as:
    A. utilization review.
    B. resource-based relative value system
    C. coordination of benefits.
    D. explanation of benefits.
    E. capitation.

Answer: **B**
Why: Resource-based relative value system (RBRVS) refers to a calculation which includes the typical charges for physician services in a specific geographic area. Charges that exceed the RBRVS limit are considered unreasonable and are not eligible for reimbursement.
Review: Yes ○   No ○

19. Medicare Part B does not cover:
    A. physician office visits.
    B. diagnostic laboratory services.
    C. hospitalization.
    D. outpatient X-rays.

Answer: **C**
Why: Part A of Medicare covers hospital charges and services except for the physician charges that are covered under Part B.
Review: Yes ○   No ○

20. Health benefits policies are purchased by an individual by paying the:
    A. premium.
    B. deductible.
    C. co-payment.
    D. coinsurance.
    E. exclusion.

Answer: **A**
Why: A premium is an annual amount charged by the insurance plan to enroll an individual for the health benefits of the policy. When an employee subscribes to health insurance through his or her workplace, a portion of the premium may be taken directly from each paycheck.
Review: Yes ○   No ○

21. A primary care physician, or PCP, is:
    A. only authorized to accept assignment of benefits.
    B. a specialist who accepts referral patients.
    C. not authorized to accept Medicare patients.
    D. a general practitioner who takes care of the routine medical needs of patients including wellness services.

Answer: **D**
Why: A PCP may be a general practitioner, pediatrician, family practitioner, or general internist who refers patients to see specialists for services as needed.
Review: Yes ○   No ○

22. A condition or circumstance for which the health insurance policy will not provide benefits is a(n):
    A. benefit.
    B. exclusion.
    C. review.
    D. waiting period.
    E. capitation.

Answer: **B**
Why: An exclusion is any condition or circumstance that is not covered by the insurance plan. For example, some insurance plans do not cover cosmetic surgical procedures.
Review: Yes ○   No ○

23. Insurance coverage that provides a specific monthly or weekly income when an individual becomes unable to work because of an illness or injury is:
   A. workers' compensation insurance.
   B. disability income insurance.
   C. TRICARE insurance.
   D. major medical insurance.

Answer: **B**
Why: Disability income insurance provides temporary or permanent income during a period when an individual cannot work because of illness or injury. This is not to be confused with workers' compensation insurance, which provides coverage of medical costs and in some cases, limited disability income incurred from work-related injuries or illness. TRICARE is an insurance plan for spouses and dependents of service men and women provided by the federal government. Major medical insurance covers the costs associated with significant illness or injury, but it does not provide income for an individual if he or she is unable to work.
Review: Yes ◯   No ◯

24. The amount of money owed by the insured to the provider at the time of service is called:
   A. capitation.
   B. exclusion.
   C. fee for service.
   D. indemnity.
   E. co-payment.

Answer: **E**
Why: A co-payment; it refers to the set amount of money that the patient is responsible to pay to the provider at the time of service.
Review: Yes ◯   No ◯

25. When a dependent child is covered by the benefit plans of both parents, determination of the primary carrier is based on the:
   A. coordination of benefits.
   B. coinsurance.
   C. assignment of benefits.
   D. birthday rule.

Answer: **D**
Why: The birthday rule is based on which parent's birthday falls earliest in the calendar year. The insurance plan carried by that parent becomes the primary carrier.
Review: Yes ◯   No ◯

26. In order to be eligible for Medicare Part C, the participant must be enrolled in
   A. Medicare Part B and Medicare Part D.
   B. a HMO plan.
   C. Medicare Part A and Medicare Part B.
   D. Medicaid.
   E. Medigap.

Answer: **C**
Why: Medicare Part C requires participants to be covered under both Medicare Part A and Medicare Part B. Medicare Part C allows the participant to choose a Medicare Advantage plan, which is HMO-type coverage. Enrollment in a HMO is not a criterion for eligibility for Medicare Part C. Medigap is a supplement to Medicare insurance that assists with the payment of coinsurance, co-payments, or deductibles.

27. The Medicare part specifically designed to provide pharmaceutical coverage is:
   A. Part A.
   B. Part B.
   C. Part C.
   D. Part D.

Answer: **D**
Why: Part A primarily covers hospitalization, Part B primarily covers outpatient care, Part C is HMO-type coverage, and Part D is designed to provide pharmaceutical coverage.
Review: Yes ◯   No ◯

28. A hospital payment system that categorizes patients by diagnosis and treatment is referred to as:
    A. ICD.
    B. CPT.
    C. UCR.
    D. HCPCS.
    E. DRG.

Answer: **E**
Why: Diagnosis-related groups (DRGs) are established by a comparison of patients with medically related diagnoses or treatments.
Review: Yes ○   No ○

---

29. UCR provider payments are based on:
    A. what the majority of physicians in a specific geographic area charge for procedures.
    B. state laws where the physician practices medicine.
    C. the maximum amount paid by other insurance companies for similar procedures.
    D. recommendations of the federal government.

Answer: **A**
Why: Usual, customary, and reasonable (UCR) charges are based on what the average or majority of physicians in a specific region would charge for the same or similar procedure. These charges are used in the calculation for RBRVS.
Review: Yes ○   No ○

---

30. When a Medicare patient is told that he or she may be responsible for payment of services not covered by Medicare, the physician's office should inform the patient and have the patient sign a form called a(n):
    A. EOB.
    B. HMO.
    C. ABN.
    D. DRG.
    E. CPT.

Answer: **C**
Why: ABN is an advanced beneficiary notice that is the formal notification to the patient that certain services may not be covered by Medicare. EOB is an explanation of benefits that were covered for services. HMO is a type of insurance plan, and DRG is a classification of diagnoses used to determine hospital payment for Medicare inpatients.
Review: Yes ○   No ○

CRITICAL THINKING CASE REVIEW

The Brandon family includes Edward, the 54-year-old father, Mary, the 42-year-old mother, Chelsey, the 8-year-old daughter, and Christopher, the 22-year-old son.

1. Edward Brandon was permanently injured while working on the railroad after 20 years of service; he is most likely eligible for which type of comprehensive health insurance?
    A. Medicare
    B. Workers' compensation
    C. CHIP
    D. Indemnity
    E. ACA plan

Answer: **A**
Why: Since Edward worked on the railroad for 20 years, he is most likely eligible for a pension. One of the Medicare eligibility criterion is railroad workers who receive a disability pension and meet criteria. Edward would have been eligible through workers' compensation for the initial injury and probably ongoing care related to the injury but not comprehensive health insurance.
Review: Yes ○   No ○

2. Mary works for a small business which provides health insurance for her, but family coverage is too expensive given her modest income; Mary's insurance is called:
   A. Medicare.
   B. workers' compensation.
   C. CHIP.
   D. commercial.

Answer: **D**
Why: Commercial insurance is private health plan through which the insured person or the insured's employer selects his or her own health-care plan.
Review: Yes ○   No ○

3. Christopher lives at home and has a low-wage part-time job which is considered a portion of the family income and puts the family above the 133% of poverty which does not qualify for Medicaid. His job does not provide health insurance. He may be eligible to purchase insurance through:
   A. Medicare.
   B. workers' compensation.
   C. CHIP.
   D. indemnity.
   E. ACA plan.

Answer: **E**
Why: Christopher is too old for CHIP (coverage up to 19 years of age), not eligible for Medicare and does not receive nor can he afford indemnity insurance through his employer. The Affordable Care Act requires most individuals with a few exceptions to have health insurance or receive a fine. There is no indication that Christopher is an exception, so the most likely insurance that he could afford would be an ACA plan.
Review: Yes ○   No ○

4. Chelsey is not eligible for coverage under her father's or mother's health insurance. Due to the family's modest income, she most likely is eligible for:
   A. Medicare.
   B. workers' compensation.
   C. CHIP.
   D. indemnity.

Answer: **C**
Why: CHIP or the Children's Health Insurance Program is the governmental program designed for children under 19 years of age who are not eligible for Medicaid but cannot afford private coverage.
Review: Yes ○   No ○

5. To compare insurance rates and to see what plans are available through the ACA, Christopher goes to the health insurance exchange known as:
   A. TRICARE.
   B. MCO.
   C. the third-party payer.
   D. PPO.
   E. the marketplace.

Answer: **E**
Why: The health-care insurance exchange is known as the marketplace. Both PPO (preferred provider organization) and MCO (managed care organization) are types of insurance plans. The third-party payer is the insurance company.
Review: Yes ○   No ○

CHAPTER
14

Medical Coding and Claims

Review Tip:

If you are not comfortable with coding, while reviewing this chapter, use the current International Classification of Diseases (ICD) editions 9 and 10 coding book, a **Current Procedural Terminology (CPT)** coding book, and a Healthcare Common Procedure Coding System (HCPCS) manual that includes Level II codes. This will simplify definitions and explanations. Further explanation of these manuals and their contents is included in this chapter.

Medical coding is a process that assigns numeric and alphabetic identifiers to illnesses and injuries, medical procedures and services, drugs, and equipment. The two major coding systems are diagnosis coding (*ICD*) and procedural coding (*CPT*). It is important that the diagnosis and the procedure be compatible. For example, a woman should have a pregnancy diagnosis to have a cesarean surgical procedure. The insurance claim is the submission of these medical codes and other information for reimbursement to the health-care provider.

The focus of this chapter is the codes for the outpatient medical practice. The organization of this chapter is similar to Chapter 13. The types of coding are described with information that has "exam probability." The "Terms" section contains the remaining information and definitions. *Do not skip it.*

PROCEDURAL CODING

The systems used for coding health-care professional services, supplies, pharmaceuticals, equipment, and other materials are referred to as *procedural coding*. These systems provide uniform methods for collecting data and determining payment. The American Medical Association (AMA) developed the *CPT* coding system, and the federal Health Care Finance Administration (HCFA) developed two additional levels. The *CPT* codes are included in the HCFA coding system and are considered Level I. Each level is described in more detail later in the chapter but is listed below to provide an overview.

- *Healthcare Common Procedure Coding System* (HCPCS [pronounced "hicpics"])—a method developed by the HCFA (now the Centers for Medicare and Medicaid Services, or CMS) for coding procedures and other services delivered to Medicare patients.
  - Level I—consists of codes for procedures and professional services; *the codes are the same as the CPT codes*
  - Level II—consists of codes for services not covered in the *CPT* codes: supplies, drugs, and other reimbursable equipment and materials

In the beginning of each year's manual, a list of symbols (Table 14-1) with the descriptor is given. The symbol provides valuable information when placed by a specific code.

CPT CODING

Each procedure code contains five numeric digits. The manual is updated annually and organized into six sections representing the major clinical areas, each with a range of five-digit numbers. The actual numbers may change, but the range is reserved for that section, whether or not all the numbers are in use. As of January 1, 2015, the following apply:

- Sections
  - Evaluation and Management: 99201 to 99499
  - Anesthesia: 00100 to 01999; 99100 to 99140
  - Surgery: 10021 to 69990
  - Radiology: 70010 to 79999
  - Pathology and laboratory: 80047 to 89398
  - Medicine (except anesthesia): 90281 to 99199; 99500 to 99607

- General steps for *CPT* coding (Box 14-1)
  1. Identify the procedure or service to be coded
  2. Locate the term(s) in the *CPT* index
  3. Review term, subterms, and code numbers for descriptions that specifically match all the components of the procedure to be coded
  4. Locate codes in the body of the manual as directed by the index; do *not* code directly from the index
  5. Read and follow any notes and cross-references
  6. Select the most descriptive and complete code
  7. Select a modifier when applicable

- Modifier—an addition to the initial *CPT* code that identifies certain circumstances (Box 14-2)
  - Common modifiers—identified by the initial *CPT* code followed by a dash and two figures (usually numbers)
    - −22—increased procedural services (services are more than usually required)
    - −24—unrelated E&M service
    - −25—significant and separate E/M service on same day by same physician
    - −26—professional component(when a service requires both a technical and professional component)
    - TC—technical component (when a service requires both a technical and professional component)
    - −32—mandated service
    - −50—bilateral procedure
    - −51—multiple procedures in the same session (first procedure without modifier; other procedures use this modifier)
    - −54—surgical care only
    - −55—postoperative care only
    - −56—preoperative care only
    - −57—decision for surgery

TABLE 14-1	*CPT* symbols and descriptors	
Symbol	Descriptor
○	New code
Δ	Revised code
><	New or revised text between triangles
+	Add on code
#	Out of numeric sequence
Ø	Multiple procedures exempting modifier -51
O	Reinstated code
↯	FDA approval pending
⊙	Moderate conscious sedation

BOX 14-1

Example of *CPT* coding process for incision and drainage of a hematoma of the skin

Follow the steps using a *CPT* code book.

1. Go to "skin" in index; read down to "incision and drainage," which gives you a range of codes or individual codes (e.g., 10040 to 10180).
2. Turn to the section with the codes suggested from the index, which will be under the "Surgery" section; "Integumentary System."
3. Read the suggested codes until you find the one that matches your procedure.
4. Read and follow any notes and cross-references (in this case, there are none).
5. Select the most descriptive and complete code, which in this case is 10140.

BOX 14-2

Examples of *CPT* coding modifiers

A cholecystectomy was performed by one physician, and postoperative management was performed by another.

Example 1

The physician performing the surgery would use the following:

CPT code: 47600-54

(47600 for the cholecystectomy and -54 as the modifier indicating the physician performed the surgery only)

Example 2

The physician providing postoperative care would use the following:

CPT code: 47600-55

(47600 for the cholecystectomy and -55 as the modifier indicating the physician is providing postoperative care only)

- Common HCPCS modifiers also used in *CPT* coding
  - −E1—upper left eyelid
  - −E2—lower left eyelid
  - −E3—upper right eyelid
  - −E4—lower right eyelid
  - −FA—left thumb
  - −F1 to −F4—left fingers, digits 2 through 5
  - −F5—right thumb
  - −F6 to −F9—right fingers, digits 2 through 5
  - −TA—left great toe
  - −T1 to −T4—left toes, digits 2 through 5
  - −T5—right great toe
  - −T6 to −T9—right toes, digits 2 through 5

(Remember that "E" represents modifier for eye, "F" for finger and "T" for toe.)

- E&M section—the E&M section is unique; in most case, it covers services (e.g., counseling) rather than actual procedures and requires specific components based on assessment and judgment; E&M codes also specify whether the patient is "new" or "established" (Box 14-3)
- Common E&M terms
  - New patient—a person who has not received care from the physician or another physician of the same specialty in the same group practice within 3 years
  - Established patient—a person who has received care from the physician or another physician of the same specialty in the same group practice within 3 years
  - Concurrent care—similar services provided to the same patient on the same day by more than one physician
  - Critical care (definition used for coding professional services)—intensive care in acute life-threatening conditions requiring constant bedside attention by the physician
  - Counseling (definition used for coding professional services)—discussion with patient or family concerning diagnosis, recommendations, risks, benefits, prognosis, options, and necessary condition-related education when it entails more than 50% of the visit
  - Consultation—services rendered by a physician whose opinion or advice is requested by another physician or agency in the evaluation or treatment of a patient's illness or suspected problem
  - Components—E&M codes usually involve five components: three major and two contributory (Table 14-2)
    - Examination (major)
    - Problem severity (major)

BOX 14-3

Example of coding for new and established patients

Coding for office or other outpatient visit of patient, which requires the following:

- A problem-focused history
- A problem-focused examination
- Straightforward medical decision-making
  Use CPT code 99201 for a new patient.
  Use CPT code 99211 for an established patient.

TABLE 14-2 ▶ **Components and levels of an E&M office visit**

			COMPONENTS			
	History	Examination	Medical Decision-Making (MDR)	Problem Severity	Coordination of Care and Counseling	Time (min)
Level 1 (minimal)	Problem focused	Problem focused	Straightforward	Minor	Consistent with the nature of the problem and the patient's or family's needs	10
Level 2 (low)	Expanded problem focused	Expanded problem focused	Straightforward	Low to moderate	Consistent with the nature of the problem and the patient's or family's needs	20
Level 3 (moderate)	Detailed	Detailed	Low complexity	Moderate	Consistent with the nature of the problem and the patient's or family's needs	30
Level 4 (moderate to high)	Comprehensive	Comprehensive	Moderate complexity	Moderate to high	Consistent with the nature of the problem and the patient's or family's needs	45
Level 5 (high)	Comprehensive	Comprehensive	High complexity	Moderate to high	Consistent with the nature of the problem and the patient's or family's needs	60

- o Medical decision-making (MDR) (major)
- o Coordination of care and counseling (contributory)
- o Time (contributory)
- Levels of care—each of the five components involves levels of care ranging from minimal to high
  - o Problem focused (PF)—minimal; only involves affected body area or one organ system
  - o Expanded PF—low; involves an affected body area or one organ system and symptoms related to other body areas
  - o Detailed—moderate; involves the affected body area or areas and related body system(s)
  - o Comprehensive—moderate to high or high; involves multiple systems or complex involvement of one organ system

HCPCS LEVEL II CODES

HCPCS Level II provides coding for services not covered in the *CPT* codes: supplies, pharmaceuticals, ambulance services, and other reimbursable equipment and materials.

The codes begin with a letter (A–V), followed by four numeric digits. A question concerning Level II codes is usually found on the exams; know the beginning letters of the main sections.

- Selected HCPCS Level II sections
  - A0000 to A0999—transportation and ambulance services
  - A4000 to A8999—medical supplies
  - E0100 to E9999—durable medical equipment
  - J0000 to J8999—drugs administered other than oral

Do not confuse HCPCS Level II codes with four-letter *ICD-9* E codes for external injuries. It is important to differentiate services and materials from the diagnosis before selecting the code.

DIAGNOSTIC CODING: *ICD-9-CM*

In 1979, the *International Classification of Diseases, Ninth Revision, Clinical Modification (ICD-9-CM)* became the primary system for coding diseases and injuries in the United States. It is published by the US Department of Health and Human Services and based on the World Health Organization's (WHO) *ICD-9*. The *ICD-9-CM* and the *ICD-9* are considered the same, and generally, the acronyms are used interchangeably.

The *ICD-9* has multiple uses.

- Purpose
  - Track disease processes
  - Classify causes of morbidity and mortality
  - Support medical research
  - Evaluate utilization of health-care resources
  - Profile physicians' services and charges
- ICD-9
  - Volumes for physician offices
    - Volume 1—tabular (numeric) listing of diseases
    - Volume 2—alphabetic listing of diseases
  - Coding digits
    - Three to five numeric digits are used for each code (three digits alone are uncommon)
    - A decimal is placed after the third digit
    - Each digit provides more specific description of the disease or condition (Table 14-3)
    - Fifth digit—identified at the beginning of the three-digit category for the disease entity (e.g., diabetes) or at the beginning of a four-digit subcategory (a further descriptor of the disease entity)
    - If there is a fifth digit listed, it is required
  - Special ICD-9 codes
    - E codes—supplementary classification of ICD-9 coding that denotes the external cause of an injury or poisoning rather than a disease; explains the mechanism of injury
    - V codes—ICD-9 coding identifying health-care encounters for reasons other than illness
  - ICD tables
    - Drugs and chemicals (use E codes)
    - Neoplasms
    - Hypertension
- General steps for ICD-9 coding

| TABLE 14-3 | Example of descriptors with five-digit ICD-9 codes |

Code	Description
250	Diabetes mellitus
250.1	Diabetes mellitus with ketoacidosis
250.13	Diabetes mellitus with ketoacidosis type 1 uncontrolled

1. Locate the term in the alphabetic index
2. Refer to the notes under the main heading
3. Read the terms in parentheses
4. Note indented subterms
5. Proceed to tabular index and instructional terms
6. Assign code

DIAGNOSTIC CODING: ICD-10-CM

In 1993, the WHO published the *International Classification of Diseases, Tenth Revision (ICD-10)*, which, at the time of this writing, is not in complete use in the United States. It is scheduled for full implementation October 1, 2015, and will replace the *ICD-9-CM*, the diagnosis-based system used in both physician offices and hospitals.

The *ICD-9* Procedural Coding System (PCS) is currently used in hospitals only and will be replaced by the *ICD-10-PCS*. The *CPT* system will continue to be used in physicians' offices for coding procedures. Documents and other materials may refer to the *ICD-9* as I-9 and the *ICD-10* as I-10. Another term is the General Equivalency Mapping (GEM), which is a crosswalk between the *ICD-9* and the *ICD-10*. The following are cited as advantages of the *ICD-10*:

- Improved ability to measure health services
- Increased sensitivity with grouping and reimbursement methods
- Enhanced ability for public health surveillance
- Decreased need for supporting documentation with claims
- Provides codes for comparing mortality and morbidity data
- Provides better data for:
  - Measuring patient care
  - Designing payment systems
  - Processing claims
  - Making clinical decisions
  - Identifying fraud and abuse
  - Conducting research
- ICD-10-CM—diagnostic coding system consisting of three to seven alphanumeric digits (characters)
  - Digit 1—alphabetic
  - Digits 2 and 3—numeric
  - Digits 4 to 7—alphabetic or numeric
  - Decimal placed after the third character

TABLE 14-4 ▶ **Example of *ICD-10* with *ICD-9* comparison**

General Description of Code	Number of *ICD-10* Codes for General Description	Example of *ICD-10* Code and Specific Description	Number of *ICD-9* Codes for Description	Example of *ICD-9* Code of Code and Specific Description
problem with breakdown of aortic graft	156	T82.310 Breakdown (mechanical) of aortic (bifurcation) graft (replacement)	1	996.1 Mechanical complication of other vascular device, implant, and graft

BOX 14-4

Changes: *ICD-9* to *ICD-10*

ICD-9-CM Diagnosis Codes
No laterality
3–5 digits
- First digit is alpha (E or V) or numeric
- Digits 2–5 are numeric
- Decimal is placed after the third character

No placeholder characters
14,000 codes
Limited severity parameters
Limited combination codes
One type of "Excludes" note
http://www.cms.gov/Medicare/Coding/ICD10.

ICD-10-CM Diagnosis Codes
Laterality—right or left account for >40% of codes
7 digits
- Digit 1 is alpha
- Digits 2–3 are numeric
- Digits 4–7 are alpha or numeric
- Decimal is placed after the third character

"X" placeholders
69,000 codes to better capture specificity
Extensive severity parameters
Extensive combination codes to better capture complexity
Two types of "Excludes" notes

A comparison of *ICD-9* and *ICD-10* codes is shown in Table 14-4 and some of the basic changes in Box 14-4. Other changes include the following:

- Laterality (which side of the body) and other location descriptors are included in the actual code, not the *CPT* modifier

- Injuries are grouped by anatomical site rather than by type of injury

- The *ICD-10* codes corresponding to *ICD-9* V codes (Factors Influencing Health Status and Contact with Health Services) and E codes (External Causes of Injury and

Poisoning) are incorporated into the main classification rather than in separate classifications as in *ICD-9* (Tables 14-4 and 14-5). Differentiating "V" and "E" codes in both the I-9 and I-10 is a potential exam question. It is not necessary to memorize the tables but to recognize the different "look" between the ICD-9 and the ICD-10

- In some instances, there are new code definitions (e.g., definition of acute myocardial infarction is now 4 weeks rather than 8 weeks)

- Category restructuring and code reorganization in a number of *ICD-10* chapters (Tables 14-5 and 14-6)

TABLE 14-5 ▶ ***ICD-9* code chapters, descriptions, and ranges**

Chapter	Description	Code Range
I (1)	Infectious and parasitic diseases	001–139
II (2)	Neoplasms	140–239
III (3)	Endocrine, nutritional and metabolic diseases, and immunity disorders	240–279
IV (4)	Diseases of the blood and blood-forming organs	280–289
V (5)	Mental disorders	290–319
VI (6)	Diseases of the central nervous system and sensory organs	320–389

Chapter	Description	Code Range
VII (7)	Diseases of the circulatory system	390–459
VIII (8)	Diseases of the respiratory system	460–519
IX (9)	Diseases of the digestive system	520–579
X (10)	Diseases of the genitourinary system	580–629
XI (11)	Complications of pregnancy, childbirth, and the puerperium	630–679
XII (12)	Diseases of the skin and subcutaneous tissue	680–709
XIII (13)	Diseases of the musculoskeletal system and connective tissue	710–739
XIV (14)	Congenital anomalies	740–759
XV (15)	Certain conditions originating in the perinatal period	760–779
XVI (16)	Symptoms, signs, and ill-defined conditions	780–799
XVII (17)	Injury and poisoning	800–999
V codes*	Identifies health-care encounters for reasons other than illness	V01–V91.99
E codes*	External cause of an injury and poisoning	E900–E999

*Do not confuse with E and V codes of *ICD-10*.

TABLE 14-6 ▶ *ICD-10* code chapters, descriptions, and ranges

Chapter	Description	Code Range
I (1)	Certain infectious and parasitic diseases	A00–B99
II (2)	Neoplasms	C00–D48
III (3)	Diseases of the blood and blood-forming organs and certain disorders involving the immune mechanism	D50–D89
IV (4)	Endocrine, nutritional, and metabolic diseases	E00–E90*
V (5)	Mental and behavioral disorders	F01–F99
VI (6)	Diseases of the nervous system	G00–G99
VII (7)	Diseases of the eye and adnexa	H00–H59
VIII (8)	Diseases of the ear and mastoid process	H60–H95
IX (9)	Diseases of the circulatory system	I00–I99
X (10)	Diseases of the respiratory system	J00–J99
XI (11)	Diseases of the digestive system	K00–K93
XII (12)	Diseases of the skin and subcutaneous tissue	L00–L99
XIII (13)	Diseases of the musculoskeletal system and connective tissue	M00–M99
XIV (14)	Diseases of the genitourinary system	N00–N99
XV (15)	Complications of pregnancy, childbirth, and the puerperium	O00–O99
XVI (16)	Certain conditions originating in the perinatal period	P00–P96
XVII (17)	Congenital malformations, deformations, and chromosomal abnormalities	Q00–Q99
XVIII (18)	Symptoms, signs, and abnormal clinical and laboratory findings; not elsewhere classified	R00–R99
XIX (19)	Injury, poisoning, and certain other consequences of external causes	S00–S99
XX (20)	External causes of morbidity	V01–Y99*
XXI (21)	Factors influencing health status and contact with health services	Z00–Z99
XXII (22)	Codes for special purposes	

*Do not confuse with E and V codes of *ICD-9*.

BOX 14-5

Can you recognize the difference in codes?

Procedural Codes

CPT or HCPCS Level 1	Five numeric digits (e.g., 99202); codes for professional services
HCPCS Level II	Letters A–V and four numeric digits (e.g., J3105); codes for nonprofessional services or materials

Diagnostic Codes

ICD-9	Three to five numeric digits with a decimal after the third (e.g., 569.82); codes that identify the patient's diagnosis
ICD-9 E codes	Letter E and three to four numeric digits with a decimal after the third digit;(e.g., E919.3); further describes the diagnostic code by reporting the external cause of an injury rather than a disease
ICD-9 V codes	Letter V and two to four numeric digits with a decimal after the second digit (e.g., V59.2); identifies health-care encounters for reasons other than illness
ICD-10 codes	Digit 1 alphabetic, digits 2 and 3 numeric, digits 4–7 alphabetic or numeric, decimal placed after the third character (e.g. M80.011D) codes that identify the patient's diagnosis beginning October 1, 2015

- Certain diseases have been reclassified to different chapters or sections in order to reflect current medical knowledge

  General steps for *ICD-10* coding:

1. Locate the term in the alphabetic index
2. Refer to the notes under the main heading
3. Read the terms in parentheses, brackets, and any instructional terms
4. Proceed to tabular index and instructional terms
5. Assign the code with the highest specificity (Caution: do not confuse the letter "O" with the number "0")

Remember, laterality (right side, left side, bilateral) is included in the code, not a modifier. Also, the *ICD-10* is much more specific and requires more detailed medical record documentation.

The exams contain critical thinking questions that require you to *differentiate* among *CPT*, HCPCS Level II, and *ICD* codes. You will not be required to know the exact code, but knowing how to recognize the types of codes will allow you to identify the correct answer. Box 14-5 assists you in this process.

CLAIMS

A *claim* is a bill sent to the insurance carrier for payment of professional services. The universal health-care insurance form is called the *CMS 1500*. (*Note:* This has a high probability to be an exam question!) It was originally designed by HCFA, now called CMS, and is used for group and individual claims. In 1990, the form was printed in red to accommodate optical scanning.

The Health Insurance Portability and Accountability Act (HIPAA) regulations regarding confidentiality must be upheld with insurance claims as with all medical documents. Extensive firewalls and other safeguards are required for electronic claims submission.

- Claims submission types
  - Paper—processed by computer; hard copy sent to the insurance carrier through the mail (this method is becoming obsolete)
  - Electronic—processed by computer and sent to the insurance carrier through an electronic data exchange, the Internet, telephone wires, or a disk
  - Digital fax—processed by computer and faxed to the insurance company, where it is read by an optical coder and transmitted into the claims system
- CMS 1500 abbreviations—use only capital letters with no punctuation
  - SSN—Social Security number
  - EIN—employer identification number
  - PIN—provider identification number
  - NPI—national provider identifier
- Dirty claims—claims held or rejected by the insurance carrier because of problems or errors such as the following:
  - Incorrect data
  - Missing data
  - Diagnosis not supporting the procedure
  - Coding errors
  - Patient ineligible for services
  - Claim to wrong carrier
  - Coding or dates not compatible with documentation

COMMON FRAUDULENT AND ABUSIVE CLAIM TERMS

Fraudulent claims (illegal) or claims that abuse the system (not illegal but wasteful use of services or billing practices and not ethical) should be reported to the specific insurance carrier or the governmental entity involved such as CMS (for Medicare or Medicaid).

- Unbundling—using several *CPT* codes to identify procedures normally covered by a single code
- Upcoding—deliberately using an incorrect code to bill at a higher rate
- Phantom billing—billing for services or supplies not provided
- Ping-ponging—unnecessary or excessive referrals of patients to other providers and back to primary office
- Yo-yoing—scheduling the patient for unnecessary follow-up visits
- Gang visits—billing for individual visits when not all the patients present during the visit received services (e.g., visiting a nursing home and not providing services for all patients who are billed)
- Split billing—billing for several visits when services were performed on one visit

OTHER FRAUDULENT CLAIM PRACTICES

- Filing a claim under another person's insurance (violation of the Red Flags Rule, Chapter 4)
- Falsifying medical records to justify higher payment
- Omitting relevant information, especially additional diagnoses
- Altering dates of service
- Altering the diagnosis

APPEALS FOR DISPUTED CLAIMS

- Process specific to the insurance carrier
- Five levels of CMS appeals
  - Predetermination
  - Reconsideration
  - Administrative Judge
  - Appeals Review Board
  - Federal Court Review

HIPAA AND COVERED ENTITIES

A *covered entity* is a medical office that performs any of the following procedures electronically:

- Files claims or managed care encounter forms
- Checks claims status
- Checks eligibility
- Checks certifications or authorizations
- Receives payment and remittance advice
- Provides coordination of benefits

A medical office is also considered a covered entity if any of the above procedures is conducted by a contracted service on the office's behalf. HIPAA requires covered entities to maintain confidentiality (see Chapter 9).

TERMS

MEDICAL CODING AND CLAIMS REVIEW

The following list reviews the terms discussed in this chapter and other important terms that you may see on the exam.

abuse an unreasonable and generally unacceptable departure from precedent and custom with one person taking advantage of another person or set of circumstances; abuse may or may not be unlawful

adverse effect a pathologic reaction to a drug that occurs when appropriate doses are given

appeal a request to an authority for a decision

benign tumor a nonmalignant lesion that is not invasive or metastatic

chief complaint a patient's statement describing symptoms and conditions that are the reason for seeking health-care services

claim a bill sent to the insurance carrier for payment related to patient care

clean claim completed insurance claim form submitted to a carrier without deficiencies or errors

CMS 1500 universal health insurance claim form used in the physician's office

comorbidity a condition that exists along with the condition for which the patient is receiving treatment

concurrent care similar services provided to the same patient on the same day by a different physician

consultation services rendered by a physician whose opinion or advice is requested by another physician or agency in the evaluation or treatment of a patient's problem

counseling discussion with patient or family concerning diagnosis, recommendations, risks, benefits, prognosis, and necessary condition-related education

critical care intensive care in acute life-threatening conditions requiring constant bedside attention by the physician

Current Procedural Terminology (CPT) coding system first published by the American Medical Association in 1966; a manual, updated annually, that contains the codes for procedures and services performed by doctors and other select medical personnel

dirty claim a claim held or rejected by the insurance carrier due to problems or errors

E code a supplementary classification of *ICD-9* coding that denotes the external cause of an injury rather than a disease

eponym the name of a disease or procedure derived from the name of a place or person

established patient a person who has received care from the physician or another physician of the same specialty in the same group practice within 3 years

etiology the cause of disease

explanation of benefits (EOB) synonymous with remittance advice (RA); a correspondence by the insurance company informing the patient and medical office the amount paid for a claim and why

fraud intentional and unlawful deception for gain that results in harm to another person or organization

gang visits billing for individual visits when not all the patients present during the visit received services

General Equivalency Mapping (GEM) a crosswalk between the *ICD-9* and the *ICD-10*

Healthcare Common Procedure Coding System (HCPCS [pronounced "hicpics"]) a method developed by the Health Care Finance Administration for coding procedures and other services delivered to Medicare patients

in situ neoplasm confined to the site of origin

International Classification of Diseases, Ninth Revision, Clinical Modification (ICD-9 or ICD-9-CM) a coding system published by the US Department of Health and Human Services to classify diseases and injuries

International Classification of Diseases, Tenth Revision, Clinical Modification (ICD-10-CM) diagnostic coding system to replace the ICD-9

International Classification of Diseases, Tenth Revision, Procedural Coding System (ICD-10-PCS) procedural coding system to replace the CPT system in hospitals

late effect a residual condition occurring after the acute phase is over

malignant tumor a neoplasm with invasive and metastatic properties

new patient a person who has not received care from the physician or another physician of the same specialty in the same group practice within 3 or more years

Not elsewhere classified (NEC) a term used in *ICD-9* coding when information is not available to code the term in a more specific category

Not otherwise specified (NOS) a term used in *ICD-9* coding for unspecified diagnosis

phantom billing billing for services or supplies not provided

ping-ponging unnecessary or excessive referrals of patients to other providers and back to primary office

point of service (POS) facility where the health-care service took place (e.g., physician's office, emergency department)

primary diagnosis the symptoms, conditions, and initial impressions diagnosed as the cause for the patient seeking health-care services

principal diagnosis the definitive diagnosis

remittance advice (RA) synonymous with explanation of benefits (EOB), correspondence by the insurance company informing the patient and medical office the amount paid for a claim and why

split billing charging for several visits when services were performed during one visit

superbill also called an *encounter form*; a charge form custom-designed for the specific medical practice; lists the *ICD-9* and *CPT* codes common to the services of that practice

unbundling using several *CPT* codes to identify procedures normally covered by a single code

upcoding deliberately using an incorrect code to bill at a higher rate

V codes *ICD-9* codes identifying health-care visits for reasons other than illness

yo-yoing scheduling the patient for unnecessary follow-up visits

REVIEW QUESTIONS

All questions are relevant for all medical assisting and medical administrative certification exams.

1. The abbreviation for the manual first published by the American Medical Association containing the codes for procedures and services performed by doctors and medical personnel is:
   A. ICD.
   B. CPT.
   C. HCPCS.
   D. DRG.

   Answer: **B**
   Why: The *Current Procedural Terminology* manual is used to determine the proper insurance codes to use when filing insurance claims for procedures and services.
   Review: Yes ○   No ○

2. The coding term used for the level of care that involves multiple systems or complex involvement of one organ system is:
   A. problem focused.
   B. expanded problem focused.
   C. detailed.
   D. minimal.
   E. comprehensive.

   Answer: **E**
   Why: Problem focused refers to minimal care involving a specific body area or one organ system. Expanded problem focused refers to the same level of care as problem focused with the addition of symptoms related to other body areas. Detailed level of care involves the affected body area(s) and related body system(s).
   Review: ○ Yes   ○ No

3. When a health professional has a discussion with a patient and his or her family concerning diagnosis, recommendations, risks, benefits, prognosis, and options, the specific coding component used is under the heading:
   A. consultation.
   B. critical care.
   C. concurrent care.
   D. counseling.

   Answer: **D**
   Why: Counseling involves meeting with a patient or the family members to discuss the patient's condition and prognosis, treatment, and concerns surrounding the treatment. This gives the patient or family member an opportunity to ask questions about the information provided by the health-care practitioner.
   Review: ○ Yes   ○ No

4. A pediatric patient comes into the office for otitis media. The physician also administers a routine childhood vaccination. What *ICD-9* diagnostic codes would be used in this situation?
   A. 99201 and 99212
   B. 86850 and E 858.1
   C. 041.5 and J 5678
   D. 382.9 and V 03.81
   E. 99201 and V 71.5

   Answer: **D**
   Why: D is the correct answer because it includes an *ICD-9* code, consisting of a three-digit number followed by a decimal and another digit, and a V code, an *ICD-9* code that identifies health-care reasons other than disease (immunization). The numbers in A are five-digit *CPT* codes; those in B are a *CPT* code and an *ICD* code related to external injuries (preceded by the letter E). C consists of an *ICD* code and a HCPCS Level III code (as recognized by the letter J and four digits); E is a combination of a *CPT* code and a V code.
   Review: ○ Yes   ○ No

5. When a claim is deliberately coded incorrectly to increase the payment, it is referred to as:
   A. superbilling.
   B. customary coding.
   C. upcoding.
   D. bundling.

Answer: **C**
Why: When a *CPT* code is manipulated to increase the amount of reimbursement, it is known as upcoding. This is an unethical practice.
Review: ○ Yes   ○ No

6. *ICD-9-CM* codes that identify health-care encounters for reasons other than illness or injury are known as:
   A. E codes.
   B. F codes.
   C. *CPT* codes.
   D. T codes.
   E. V codes.

Answer: **E**
Why: V codes are used to identify reasons other than illness or injury and to identify patients whose injury or illness is influenced by special circumstances or problems.
Review: ○ Yes   ○ No

7. The coding system published by the US Department of Health and Human Services used to categorize diseases and injuries is the:
   A. *Physician's Desk Reference.*
   B. *Current Procedural Terminology.*
   C. *International Classification of Diseases.*
   D. Relative Value Study.

Answer: **C**
Why: The *International Classification of Diseases, Ninth Revision, Clinical Modification (ICD-9-CM)* manual is a numeric code system for diagnoses of diseases and injuries.
Review: Yes ○ Yes   ○ No

8. CMS developed codes for use when specific services, materials, drugs, and procedures are not listed in the *CPT* code book. These are known as:
   A. RVU.
   B. HCPCS.
   C. DRG.
   D. E codes.
   E. E&M codes.

Answer: **B**
Why: HCPCS, the CMS Common Procedure Coding System, was developed to accommodate coding areas not already specified in the *CPT* code book. These services, materials, drugs, and procedures are provided to Medicare patients.
Review: ○ Yes   ○ No

9. The largest of the six major sections of the *CPT* manual, which contains codes from 10021-69990, is:
   A. medicine.
   B. anesthesia.
   C. radiology.
   D. surgery.

Answer: **D**
Why: The six sections of the *CPT* manual are as follows: Evaluation and Management, 99201 to 99499; Anesthesia, 00100 to 01999; Surgery, 10021 to 69990; Radiology, 70010 to 79999; Pathology and Laboratory, 80047 to 89398; and Medicine, 90281 to 99199.
Review: Yes ○   No ○

10. When a physician requests the services of another physician whose opinion or advice assists in the evaluation or treatment of a patient's illness or suspected problem, the component section used is titled:
    A. critical care.
    B. consultation.
    C. counseling.
    D. concurrent care.
    E. comorbidity.

Answer: **B**
Why: A consultation is the process of seeking the advice or opinion of another physician or specialist to aid in the diagnosis or evaluation of a patient's disease or condition.
Review: ○ Yes   ○ No

11. Of the following, which is not one of the purposes of diagnostic coding?
  A. To track disease processes
  B. To support medical research
  C. To provide increased revenue for the physician or medical practice
  D. To classify the causes of morbidity and mortality

Answer: **C**
Why: Diagnostic coding helps establish statistics and demographic information about diseases and illness. Diagnostic coding is not a mechanism to increase a physician's income.
Review: ○ Yes   ○ No

12. When a patient has received an external injury, which type of code is used to explain the mechanism of the injury using the *ICD-9*?
  A. V code
  B. *CPT* code
  C. UCR code
  D. E code
  E. NOS

Answer: **D**
Why: E codes are supplemental codes that are used to code external injuries rather than diseases.
Review: ○ Yes   ○ No

13. Which *CPT* code identifies a sigmoidoscopy?
  A. 531.03
  B. 453.30
  C. 45330
  D. 685

Answer: **C**
Why: Answer C is correct because it is the only five-digit number that is characteristic of a *CPT* code.
Review: ○ Yes   ○ No

14. The *CPT* code used for a cholecystectomy, along with the modifier indicating that the physician provided only preoperative care, is which of the following?
  A. 47600
  B. 99201
  C. J3105
  D. 47600-V59.2
  E. 47600-56

Answer: **E**
Why: Answer E is a *CPT* code indicating a procedure and includes a dash and a two-digit modifier that identifies a specific circumstance. A and B are *CPT* codes without modifiers. C is a HCPCS Level II code, recognized by the letter J followed by four digits. D is a *CPT* code with an attached *ICD* code, which is never done.
Review: ○ Yes   ○ No

15. The components used to determine the level of E&M code applicable include the following *except* the:
  A. comprehensive depth of the patient history.
  B. problem severity.
  C. amount of time spent with the patient.
  D. number of procedures ordered for the patient.

Answer: **D**
Why: The E&M, or Evaluation and Management, codes require assessment of the visit and judgment of the provider as to the depth of the visit, complexity of the illness, and amount of time involved in treatment of the patient.
Review: ○ Yes   ○ No

16. The Health Care Finance Administration is now named:
  A. Centers for Disease Control and Prevention.
  B. Department of Health and Human Services.
  C. Centers for Medicare and Medicaid Services.
  D. National Institutes of Health.
  E. American Medical Association.

Answer: **C**
Why: The Health Care Finance Administration (HCFA) has been renamed the Centers for Medicare and Medicaid Services, or CMS. This is the federal government agency that oversees the regulations and policies for Medicare and Medicaid.
Review: ○ Yes   ○ No

17. The patient's statement describing symptoms and conditions that are the reason for seeking health-care services is the:
   A. adverse effect.
   B. primary concern.
   C. objective finding.
   D. chief complaint.

Answer: **D**
Why: The chief complaint is the primary reason that brings the patient to the health-care provider for treatment. The insurance company requires this information to appear on the claim form.
Review: ○ Yes   ○ No

18. When a patient has a condition that coexists with his or her primary condition and complicates the treatment and management of the primary condition, it is referred to as:
   A. late effect.
   B. comorbidity.
   C. etiology.
   D. critical care.
   E. concurrent care.

Answer: **B**
Why: Comorbidity occurs when the patient experiences a complication in the treatment plan resulting from a condition other than the primary condition. This may actually lengthen a hospital stay.
Review: ○ Yes   ○ No

19. **Etiology** is a term meaning:
   A. residual condition.
   B. metastatic disease.
   C. cause of the disease.
   D. prognosis of a disease.

Answer: **C**
Why: Etiology is the study of all factors that may be involved in the development of a disease.
Review: ○ Yes   ○ No

20. The coding abbreviation NOS means:
   A. Not otherwise specified.
   B. No objective signs.
   C. Nonspecific objective symptoms.
   D. Nonorganic syndrome.
   E. Not otherwise classified.

Answer: **A**
Why: NOS means "not otherwise specified," a term used in the *ICD-9-CM* coding system to indicate an unspecified diagnosis.
Review: ○ Yes   ○ No

21. When coding, the term describing a cancer that has not invaded neighboring tissues is:
   A. metastatic.
   B. carcinoma.
   C. in situ.
   D. benign.

Answer: **C**
Why: In situ refers to a neoplasm or new growth (tumor) that is confined to the site of origin and has not spread or metastasized.
Review: ○ Yes   ○ No

22. The coding abbreviation NEC is used:
   A. if information is unavailable for more specific coding.
   B. to describe external injuries.
   C. to abbreviate normal causes for the disease.
   D. when the patient is newly established.
   E. if the patient has extensive injuries.

Answer: **A**
Why: NEC means "not elsewhere classified." This term is used in *ICD-9-CM* coding when information necessary to code the disease or injury in a more specific category is not available.
Review: ○ Yes   ○ No

23. The reference manual used to code a
cholecystectomy is:
  A. PDR.
  B. *ICD*.
  C. *CPT*.
  D. HCFA.

Answer: **C**
Why: The *CPT* manual is the *Current Procedural
Terminology* book that contains procedures, including surgeries. A cholecystectomy is the surgical
removal of the gallbladder. If disease of the gallbladder—cholecystitis or cholelithiasis—needs to
be coded, the *ICD* manual is used.
Review: ◯ Yes   ◯ No

24. If a patient's current injury is a fracture of
the left ankle but he or she then experiences
a malunion of this fracture, this is referred to
as a(n):
  A. principal diagnosis.
  B. secondary complaint.
  C. adverse effect.
  D. concurrent care.
  E. late effect.

Answer: **E**
Why: A late effect is a problem that occurs after the
original problem. A malunion of a fracture means
the fracture did not heal properly.
Review: ◯ Yes   ◯ No

25. A claim that is submitted to the carrier
without deficiencies or errors is called a:
  A. common claim.
  B. customary claim.
  C. managed claim.
  D. clean claim.

Answer: **D**
Why: A clean claim means that the completed insurance claim form contains all the necessary information without deficiencies so it can be processed
and paid promptly.
Review: ◯ Yes   ◯ No

26. A physician charging an unreasonable
amount for a procedure is most likely an
example of:
  A. fraud.
  B. abuse.
  C. upcoding.
  D. phantom billing.
  E. unbundling.

Answer: **B**
Why: Abuse is an unreasonable and generally unacceptable departure from precedent and custom,
with one person taking advantage of another person. Fraud is intentional deceit resulting in harm
and unlawful. Upcoding is selecting a higher level
of care than actually provided. Phantom billing
is charging for services that were not rendered.
Unbundling is billing separately for services that
should have been billed under one code for the sole
purpose of making more money.
Review: ◯ Yes   ◯ No

27. Phantom billing is an example of:
  A. fraud.
  B. abuse.
  C. upcoding.
  D. unbundling.

Answer: **A**
Why: Phantom billing is charging for services that
were not provided and is an unlawful intentional
deceit.
Review: ◯ Yes   ◯ No

28. All *ICD-10-CM* codes contain:
  A. three to five numeric digits.
  B. three to five alphanumeric digits.
  C. three to seven numeric digits.
  D. three to seven alphanumeric digits.
  E. seven alphanumeric digits.

Answer: **D**
Why: ICD-10-CM codes contain three to seven al-
phanumerical digits because that is how the coding
system is designed.
Review: ◯ Yes   ◯ No

29. The final appeal for a denied CMS claim is determined by the:
   A. Attorney General.
   B. Supreme Court.
   C. Administrative Judge.
   D. Federal Court Review.

Answer: **D**

Why: The Attorney General and the Supreme Court do not become involved in Medicare/Medicaid claims. The fourth level of appeal is with an Administrative Judge, and the final level of appeal is the Federal Court Review.

Review: ○ Yes   ○ No

---

30. The *ICD-10* is scheduled for full implementation in the United States on:
   A. April 15, 2014.
   B. December 31, 2014.
   C. January 1, 2015.
   D. April 15, 2015.
   E. October 1, 2015.

Answer: **E**

Why: October 1, 2015, is the date designated by the federal government to provide organizations with enough time for implementation. October 1 is also the beginning of the federal fiscal year.

Review: ○ Yes   ○ No

CRITICAL THINKING CASE REVIEW

The office of Angland General and Internal Medicine is training staff on the *ICD-10* diagnostic coding system. The practice manager is aware that there will be a crossover period with claims and RAs that contain either the *ICD-9* or the *ICD-10*. To deal with insurance companies and patients, it is important that the staff is familiar with both systems.

1. An RA explains the amount the insurance company paid and why. RA refers to:
   A. return amount.
   B. return advice.
   C. remittance advice
   D. remittance amount.
   E. refund advice.

Answer: **C**

Why: RA stands for remittance advice or explanation of benefits (EOB), which is the correspondence sent by the insurance company to the medical office and the patient informing them of the amount paid and why.

Review: ○ Yes   ○ No

---

2. Under the *ICD-9*, a code for a diagnosis regarding a well-baby visit might be:
   A. V20.2.
   B. Z00.129.
   C. E20.2.
   D. 99382.

Answer: **A**

Why: Under the *ICD-9* system, a diagnosis associated with a visit for other than sickness or injury, such as well-child visits, is under V codes. While the 99382 code may be associated with a well-child visit, it is a procedural code (*CPT*), not a diagnostic code.

Review: ○ Yes   ○ No

---

3. The V code using the *ICD-9* system refers to a visit for other than sickness or injury. Under the *ICD-10* system, the same code refers to an external cause of morbidity. During the cross over period of the two systems it is also important to:
   A. assure the documentation in the medical record is correct.
   B. check that the insurance claim is for the correct patient.
   C. inspect the date of service for the claim.
   D. analyze the diagnosis and the procedure for compatibility.
   E. assure that you are compliant with HIPAA.

Answer: **C**

Why: All the answers are correct, but in the case where you have two codes that could be either an *ICD-9* or an *ICD-10*, it is important to look at the date of service. Before October 1, 2015, the *ICD-9* would be used, and on or after October 1, 2015, the *ICD-10* would be used. After you establish the date, then the information in the medical record should be used to determine the correct code.

Review: ○ Yes   ○ No

4. Under the *ICD-10*, a code for a diagnosis regarding a well-baby visit might be:
   A. V20.2.
   B. Z00.129.
   C. E20.2.
   D. 99382.

Answer: **B**
Why: Under the *ICD-10*, the Z codes are used for factors influencing health status and contact with health services and replace the majority of the V codes under *ICD-9*.
Review: ○ Yes   ○ No

5. After October 1, 2015, the *CPT* codes for medical offices will:
   A. use the *CPT-10* system.
   B. use the HCPCS level II.
   C. be determined by the AMA.
   D. be determined by CMS.
   E. remain the same.

Answer: **E**
Why: While the procedural codes for inpatient hospital patients will change October 1, 2015, at this time CMS is not requiring a change to the current *CPT* coding system for medical offices.
Review: ○ Yes   ○ No

Financial Practices

Chapters 13 and 14 described how physician fees are established and reimbursement is obtained through insurance companies using claims and coding. This chapter concentrates on the day-to-day financial practices in the medical office.

ACCOUNTS

Accounts are records of financial transactions and the resulting balances during a fiscal period, usually January 1st through December 31st. The medical office primarily deals with two types of accounts: *accounts receivable*, which is the money owed to the practice (e.g., patient bills), and *accounts payable*, which is the money the practice owes (e.g., rent, utilities, medical supplies, payroll; refer to Fig. 15-1). The following accounting functions may apply to both accounts receivable and accounts payable.

- Accounting functions
  - Entries—recording of each transaction
  - Postings—transferring information from the journal (day sheet) to the accounts receivable ledger or to the individual patients' ledgers

Typical Medical Office Expenditures

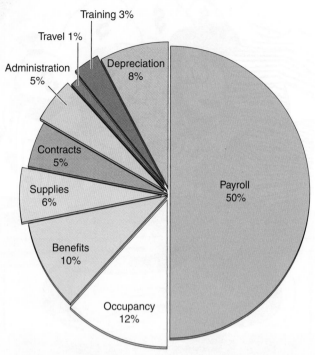

FIGURE 15-1 Typical medical office expenditures.

- Adjustments—changes made to the amount of money owed for reasons other than additional services or payments, such as fee discounts or refunds
- Billings—records of charges sent to the patient in the form of statements to indicate balance due and to request payment; most practices bill on a monthly cycle or after the patient's insurance pays
- Balancing—ensuring accuracy in totals by comparing them with preestablished criteria (e.g., in accounts receivable, the total of balances from individual patient statements must equal the total of accounts receivable recorded in the journal)
- Accounts receivable
  - Components
    - Day sheet—a daily record of the services rendered, charges made, and payments received; may be a manual or a computerized system
    - Journal—a chronologic collection of the day sheets with running totals for a specific period
    - Accounts receivable ledger—a listing by individual patient names of all monies owed to the practice
    - Patient ledger—a patient statement or itemized statement that is an individual form of each patient's accounts receivable activities; often used as the patient bill
    - Charge slip—a form given to the patient to indicate the charges for the service(s); may be a copy of the superbill or the patient ledger

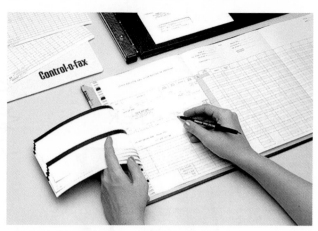

FIGURE 15-2 Pegboard system.

  - Receipt—a numbered form given to the patient indicating the payments he or she made that day
  - Pegboard system—a system of layered forms that allows all transactions to be completed at one time (Fig. 15-2); composed of day sheet, patient ledger, charge slips, receipts, and day sheet–sized board with pegs to hold forms in place; still in use in some small practices
- Age of accounts receivable—the period between when the service is rendered and the bill is paid, usually in 30-day intervals; computerized financial programs will process statements calculating the amount of money that is owed on the account for 30, 60, 90, or 120 days since the date of service; also known as *aging analysis*
- Trial balance—an accounting of all the debits and credits for the medical practice done at regular time periods or randomly if an error is suspected to assure all totals are correct; this is in addition to the final balance for the time period.
- Collections—efforts to obtain money owed to a medical office
  - Office efforts can include payment by cash, check, or debit or charge card remitted at the time of service
  - Payment plans with or without interest
  - Prepayment plans when a noncovered usually expensive procedure is scheduled
  - Payment through billing (by the office or a contracted service)
  - Billing cycles—all patients on the same day each month or by rotating patients for billing on different days of the month based on preestablished criteria, such as billing those whose names begin with the same letters on the same day of the month

- Telephone calls and letters for aging bills
  - Collection agency—an outside company, independent of the medical practice, that is contracted by the medical practice to attempt to obtain payment of delinquent bills after internal efforts or other contracted services have failed; *a medical practice should not make further efforts to collect a bill after the account is turned over to the collection agency*; collection agencies are usually paid 50% of the amount collected
  - Small claims court—a less formal court setting that allows the parties to represent themselves in civil disputes involving small amounts; the amount is designated by the court and is generally less than $5,000
  - Bankruptcy—if a patient declares bankruptcy, the medical office must attempt to collect unpaid bills through the court-appointed representative
  - Deaths—unpaid bills of deceased patients **should be collected through the patient's estate**
- Accounts payable
  - Purchase order—a document sent to a vendor via mail, fax, or the Internet to purchase supplies and equipment for the medical office
  - Invoice—a bill sent from the vendor stating what was purchased and the charges
  - Materials—items received from the vendor should be verified with the invoice or packing list and purchase order
  - Bill—statements sent to the medical office requesting payment for materials or services
  - Payment—money remitted by the medical office for materials or services
  - Petty cash—a small sum of money (usually less than $200), kept separate from the cash drawer, *used for incidental expenses* (e.g., postage due)

ASSETS AND DEBITS

As with all businesses, the medical office has assets and debits.

- **Assets**—property owned by the organization that is available to meet debts and commitments
- **Debit**—an amount deducted; do not confuse this with a debt
- **Bookkeeping accounting**—a separate process that differs from balancing accounts receivable and accounts payable; do not spend time trying to understand this complicated process but be aware that the assets and debits must always balance

BANKING

Although much of banking has moved to electronic processes, people continue to pay in cash and hard copy checks, which may qualify for a discount in some offices.

- Checks
  - Payee—the person to whom the check is written; the person receiving the money
  - Payer—the person or organization giving the money to the payee
  - Acceptable checks—cashier's check, traveler's check, certified check, personal check with proper identification, money order
  - Unacceptable checks—third-party checks (except from the patient's insurance company), payroll checks, personal checks without identification if unfamiliar with the person and his or her financial history with the medical practice
  - Voided check—a check written by the practice but not used because of error or other reason; write *VOID* across the front and keep with canceled checks in the proper numeric sequence
  - Lost or stolen check—the bank should be notified immediately and a notation made in the checkbook
  - Endorsement—signing the back of a check as the payee for the amount represented on the front of the check
    - Blank endorsement—only the signature of the payee on the back of the check (can be easily cashed by anyone)
    - Restrictive endorsement—signature of the payee with instructions, such as "for deposit only"
  - Nonsufficient funds (NSF)—indicates that the checking account on which the check is written does not hold enough money to honor the amount of the check; medical offices usually add a charge to the balance to cover the associated bank charges
- Deposits—checks and cash paid to the medical office and placed in a checking account at the bank; usually deposits are made daily
  - Deposit slip—a form completed with the deposit listing all checks and cash and the total amount deposited; contains account number and other identifying information
  - Check register (checkbook)—a book or computer program maintained by the office listing in chronologic order all checks written, deposits made, and an ongoing balance; used to reconcile bank statement
- Bank statements—reports sent by the bank or accessed online listing the monthly account activities,

BOX 15-1

Example of main components of checking account reconciliation

1. Beginning balance	$25,000.00
2. Total deposits	+$45,000.00
3. Total checks cleared	−35,000.00
4. Total checks outstanding	−10,000.00
5. Charges	00.00
Ending balance	$25,000.00

To determine the ending balance, add lines 1 and 2, and then subtract lines 3, 4, and 5 from the total of lines 1 and 2.

including checks written and cashed, deposits, bank charges, and balances

- Reconciliation (balancing or trial balancing)—process of verifying that the information on the bank statement tallies with the information in the check register (Box 15-1)
- Line of credit—a financial agreement between a bank or financial institution and a borrower establishing the maximum amount of money the borrower can obtain through a loan; the total amount of the funds may be borrowed at one time or in increments as needed until the maximum amount has been reached

TRUTH IN LENDING ACT

The *Truth in Lending Act* (TILA) of 1968, similar to informed consent for medical treatment, protects the consumer by requiring the informed use of consumer credit with all costs calculated and all terms disclosed. It also prohibits unsolicited credit cards. *Regulation Z* is how the Truth in Lending Act is referred to in the Federal Register and sometimes used synonymously.

FAIR DEBT COLLECTION PRACTICES ACT

Enacted in 1977, the *Fair Debt Collection Practices Act* was established to eliminate abusive, deceptive, and unfair debt collection. The major guidelines for bill collection include the following:

- Only call between the hours of 8:00 AM to 9:00 PM. Outside of these hours is considered harassment
- Avoid false threats or inappropriate language

- Discuss the debt only with the person responsible for the payment; in some cases this may be an attorney or bank
- Avoid any form of misrepresentation such as posing as a government agent
- Avoid any perceived violence

COMMON TAXES

The federal and state governments require medical offices to pay specific taxes. The most common and "exam probable" taxes follow:

- Federal income tax—a specified percentage of income withheld based on the total amount earned
  - W-2 form—a federal tax form prepared for each office employee containing all income and deductions for the previous calendar year
  - W-4 form—a federal tax form completed and signed by each employee at the time of hire that contains the number of tax exemptions he or she claims
- Federal Insurance and Contribution Act (FICA)—a percentage of income withheld from each employee's paycheck for Social Security and Medicare
- Federal Unemployment Tax Act (FUTA)—a percentage of each employee's income paid by the employer into an unemployment fund

INCOME

The amount of money a medical practice earns is the *income* (accounts receivable, interest, etc.). The practice also incurs expenses such as wages, taxes, supplies, equipment, and utilities (accounts payable). Certain additional deductions (e.g., bad debts) are allowed in addition to expenses. These are deducted from the total income.

- Gross income—total amount of earned income for the medical practice before deductions
- Net income—amount of earned income for the medical practice after deductions (Box 15-2)

BOX 15-2

Example of gross and net income difference

Gross income	$250,000
Deductions & expenses	−75,000
Net income	$175,000

TERMS

FINANCIAL PRACTICES REVIEW

The following list reviews the terms discussed in this chapter and other important terms that you may see on the exam.

accounts records of financial transactions and the resulting balances during a fiscal period, usually January 1st through December 31st

accounts payable the money the practice owes (e.g., rent, utilities, medical supplies, payroll)

accounts receivable the money owed to the practice, such as patient bills

accounts receivable ledger listing by individual patient name of all monies owed to the practice

adjustments changes to the amount of money owed for reasons other than additional services or payments (e.g., fee discounts, refunds)

age of accounts receivable (aging analysis) the period between when the service is rendered and the bill is paid, usually in 30-day intervals; computerized financial programs will process statements calculating the amount of money that is owed on the account for 30, 60, 90, or 120 days since the date of service

asset anything of value owned by an individual or business

balancing ensuring accuracy in totals by comparing them with preestablished criteria; in accounts receivable, the total of balances from individual patient statements must equal the total of accounts receivable recorded in the journal

blank endorsement only the signature of the payee appears on the back of the check

credit value added to an account, usually in the form of payment for a debt owed to that party

currency official paper money of a country

day sheet a daily record of the services rendered, charges made, and payments received; may be a manual or computerized system

debit value subtracted from the companies' assets

endorsement signing the back of a check as the payee for the amount represented on the front of the check

entry the recording of each transaction on the appropriate forms or components

gross income the total amount of income for the medical practice before deductions

income the amount of money a medical practice earns

invoice a bill sent from a vendor stating what was purchased and what the charges are

journal a chronologic collection of day sheets with running totals for a specific period

liability obligation; debt of the individual or business

line of credit a financial agreement between a bank or financial institution and a borrower establishing the maximum amount of money the borrower can obtain through a loan

monthly trial balance a list and total of all the debit and credit accounts for the medical practice

net income the amount of income for the medical practice after deductions

patient ledger a patient statement that is an individual form of each patient's accounts receivable activities; often used as the patient bill

payee the person to whom the check is written; the person receiving the money

payer the person or organization giving the money to the payee

pegboard system a system of layered day sheets, patient ledgers, charge slips, and receipts; allows all entries to be made with one transaction

petty cash a small sum of money (usually less than $200), separate from the cash drawer, used for *incidental* expenses

posting transferring information from the journal (day sheet) to the accounts receivable ledger or to the individual patients' ledgers

purchase order a document sent to a vendor via mail, fax, or the Internet to purchase supplies and equipment for the medical office

reconciliation the process of verifying that the information on the bank statement agrees with the information in the check register

Regulation Z the Truth in Lending Act as recorded in the Federal Register

restrictive endorsement signature of the payee with instructions (e.g., "for deposit only")

superbill (encounter form) a provided form that has all the necessary information to file an insurance claim related to that office visit

Truth in Lending Act (TILA) established in 1968, protects the consumer by requiring the informed use of consumer credit with all costs calculated and all terms disclosed

REVIEW QUESTIONS

All questions are relevant for all medical assisting and medical administrative certification exams.

1. The patient's bill or statement is also referred to as the patient's:
   A. receipt.
   B. charge slip.
   C. ledger.
   D. posting.

   Answer: **C**
   Why: A patient's ledger is an individual form containing each patient's accounts receivable activities.
   Review: ○ Yes   ○ No

2. The listing by individual patient names of all monies owed to the practice is the:
   A. receipt.
   B. charge slip.
   C. day sheet.
   D. accounts payable roster.
   E. accounts receivable ledger.

   Answer: **E**
   Why: Accounts receivable refers to the money owed to the practice by patients. These amounts are recorded in a ledger called the accounts receivable ledger.
   Review: ○ Yes   ○ No

3. A check written from an account that does not have enough money for the amount of the check is called a(n):
   A. voided check.
   B. NSF check.
   C. blank check.
   D. third-party check.

   Answer: **B**
   Why: When there is not enough money in an account to cover the amount of a check, the bank account has nonsufficient funds (NSF) to cover the check.
   Review: ○ Yes   ○ No

4. The Federal Insurance and Contribution Act was created to sponsor:
   A. unemployment.
   B. life insurance.
   C. Social Security and Medicare.
   D. workers' compensation.
   E. Medicare.

   Answer: **C**
   Why: The Federal Insurance and Contribution Act (FICA) requires deduction from an employee's pay to cover the cost of sponsoring Social Security and Medicare.
   Review: ○ Yes   ○ No

5. The process of verifying that the information on the bank statement agrees with the information in the check register is:
   A. registering.
   B. accounting.
   C. reconciling.
   D. examining.

   Answer: **C**
   Why: Reconciliation is the process of making things right. The balance in the checkbook should equal the balance on the bank statement after adjustments have been made for outstanding checks and deposits.
   Review: ○ Yes   ○ No

6. When a discount or refund is applied to an account, this is referred to as a(n):
   A. charge.
   B. adjustment.
   C. payable.
   D. receivable.
   E. withholding.

   Answer: **B**
   Why: When a medical practice applies a discount or refunds money to an account, it is making an adjustment to the total amount owed by the client. Another example is when a client pays his or her balance in full and then the medical practice receives an insurance payment to cover some or all of the visit; the patient should be refunded the overpayment.
   Review: ○ Yes   ○ No

7. Activities that an office can do to assist in the collection of money owed the practice include:
   A. allowing patients to pay for services when they get paid.
   B. requiring all patients to pay cash when services are rendered and not providing any payment plans.
   C. asking patients at the time of service if they want to pay for the services by cash, check, or charge.
   D. sending billing notices to patients on a quarterly basis.

Answer: **C**
Why: Patients should be asked at the time of service what method of payment they want to use to pay for the services. This allows the office to establish that it is necessary to pay for services at the time they are rendered. If a patient is unable to pay in full, billing for the balance should be done on a monthly basis.
Review: ○ Yes ○ No

8. When a patient declares bankruptcy, the medical office must:
   A. turn over the patient's balance owed to a collection agency.
   B. write off the balance of the account.
   C. sue the patient for the balance owed on the account.
   D. collect unpaid bills through the court-appointed representative.
   E. set up a loan repayment plan with interest.

Answer: **D**
Why: After bankruptcy has been declared, the office is not allowed to contact the patient directly but must attempt to collect any debt through the court-appointed representative.
Review: ○ Yes ○ No

9. The form enclosed with merchandise ordered from a vendor that states the contents of the package and the amount owed is a(n):
   A. ledger.
   B. invoice.
   C. purchase order.
   D. receipt.

Answer: **B**
Why: The invoice usually accompanies the merchandise and includes the total amount due on the order. A ledger is a list of the accounts receivable activities for a patient or a company. A purchase order is a document sent to a vendor to purchase supplies and equipment for the medical office. A receipt is given as proof of payment.
Review: ○ Yes ○ No

10. If a check is written but not used, what is written across the front of the check?
   A. Void
   B. Nonsufficient funds
   C. Do not use
   D. Error
   E. Reconcile

Answer: **A**
Why: The word "void" means useless or invalid. A voided check should be filed with the canceled checks for tracking purposes.
Review: ○ Yes ○ No

11. The amount of money earned before taxes or deductions are taken out is called:
   A. net income.
   B. total income.
   C. prior earnings.
   D. gross income.

Answer: **D**
Why: The gross income refers to the entire amount of money earned by an employee or the amount of income in a business before expenses, deductions, or taxes have been subtracted.
Review: ○ Yes ○ No

12. The cash kept on hand in a business practice used for incidental purchases is called:
A. purchase order.
B. petty cash.
C. ancillary money.
D. spending money.
E. currency.

Answer: **B**
Why: "Petty" refers to a small amount. Petty cash is usually around $200 cash and is used to purchase items that are needed on a daily basis that are paid for right away. Postage stamps, coffee supplies, office supplies, and so on are often bought with petty cash.
Review: ◯ Yes   ◯ No

13. The money owed by the physician for items such as rent, utilities, and payroll is referred to as:
A. financial responsibility.
B. accounts receivable.
C. business expenses.
D. accounts payable.

Answer: **D**
Why: Accounts payable refers to the amount of money the physician or business owner needs to pay out for expenses of the business.
Review: ◯ Yes   ◯ No

14. To balance a checkbook, you must have:
A. a copy of all the bills paid in the month to verify all checks written.
B. paycheck stubs to prove deposits made.
C. the monthly bank statement.
D. a copy of all endorsed checks.
E. day sheets.

Answer: **C**
Why: The bank sends a monthly statement that lists all deposits made, checks written and cashed, bank charges and fees, and the beginning and ending balance on the account for the month. This statement is used to compare with the check register to balance it.
Review: ◯ Yes   ◯ No

15. The signature of the payee of a check with instructions stating "for deposit only" is an example of a(n):
A. blank endorsement.
B. unlimited endorsement.
C. restrictive endorsement.
D. registered endorsement.

Answer: **C**
Why: A check that has a signature and "for deposit only" on the reverse side indicates that it can only be deposited into the account of the payee, making it a restrictive endorsement. If the payee signs the check without writing any restrictions, it can be cashed by anyone if lost or stolen.
Review: ◯ Yes   ◯ No

16. The monitoring of unpaid accounts to determine how overdue the accounts are is called:
A. posting.
B. calendar tracking.
C. collections.
D. overdue auditing.
E. aging accounts.

Answer: **E**
Why: Aging of accounts is a way to monitor the ability of offices to collect money on unpaid accounts. Usually, the practice will measure in 30-day intervals up to 120 days.
Review: ◯ Yes   ◯ No

17. The most common schedule of billing patients is:
A. weekly.
B. monthly.
C. bimonthly.
D. quarterly.

Answer: **B**
Why: Monthly billing is the most accepted method of billing because it is highly effective in collection of unpaid debts. Most people pay bills based on monthly income and, if budgeted properly, will schedule payments on owed accounts monthly.
Review: ◯ Yes   ◯ No

18. When the medical assistant is given the task of trying to collect payment on an account, it is appropriate practice to first:
   A. contact the client's employer.
   B. contact the client at home before 8:00 AM.
   C. leave a message on the client's answering machine about possible lawsuits or small claims court activity if he or she does not call you back.
   D. contact the client about the overdue bill through a mailed letter or notice attached to his or her bill.
   E. visit the patient at his or her home to discuss a payment plan.

Answer: **D**
Why: It is improper collections activity to contact someone before 8:00 AM or after 9:00 PM. It is also inappropriate to visit patients at their homes or to contact a client's employer. Threatening calls are a form of harassment and intimidation and should not be made. Initially, the office should try to collect the money through written correspondence. This method also provides a paper trail for tracking if further collection methods need to be tried.
Review: ○ Yes   ○ No

19. When a charge is made to an account, it is called a(n):
   A. posting.
   B. credit.
   C. debit.
   D. adjustment.

Answer: **C**
Why: A debit is a charge to an account and represents what is owed. Posting is the process of transferring information from a day sheet to an accounts receivable ledger or to an individual patient's ledger. A credit is the same as a payment, or applying money to an account to lower the balance owed. An adjustment is a change made to the amount of money owed for reasons other than additional services or payments.
Review: ○ Yes   ○ No

20. A preprinted form that has the basic office charges listed and space for the patient's current charges is an example of a(n):
   A. ledger.
   B. journal.
   C. day sheet.
   D. superbill.
   E. invoice.

Answer: **D**
Why: A superbill is usually a three-copy form that has all the necessary information for the patient to use in filing an insurance claim. It states the coding for the office visit with diagnosis and the amount charged for the services during the visit. Most superbills also have a place to put information about the patient's return or follow-up visit.
Review: ○ Yes   ○ No

21. An example of a debit adjustment is:
   A. applying a professional discount to the account.
   B. posting the payment made from the patient's insurance company.
   C. return of a nonsufficient fund check from a patient's bank.
   D. removing a charge from a patient's account that was placed there by mistake.

Answer: **C**
Why: A debit adjustment increases or adds to the patient's account balance. When a patient's check is not honored by the bank because there are not enough funds in the account to cover the amount, the office will apply the amount of the check back to the account. The payment is eliminated, and the patient owes the amount of the check plus an additional fee.
Review: ○ Yes   ○ No

22. When a check is received in the office, the medical assistant should first:
   A. place the check in a cash lockbox.
   B. endorse the check in writing or with a rubber stamp reading "for deposit only."
   C. contact the bank to verify the funds are in the account.
   D. enter the receipt of the check in the patient's medical chart.
   E. process a receipt to send to the patient.

Answer: **B**

Why: Checks received in the office should be immediately endorsed "for deposit only" so no one would be able to cash the checks if the checks were lost or stolen.

Review: ○ Yes   ○ No

23. To reconcile a checking account, you must:
   A. ensure that the information on the bank statement agrees with the information in the check register.
   B. add to the checkbook balance any monthly fees or bank charges that are listed on the bank statement.
   C. add any outstanding checks to the bank statement balance.
   D. add to the bank statement the amount of interest earned on the account that month.

Answer: **A**

Why: The purpose of reconciling a checking account is to ensure that the information contained on the bank statement agrees with the information in the check register. Steps in reconciling that account include subtracting monthly fees or charges from the checkbook balance, subtracting outstanding checks from the bank statement balance, and adding the amount of interest earned to the checkbook balance.

Review: ○ Yes   ○ No

24. The amount of money an employee is paid after taxes are withheld is called:
   A. gross income.
   B. tax withholding.
   C. wage.
   D. net income.
   E. deduction.

Answer: **D**

Why: The gross income is the amount of money earned before tax withholding. The wage is the amount of money earned by the employee, usually based on an hourly rate. Net income is known as "take-home" pay after all the taxes and other deductions have been subtracted from the gross amount. A deduction is any amount of money taken out of the total income. Deductions may include state and federal taxes and insurance premiums.

Review: ○ Yes   ○ No

25. At the end of each calendar year, the employer is required to provide a statement to each employee of the year's total gross income and the taxes withheld. This form is the:
   A. W-4.
   B. W-2.
   C. FICA.
   D. FUTA.

Answer: **B**

Why: The W-4 form is the Employee's Withholding Allowance Certificate. The employee completes this form when employed and specifies the amount of deductions claimed for tax purposes. A W-2 form is issued to the employee at the end of each year to show the amount of money the employee earned during the year. It is required as proof of income when filing income tax. The Federal Insurance and Contribution Act (FICA) was developed to sponsor Social Security and Medicare. The Federal Unemployment Tax Act (FUTA) requires employers to pay a percentage of each employee's income to sponsor an unemployment fund.

Review: ○ Yes   ○ No

26. If a medical practice periodically had unexpected expenses and needed a loan, the practice owner could apply for:
    A. additional petty cash.
    B. a withholding allowance.
    C. an endorsement.
    D. reconciliation.
    E. a line of credit.

Answer: **E**

Why: A line of credit is an established amount of money that a bank will loan a borrower. It can be used all at one time or in increments as needed. Petty cash is a small amount of cash kept on hand in the office for small purchases. Withholding allowance refers to money held out of earnings for tax purposes. Endorsement is the act of signing the back of a check as the payee for the amount represented on the front of the check. Reconciliation is the process of verifying that the information on the bank statement agrees with the information in the check register.

Review: ○ Yes   ○ No

27. A chart or table that includes a list and total of all the debit and credit accounts for a medical practice is a(n):
    A. check register.
    B. pegboard day sheet.
    C. aging analysis.
    D. monthly trial balance.

Answer: **D**

Why: A monthly trial balance is a chart of all the debits and credits for the practice and is used to ensure that the practice debits equal the credits. A check register is a log of all the activity of the checking account. A pegboard day sheet lists patient charges and payments made in a single day for the practice. Aging analysis is the process of determining the period between when the service is rendered and the bill is paid, usually in 30-day intervals.

Review: ○ Yes   ○ No

CRITICAL THINKING CASE REVIEW

Taylor Sylvester is a certified medical administrative specialist working at Family Medical Associates. Taylor was calling patients at 7:30 AM to remind them of upcoming appointments.

1. One of the patients, Mr. Matthew had an outstanding balance. The CMAS used this opportunity to remind him of it. Mr. Matthew accused the office of violating the Fair Debt Collection Practices Act. Was this a violation?
    A. Yes, because the call was made before 8:00 AM.
    B. Yes, because the intent was to pursue the unpaid bill.
    C. No, because the primary intent of the call was an appointment reminder.
    D. No, because the Fair Debt Collection Practices Act applies only to collection agencies.
    E. No, because Taylor did not threaten Mr. Matthew.

Answer: **A**

Why: The primary intent of the call was to remind the patient of an upcoming appointment, not to collect an unpaid bill and no effort was made to prohibit the patient from keeping his appointment. It would be similar to informing the patient of a co-pay. The Fair Debt Collection Practices Act applies to anyone collecting a debt, and threatening a person is only one part of the law. However, it is not considered a standard practice to call patients prior to 8:00 a.m. for any reason.

Review: ○ Yes   ○ No

2. After the reminder calls, Taylor was preparing the bank deposit from the previous day's checks. He noticed one check made out to Family Medical Associates but with a restricted endorsement on the back with the name of a physician who was not known to that practice. The correct procedure would be to:
   A. deposit the check in the bank.
   B. return the check to the payer.
   C. return the check to the payee.
   D. void the check.

Answer: **B**

Why: A restricted endorsement is the instructions of the payee (the person receiving the check—Family Medical Associates) to the bank for cashing the check. If the endorsement was made by a third party other than the payee, the check should be returned to the payer (patient) and a new one issued.

Review: ○ Yes   ○ No

---

3. Family Medical Associates gives a 5% discount for patients who pay by check or in cash. This discount is not extended to debit or credit card payments because:
   A. the card may be fraudulent.
   B. the card does not guarantee payment.
   C. the bank takes longer to process card payments.
   D. the bank charges the medical office for processing card payments.
   E. the patient may owe money on the card.

Answer: **D**

Why: There is a charge to the medical office, usually 2% to 5% for setting up and processing debit or credit card payments. The cash and checks save the office that amount which it passes on to the patient.

Review: ○ Yes   ○ No

---

4. Taylor is helping to process a new employee who must complete a:
   A. W-2 form.
   B. W-4 from.
   C. FICA form.
   D. FUTA form.

Answer: **B**

Why: The employee must complete a W-4 form which indicates the number of tax exemptions he or she wishes to claim. The W-2, FICA, and FUTA are the responsibility of the employer.

Review: Yes ○ No ○

---

5. Taylor received a raise and noticed on his pay slip that his FICA had gone up. This is because:
   A. FICA is a percent of your income.
   B. he did not pay all his taxes last year.
   C. his health-care insurance rates were increased.
   D. the government probably raised taxes.
   E. the medical office made an error.

Answer: **A**

Why: Since FICA is a percent of a person's income, if the income goes up, the FICA also goes up. For example, if a person is making $45,000 a year and the FICA is 15%, the FICA is $6,750 (before deductions). If the pay is increased to $48,000 and the FICA is 15%, it goes up to $7,200 (before deductions).

Review: ○ Yes   ○ No

CHAPTER

16

Administration and Compliance

Review Tip:

If your medical office manager or administrator is not aware that you are preparing to take the national exam, this may be an opportunity to tell him or her of your plans. Ask for any encouragement or advice that he or she may have and discuss sections of this chapter that may not be clear to you or how they are organized at your place of employment. Also, review Chapter 4, Law and Ethics, which contains pertinent laws, risk management, and some compliance related to material in this chapter.

ORGANIZATION

According to the Merriam Webster Dictionary, an organization is defined as "a company, business, club, etc., that is formed for a particular purpose." This includes the medical offices. Every medical office has an organizational model that may or may not be represented by a formal **organizational chart**. The chart shows the supervisory structure and reporting relationships between different functions and positions—who is responsible for whom and what. In most states, the medical assistant is under the direct supervision of the physician and/or **midlevel providers**, such as the physician assistant or nurse practitioner, for direct patient care activities. The practice manager is usually responsible for interviewing, hiring, firing, scheduling (Fig. 16-1), evaluating, assuring training, and credentialing of medical assistants, which are all considered administrative functions and not direct patient care functions. Figure 16-2 is a simplified organizational chart of a physician-owned practice. A physician-owned medical practice often has the legal designation of a professional corporation (PC).

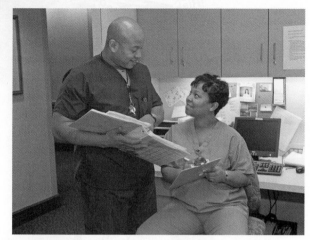

FIGURE 16-1 The practice manager reviews the medical assistant's schedule with her.

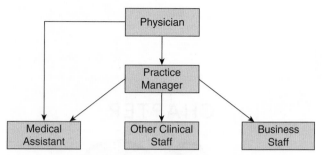

FIGURE 16-2 Organizational chart of physician-owned medical practice.

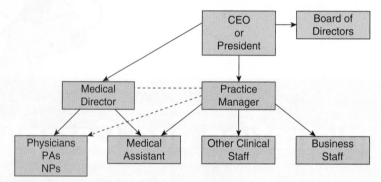

FIGURE 16-3 Organizational chart of corporate-owned medical practice.

Figure 16-3 shows a simplified organizational chart of a corporate-owned medical facility. The company may be for profit or nonprofit. The practice manager is in charge of the day-to-day operations, with the exception of the direct patient care functions of the medical assistants, the physicians, and the midlevel providers who are accountable to the medical director. The dotted lines between the practice manager and the medical director indicate equality in rank and collaboration between the roles. The dotted line from the practice manager to the other physicians indicates collaboration. For example, the practice manager may ensure the physicians are properly credentialed. The medical director has the majority of the responsibilities for the physicians such as supervision and evaluations. The president, practice manager, medical director, and other physicians and staff are employees of the company and paid by the company. A board of directors is ultimately responsible but is not involved in the daily operations of the company.

The organizational charts reflect the **chain of command**, which demonstrates how each position is accountable to those directly superior and how the authority passes from one link in the chain to the next, or from the top to the bottom. Today's businesses, including medical offices, operate using a chain of command. It is important for employees to understand the chain of command and stay within it.

MORE ABOUT COMMUNICATION

Chapter 7 discusses general communication techniques and communication with patients, persons with special needs, and some coworkers. Other routine individuals and groups with whom the staff in the organization communicates on a regular basis are given below:

- Patients
- Physicians (within the practice and in other practices)
- Hospitals
- Insurers
- Vendors
- Employers
- Contractors
- Governmental agencies
- Other regulatory and professional agencies
- Educational facilities
- Bankers
- Attorneys
- Community organizations

All forms of communication should be appropriate, respectful, timely, and Health Insurance Portability and Accountability Act (HIPAA)-compliant. Many offices have policies and procedures (P&Ps) related to communication, especially electronic communication.

STAFF COMMUNICATION

The following are communication modalities often used with staff.

- Staff meetings
- **In-service**—facilitating and communicating education and training conducted in the facility
- E-mail—a large number of offices have e-mail for each employee or group of employees
- Newsletters—provide information on what is going on in the practice, new P&Ps or requirements, accomplishments and awards, and internal and community events; also often highlight staff members or departments
- Bulletin boards—usually located in the staff lounge; should not contain any confidential or sensitive information because janitorial staff and others outside of the practice may have access
- Communication books—becoming replaced with electronic communication; a notebook or binder with information the manager wants to inform the staff about is kept in a central location; employees may be required to initial each entry to assure it was read
- Suggestion box—staff submit ideas in a box with a name or anonymously

COMPLIANCE

To once again quote the Merriam Webster Dictionary, **compliance** is "the act or process of doing what you have been asked or ordered to do." Each medical organization is expected to be compliant with legal requirements and the requirements and standards for medical and business practices. In some organizations, this is the responsibility of the administrator or directors of specific departments or a specially designated compliance officer. The responsibility involves many systems and processes. Some of the more common ones are assuring that

- Policy and procedure manuals are developed, maintained, reviewed, and updated (usually annually)
- Physicians and midlevel providers are properly licensed
- Physician and midlevel provider Drug Enforcement Administration (DEA) forms are up to date
- Medical assistants, phlebotomists, coders, and other personnel are properly trained and certified or credentialed according to federal, state, and professional standards
- Required licenses to operate the facility, such as local business licenses, are up to date
- Centers for Medicare and Medicaid Services (CMS) and accrediting approvals are in place and up to date
- HIPAA and Meaningful Use conditions are met and maintained
- Insurance requirements such as malpractice and liability contracts are up to date and reflect current values
- Contracts with health insurance companies, laboratories, attorneys, and other services necessary to conduct business are in place
- Required reporting to authorities, such as communicable diseases, is being done

OTHER BUSINESS FUNCTIONS

The contemporary medical office relies on technology for communication, appointment scheduling, coding, billing, diagnostic test ordering and reporting, prescription refills, and the electronic health record. These areas require highly specialized skills to install and maintain such as:

- Evaluating and purchasing or leasing the systems and equipment that fit the needs and budget of the practice
- Facilitating the installation and staff training
- Overseeing the ongoing operations

Other business functions include assuring the following:

- Efficient mail and shipping services
- Inventory and supply purchase
- Office polices and patient's rights and responsibilities are available; frequently in a patient information packet
- Appropriate market and public relation strategies such as websites, brochures, and community events

HUMAN RESOURCES

Human resources (HR), personnel services, or people services refers to how employees are managed by the business and deals with the following.

- Writing job descriptions
- Recruiting staff
- Verifying qualifications and credentials
- Interviewing (Box 16-1)
- Hiring and terminating following designated P&Ps
  - Performing staff evaluations and an improvement process as necessary
  - Orienting new staff

BOX 16-1

Interviewing topics to avoid

The US Equal Employment Opportunity Commission (EEOC) prohibits discrimination in hiring. The following topics should be avoided when interviewing a job applicant to assure the applicant's rights are not violated:

Race

Sex

Color

Disability

(may ask if the applicant has anything that may prevent him or her from fulfilling the job requirements)

Religion

Birthplace

National origin

(may ask for proof that the applicant has authorization to work in the United States)

Marital/family status

(do not ask if the applicant has children)

Age

(may ask for proof that applicant is over 18 years of age if appearance justifies it and necessary for position)

IF THE APPLICANT HAS OR HAS HAD EEOC MATTERS

- Managing salaries, payroll, and benefits, including following workers' compensation cases of office employees
  - Developing, enforcing, and updating P&Ps for personnel issues including the following:
    - **Employee grievance process**—a formal step-by-step process for an employee to submit a complaint to his or her employer
    - **Sexual harassment**—unwelcome behavior from anyone in the workplace including vendors or patients whose actions, communications, or manners ridicule, degrade, or make an employee uncomfortable including offensive jokes, names, nicknames, and pictures or objects
    - **Cultural competence**—behaviors, attitudes, and policies that support working well with diverse populations in cross-cultural situations
    - **Conflict of interest (COI)**—a situation when a person's personal interest has the potential to influence his decision-making to further his own gain rather than the good of the party he or she is representing; an example is a medical assistant recommending to a patient a product when the vendor for that product is a spouse
- Publication of an **employee handbook**—a manual given to each employee that explains a company's major P&Ps, employee benefits, and expected behaviors; and reflects compliance with employment laws
- Maintaining staff records such as performance evaluations, trainings, and employee health requirements
- Assuring compliance with federal, state, and local income taxes and other regulations related to personnel
- Mediating appropriate issues between staff members

HEALTH AND SAFETY

Regulations from the Occupational Safety and Health Act (OSHA), other federal agencies, and state and local authorities regarding a safe health care and work environment must be followed. Compliance is assured by

- Developing P&Ps, which are then incorporated in a safety manual, including reporting unsafe activities and behaviors as described in The Joint Commission guidelines:
  - internally, to the appropriate supervisor or compliance officer; if no action,
  - externally to the appropriate agency such as the state medical board or OSHA and
  - full disclosure to the patient regarding errors in treatment. This should be done through the doctor or practice manager; seek legal advice if this does not happen.
- Establishing systems to accommodate P&Ps, for example, establishing a contract with a biohazardous waste company that includes containers, a schedule, and removal
- Educating and training staff on the P&Ps
- Making supplies and equipment available such as personal protective equipment
- Monitoring observance of the P&Ps

Health and safety also incorporate emergency preparedness plans with directions for office evacuation and posted information. Chapter 25, Emergency Preparedness, provides detailed information.

THE PHYSICAL FACILITY

The physical facility or plant is the building or buildings, offices, parking structures, furniture, and mechanical systems (elevators, electrical, heating, cooling, plumbing, etc.) that make up the medical practice. An efficient workplace requires the following:

- Appropriate utilization of space
- Payment of mortgage or rental, utilities, etc. (accounts payable)
- Selection and purchase or lease of capital equipment such as copy machines and telephone systems
- Establishment of contracts and oversight of janitorial, biohazardous waste disposal, and other services
- Maintenance of elevators and heating, air conditioning, and other equipment; parking lot
- Replacement of worn furniture, carpeting, etc.
- Compliance with Americans with Disabilities Act (ADA)
- Availability of adequate supplies and materials
- Emergency repairs such as clogged drains
- Security
- Landscape maintenance
- Plans for future needs

TERMS

ORGANIZATION AND COMPLIANCE REVIEW

The following list reviews the terms discussed in this chapter and other important terms that you may see on the exam.

chain of command demonstrates how each rank is accountable to those directly superior and how the authority passes from one link in the chain to the next, or from the top to the bottom; reporting hierarchy

compliance the act or process of doing what you have been asked or ordered to do

Conflict of interest (COI) a situation when a person's personal interest has the potential to influence his decision-making to further his own gain rather than for the good of the party he or she is representing

cultural competence behaviors, attitudes, and policies that support working well with diverse populations in cross-cultural situations

employee grievance a formal step-by-step process for an employee to submit a complaint to his or her employer

employee handbook a manual given to each employee that explains a company's major policies and procedures, employee benefits, and expected behaviors and to ensure compliance with employment laws

in-service education and training conducted in the facility

midlevel providers generally, physician assistants and nurse practitioners examine, diagnose, and provide some treatments that must be signed off by a supervisor

minutes the meeting record; contains the date and time, who was present and absent, what was discussed, and who is responsible for any actions

organizational chart a model showing the supervisory structure and reporting relationships between different functions and positions; who is responsible for whom and what

sexual harassment unwelcome behavior from anyone in the workplace including vendors or patients whose actions, communications, or manners ridicule, degrade, or make an employee uncomfortable including offensive jokes, names, nicknames, and pictures or objects

REVIEW QUESTIONS

All questions are relevant for all medical assisting and medical administrative certification exams.

1. The model that shows the chain of command is called the:
   A. practice management.
   B. staff assignments.
   C. practice ownership.
   D. organizational chart.
   E. corporate plan.

   Answer: **D**
   Why: An organizational chart contains the formal supervisory structure and reporting relationships between different functions and positions of the management and staff. This is referred to as the chain of command.
   Review: Yes ○   No ○

2. The hiring and firing role comes under the category of:
   A. health and safety.
   B. communications.
   C. human resources.
   D. quality improvement.

   Answer: **C**
   Why: Human resources is a common term involving services directly related to the people or staff in the organization. Hiring and firing are directly related to staff. Health and safety, communications, and quality improvement involve patients and other entities outside of the organization.
   Review: Yes ○   No ○

3. If a medical practice has a health and safety violation, the organization involved would be:
   A. CDC.
   B. SDS.
   C. CMS.
   D. ADA.
   E. OSHA.

   Answer: **E**
   Why: Workplace health and safety is under the Occupational Safety and Health Administration. The CDC is involved with public health, and the CMS is involved with Medicare and Medicaid health insurance.
   Review: Yes ○   No ○

4. Management of the physical plant involves:
   A. leasing the facility.
   B. selecting the EHR system.
   C. complying with CMS.
   D. managing payroll.
   E. mailing and shipping.

   Answer: **A**
   Why: The physical plant, also referred to as the physical facility, makes up the building and the systems, equipment, and supplies that are directly involved in the functioning of the building, whether it is associated with a medical practice or another business such as an attorney's practice.
   Review: Yes ○   No ○

5. Which of the following would not likely constitute an act of sexual harassment?
   A. Complimenting a coworker about a new haircut.
   B. Displaying a calendar with scantily clad men and women.
   C. Requesting a date with a subordinate employee in exchange for a better work schedule.
   D. E-mailing off color jokes to coworkers because they are so funny and always get a laugh.

   Answer: **A**
   Why: As long as the compliment about a new haircut is sincere and appropriate, it should not lead to sexual harassment. The other examples are definitely ones that could be offensive to coworkers. Employees need to understand that sexual harassment might include any behavior that makes the workplace an unpleasant and uncomfortable environment for another person.
   Review: Yes ○   No ○

6. Which of the following specifically refers to the process of discovering and preventing problems that may lead to harm and loss for the practice?"
   A. Policies and procedures
   B. Organizational chart
   C. Risk management
   D. Physical plant
   E. Human resources

Answer: **C**
Why: Risk management is a process to routinely assess, identify, correct, and monitor any potential problems to prevent harm and loss.
Review: Yes ○   No ○

7. Compliance is best defined as
   A. performing all tasks requested by the employer regardless of the scope of practice.
   B. notifying a patient of all test results.
   C. working well with the entire office staff.
   D. the act or process of doing what you are required to do.

Answer: **D**
Why: In the health-care workplace, the term "compliance" typically refers to following rules and policies set forth by a regulatory agency, for example, OSHA and HIPAA.
Review: Yes ○   No ○

8. Which of the following would not be found in an employee handbook?
   A. The dress code for all employees
   B. How an employee can accrue vacation time
   C. Staff meeting minutes
   D. The company's policy on sick time
   E. The organization's mission statement

Answer: **C**
Why: An employee handbook is provided to all new employees and explains the company's policies and procedures that apply to all employees. Staff meeting minutes are not published in the handbook. Items found in a typical handbook include the employee dress code, sick time, and vacation policies. The mission statement is usually found in the beginning of the handbook.
Review: Yes ○   No ○

9. The physical plant or facility must comply with the requirements set forth by:
   A. ADA.
   B. HIPAA.
   C. CMS.
   D. SDS.

Answer: **A**
Why: The physical plant refers to the building, parking area, hallways, elevators, and so on. All of these structures are expected to meet the specifications of the Americans with Disabilities Act (ADA), which requires adequate access to people with special needs.
Review: Yes ○   No ○

10. Which of the following functions would not be the responsibility of the human resources department of a medical practice?
    A. Verifying credentials of employee candidates
    B. Establishing hiring policies
    C. Determining the medical assistant scope of practice
    D. Managing payroll and benefits
    E. Terminating employees

Answer: **C**
Why: Although there are basic duties and tasks that most medical assistants can do, the medical assistant scope of practice is established by each state according to the medical practice acts.
Review: Yes ○   No ○

11. Training of employees conducted in the workplace is referred to as:
    A. staff meetings.
    B. seminars.
    C. in-service.
    D. supervision.

Answer: **C**
Why: A staff meeting is a get together of all members of the practice to discuss various topics with a planned agenda. A seminar is an educational program attended outside of the office and usually conducted by a professional organization. Supervision is what the person above you on the chain of command does.
Review: Yes ○   No ○

12. All of the following are common methods used to communicate with staff EXCEPT:
    A. bulletin boards.
    B. e-mails.
    C. communication books.
    D. newsletters.
    E. certified letters.

Answer: **E**
Why: The organization would not normally send a staff member a certified letter unless he or she was unable to reach the person using the common methods. Certified mail is used to reach patients with important information that may require documentation that it was received.
Review: Yes ○   No ○

13. Which of the following represents a conflict of interest in the medical office?
    A. A physician refers a patient to a well-known specialist.
    B. The office manager asks an employee where she has her haircut.
    C. A medical assistant encourages patients to make appointments with her husband, a massage therapist.
    D. An employee provides coworkers with discount coupons from the newspaper for a local fast food restaurant.

Answer: **C**
Why: It would be inappropriate for an employee to solicit services or products for financial gain. The other answers provided are appropriate and do not constitute a conflict of interest.
Review: Yes ○   No ○

14. The quality or characteristics of all communications within the health-care field must be all the following EXCEPT:
    A. appropriate.
    B. respectful.
    C. timely.
    D. electronic.
    E. compliant.

Answer: **D**
Why: Electronic communication is an acceptable form of communication, but it is not the only type that can be used. Communication should always be appropriate, respectful, timely, and compliant.
Review: Yes ○   No ○

15. Which of the following does NOT represent the concept of cultural competence?
    A. A medical assistant will only work with persons who share the same religious beliefs.
    B. A Hispanic physician who hires non-Hispanic medical assistants.
    C. An Asian patient seeks medical care from a physician who is Caucasian.
    D. A medical clinic is located within a culturally diverse neighborhood.

Answer: **A**
Why: Cultural competence refers to behaviors, attitudes, and policies that support working well with diverse populations in cross-cultural situation. A medical assistant needs to be aware that there are many different cultures and religious beliefs that will be encountered in the medical field. Diverse populations exist among patients as well as staff members.
Review: Yes ○   No ○

16. Compliance with OSHA, federal, state, and local regulations can be assured by all the following EXCEPT:
    A. withholding information from patients regarding errors in treatment.
    B. making PPE available to employees.
    C. reporting incidents to the compliance officer.
    D. educating and training all employees on policies and procedures.
    E. contracting with a biohazardous waste company.

Answer: **A**
Why: The Joint Commission guidelines require full disclosure of all patient errors in treatment. OSHA requires the employer to supply PPE for all employees performing tasks that may result in possible exposure to blood-borne pathogens. All employees are required to receive education and training about the OSHA blood-borne pathogen standard. OSHA also requires that biohazardous waste is disposed of in an acceptable and safe manner such as contracting with a waste management company.
Review: Yes ○   No ○

17. A question that you would not ask during an interview would be whether the applicant:
    A. is certified in his or her field.
    B. has a college degree.
    C. is able to work on Sundays.
    D. has a religious affiliation.

Answer: **D**
Why: Whether the person has a certification or went to college could very well be a job requirement or preference. If the office is open on Sundays or may hold special events on Sundays, such as immunization clinics prior to the beginning of school, then asking the applicant if he or she is able to work on Sundays is appropriate. It is never appropriate to ask about an applicant's religious affiliation.
Review: Yes ○   No ○

18. Which of the following represents mid-level providers?
    A. Medical assistant and physician
    B. Practice manager and medical assistant
    C. Physician's assistant and nurse practitioner
    D. Practice manager and physician's assistant
    E. Physician and physician's assistant

Answer: **C**
Why: The medical assistant and practice manager are not classified as providers. A midlevel provider is not a physician but is someone authorized through licensure to treat patients.
Review: Yes ○   No ○

19. Which of the following is a responsibility of the practice manager?
    A. Obtaining patient vital signs
    B. Ensuring all surgical instruments are sterilized prior to use
    C. Verifying credentials of medical assistants
    D. Calling prescription refills to the pharmacy

Answer: **C**
Why: A practice manager is responsible for the day-to-day administrative operations of the medical practice. They are not usually involved in any direct patient care activities.
Review: Yes ○   No ○

20. An organizational chart reflects all the following EXCEPT:
    A. the supervisory structure of the organization.
    B. the hiring policies of the organization.
    C. the reporting relationship of the members of the organization.
    D. the departments within the organization.

Answer: **B**
Why: An organizational chart is a flow chart that lists the various departments of an organization, the supervisors, and the persons that report to them. It is an easy way to initially understand the structure of the organization.
Review: Yes ○   No ○

21. A meeting record (minutes) would contain all the following EXCEPT:
   A. the date meeting was held.
   B. attendees to the meeting.
   C. a list of action items.
   D. a list of the patients seen that week.
   E. the time the meeting was held.

Answer: **D**
Why: Meeting minutes would not include a list of patients who were scheduled or seen within the week of the meeting. Only items specific to the meeting are included in the minutes. These items include the date and time of the meeting, the discussion and action items, and the list of those in attendance.
Review: Yes ○   No ○

22. If an incident occurs in the medical office that results in a legal action, the organization is expected to:
   A. keep it a secret.
   B. place the information in the staff newsletter.
   C. maintain records of the occurrence.
   D. go to court.

Answer: **C**
Why: The designated person by the organization such as a manager or quality assurance director is expected to discuss the incident with the appropriated parties involved and keep it to himself or herself. It should not be discussed in the staff newsletter because a newsletter is not confidential. The organization is expected to keep accurate records on the incident and save medical records that may be involved.
Review: Yes ○   No ○

23. A function of managing the physical facility may be to:
   A. purchase pharmaceuticals.
   B. contract for landscaping maintenance.
   C. upgrade the electronic health record system.
   D. replace the electrocardiogram (ECG) machine.
   E. evaluate a new payroll service.

Answer: **B**
Why: Landscaping maintenance is a function of the physical facility. Purchasing pharmaceuticals, upgrading the electronic health record, and replacing the ECG machine are related to direct patient care services. Payroll is a human resources function.
Review: Yes ○   No ○

CRITICAL THINKING CASE REVIEW

Anthony Amadore is the new practice manager for Family Medical Associates, a general practice office with 4 physicians and 12 staff members.

1. When Anthony arrived, he discovered that the organization did not have an employee handbook, a website, marketing brochure, travel policies, or flexible staffing hours. His priority should be:
   A. the employee handbook.
   B. a website.
   C. a marketing brochure.
   D. travel policies.
   E. flexible staffing hours.

Answer: **A**
Why: The employee handbook is an important human resources publication to concisely clarify for employees what is expected of them and to inform them of their benefits. These are important issues for the employer and employee. The organization has been operating without a website or a brochure or travel policies, and there is no indication of an urgent need. Flexible hours may or may not be a need or desire, but an employee manual is a human resources standard.
Review: Yes ○   No ○

2. As the practice manager, Anthony may do all the following EXCEPT:
   A. supervise the CMAS while doing procedures.
   B. supervise the CMA while doing procedures.
   C. schedule the CMAS.
   D. schedule the CMA.

Answer: **B**
Why: Only the physician or a midlevel provider as allowed by the state in which he or she practices may supervise the medical assistant's performance of a clinical procedure. The practice manager may supervise the CMAS during his or her procedures and may schedule both the CMAS and the CMA.
Review: Yes ○   No ○

3. Anthony also serves as the compliance officer which means that he:
   A. is also serving as a federal officer.
   B. is responsible to assure governmental and certifying agencies and requirements are met.
   C. must personally supervise the training of all staff on policies and procedures.
   D. must assure all accounts payable such as mortgage, utilities, and salaries are paid.
   E. must go to court if there are any legal actions against the organization.

Answer: **B**
Why: The compliance officer is responsible to assure governmental and certifying agencies and requirements are met. This includes HIPAA, Meaningful Use, OSHA, etc. While he must assure that staff is properly trained, he may designate that job to others. As practice manager, he is responsible for accounts payable but not as the compliance officer. If the organization is required to go to court, Anthony **may** *not* **must** go. Watch the words that are used in questions!
Review: Yes ○   No ○

4. If Anthony, as the compliance officer for Family Medical Associates, was also a federal officer involved in health care, this would most likely be a(n):
   A. HIPAA violation.
   B. EOB.
   C. COI.
   D. ADA violation.

Answer: **C**
Why: A COI or conflict of interest is defined as a situation when a person's personal interest has the potential to influence his decision-making to further his own gain rather than for the good of the party he or she is representing. In this case, he would be representing both agencies—the medical office and federal agencies that oversee the medical office which is in conflict, since he cannot represent both simultaneously. It would be similar to an attorney for a client also being the judge.
Review: Yes ○   No ○

5. A medical assistant working at Family Medical Associates made an error in patient care. Under TJC and some federal agency guidelines, the practice is obligated to:
   A. notify the office's malpractice attorney.
   B. fire the medical assistant.
   C. disclose the error to the patient.
   D. avoid insurance fraud.
   E. report patient abuse.

Answer: **C**
Why: TJC or The Joint Commission include in their guidelines full disclosure of errors in patient care. Dependent on the error and any damage to the patient, the malpractice attorney should be notified and the medical assistant may be fired, but C is the best answer. In general, insurance fraud should be avoided and patient abuse reported, but they do not apply to this scenario.
Review: Yes ○   No ○

Clinical Practice

Clinical Practice

17

Microorganisms and Asepsis

MICROORGANISMS

Microorganisms, or microbes or germs, are living organisms that are too small to see with the naked eye. These organisms surround us and are part of every living process. Some of these microbes cause disease, and others cause disease only under certain circumstances; for example, *Escherichia coli* (*E. coli*), which is found normally in the intestinal tract, may cause illness if the number of bacteria increases or even sepsis if introduced into the bloodstream.

COMMON PATHOGENS

Pathogens are microorganisms that cause infectious disease.

- Blood-borne pathogen—any type of pathogen that lives in and is transmitted through blood
  - Bacteria (singular *bacterium*)—one-celled microorganisms; may be found singularly or in chains

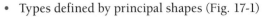

FIGURE 17-1 Bacteria can be classified according to shape. Cocci are round, and can be found as diplococci, staphylococci, or streptococci. Bacilli are rod shaped. Spirilla are spiral-shaped.

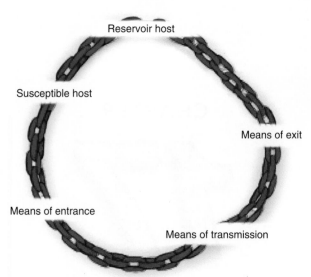

FIGURE 17-2 Chain of infection.

- Types defined by principal shapes (Fig. 17-1)
  - Spherical (cocci; singular *coccus*; Latin, meaning "berry")—examples are streptococci, staphylococci, pneumococci
  - Rod (bacilli; singular *bacillus*; Latin, meaning "little staff")—examples are *Bacillus anthracis* (cause of anthrax), *Mycobacterium tuberculosis* (cause of tuberculosis), *Bacillus tetanus* (cause of tetanus)
  - Spiral (spirilla or spirochete; singular *spirillum*; Latin, meaning "spiral"); corkscrew-shaped; an example is *Helicobacter pylori* (one cause of chronic gastritis)
  - Spores—encapsulated (shell or capsule) bacteria in an inactive or resting state; in the medical office, spores are killed only by autoclaving
- Types defined by air need
  - Aerobic—bacteria that require oxygen for survival
  - Anaerobic—bacteria that live without oxygen
- Virus—extremely small microbes that pass through most filters; examples of viral diseases include measles, mumps, rubella, herpes, hepatitis B (HBV), hepatitis C (HCV), human immunodeficiency virus (HIV), and influenza
- Fungus (plural *fungi*)—microbes that grow on other organisms, causing diseases such as tinea (ringworm), candidiasis (thrush), histoplasmosis, or coccidioidomycosis
- Protozoa—simplest form of animal pathogen; parasites; examples of diseases caused by protozoa are malaria, giardiasis, and *Trichomonas* (one cause of vaginitis)

PORTALS OF ENTRY

Portals of entry are the ways microorganisms enter the body.

- Upper respiratory system—nose, mouth (air); diseases such as influenza, measles, and the common cold
- Gastrointestinal system—mouth, rectum (food and water); diseases such as enteritis, hepatitis A, salmonella
- Integumentary system—any break in the skin or mucous membrane; diseases such as methicillin-resistant *Staphylococcus aureus* (MRSA), impetigo, HIV, HBV
- Eyes and ears (special senses); diseases such as otitis media, conjunctivitis
- Vascular system—through blood supply; diseases such as HBV and HIV causing acquired immunodeficiency syndrome (AIDS)

CHAIN OF INFECTION

The **chain of infection** illustrates the elements necessary for disease to spread (Fig. 17-2). Breaking the chain of infection along any of its links helps to prevent and to decrease infectious diseases.

1. Reservoir host—initial carrier of the microbe; may be a person, an animal, an insect
2. Means of exit—method of leaving the reservoir host (e.g., sneezing, coughing, feces, blood)
3. Means of transmission—method of moving from the exit of the reservoir host to the entrance of the susceptible host, such as air, contaminated materials called **fomites** (such as food or water), or soiled hands
4. Means of entrance (refer to portal of entry)—routes by which microorganisms enter the body

5. Susceptible host—person with no previous immunity or with weakened immunity resulting from illness, injury, or poor nutrition, or if the pathogen is too virulent (strong) for a normal immune system to resist

IMPORTANT TERMS ASSOCIATED WITH INFECTIOUS DISEASES

- **Contagion**—the spread of disease by direct or indirect contact with a pathogen
- **Localized**—infection confined to one area of the body (e.g., a pustule)
- **Generalized or systemic**—infection spread throughout the body (e.g., septicemia)
- **Endemic**—the usual amount of a specific disease present in a community
- **Outbreak**—an excess of the normal occurrences of a specific disease
- **Epidemic**—an increase in the normal number of cases of a specific disease occurring in a defined geographic area or locale
- **Pandemic**—an epidemic that has spread over several countries or continents, usually affecting a large number of people
- **Emerging infections**—recently appearing infectious diseases in a population or diseases that are rapidly increasing or threatening to increase in the near future

BIOCHEMICAL AGENTS TO COMBAT PATHOGENS

- Antibiotics—substances ingested, injected, or applied to a living being that have the power to inhibit the growth of or to destroy pathogens
- Chemotherapy—ingestion, injection, or application of chemical agents in treating disease
- Immunizations—biologic or chemical agents that create immunity to specific diseases when ingested or injected (see Box 6-7, "Types of Immunity," and Box 6-8, "Common Vaccine-Preventable Diseases," in Chapter 6)

ASEPSIS

Asepsis is the absence or the control of microorganisms.
- The Centers for Disease Control and Prevention (CDC) establishes many of the standards for asepsis
- The US Occupational Safety and Health Administration (OSHA) oversees or enforces many of these standards or guidelines as related to the workplace

PURPOSES OF ASEPSIS

- Protect patient/public
- Protect health-care worker
- Prevent infectious disease from starting
- Stop infectious disease from spreading

TYPES OF ASEPSIS

- **General asepsis**—common techniques and procedures to reduce the number of pathogenic microorganisms in the normal environment and to decrease the opportunity for further spread (Fig. 17-3)
- **Medical asepsis (clean technique)**—techniques and procedures to reduce the number of microorganisms in a health-care environment and decrease opportunities for further spread
- **Surgical asepsis (sterile technique)**—techniques and procedures to eliminate *all* microorganisms in an environment

COMMON METHODS OF ASEPSIS

Frequent handwashing is the most effective aseptic practice.
- Medical handwashing
  1. Remove jewelry (wedding and engagement rings usually remain)
  2. Use hand- or foot-controlled faucet
  3. Wash hands and wrists for 2 to 3 minutes
  4. Use brush and cuticle stick on nails
  5. Hold hands in downward position while rinsing
  6. Dry hands with paper or clean cloth towel
  7. Turn off hand faucets with paper or clean cloth towel
  8. Lotion may be applied
- Surgical handwashing
  1. Remove all jewelry
  2. Use foot- or knee-controlled faucet
  3. Wash hands, wrists, and forearms for 10 minutes with brush (first surgical scrub of day)
  4. Use cuticle stick on nails
  5. Hold hands in upward position while rinsing
  6. Dry with sterile towel
  7. Do not apply lotion
  8. Keep hands upright and do not touch anything until sterile gloves are applied
- Handwashing with an alcohol hand disinfectant (AHD) or alcohol-based gel
  - When water is not available and hands are not visibly dirty or contaminated, use a 60% to 95% alcohol-based gel or disinfectant

Stop the spread of germs that make you and others sick!

Cover your Cough

Cover your mouth
and nose with a
tissue when you
cough or sneeze
or
cough or sneeze into
your upper sleeve,
not your hands.

Put your used tissue in
the waste basket.

Clean your Hands after coughing or sneezing.

Wash hands
with soap and
warm water

or

clean with
alcohol-based
hand cleaner.

 MINNESOTA MDH DEPARTMENT OF HEALTH   STOP Minnesota Antibiotic Resistance Collaborative   APIC ASSOCIATION FOR PROFESSIONALS IN INFECTION CONTROL AND EPIDEMIOLOGY, INC   DMACC DES MOINES AREA COMMUNITY COLLEGE Life's Calling™

FIGURE 17-3 Common practices to stop the spread of disease.

- Pump or pour the substance into the palm
- Rub the hands together ensuring the solution covers all surfaces of the back and palms of the hand including between the fingers and fingernails until the solution is evaporated

■ Common medical office practices in addition to frequent handwashing:

- Requiring employees to have specific disease–preventable immunizations such as annual flu shots
- Instructing coughing staff and patients to wear masks
- Having appropriate personal protective equipment (PPE) available, including gloves and masks at the front desk
- Avoiding stuffed animals or other toys that cannot be easily and frequently cleaned
- Cleaning with approved products, especially restrooms

■ Antiseptics—bacteriostatic chemical cleaning agents used on skin to remove and to inhibit the growth of bacteria; these agents do not destroy all pathogens

■ Disinfectants—bacteriostatic chemical agents used to clean and to decrease the pathogens on inanimate objects (e.g., surgical instruments, countertops); these agents do not destroy all pathogens

■ Sterilization—process of destroying all living organisms

- Gas—used for wheelchairs, beds, and other large equipment; very toxic
- Dry heat—used for instruments that corrode easily; requires at least 1 hour at 320°F
- Chemical (cold sterilization)—used for heat-sensitive equipment such as fiber-optic endoscopes; equipment is soaked in closed containers with strong agents (e.g., glutaraldehyde); specific time recommendations are determined by the manufacturer of the chemical agent
- Steam heat (autoclave)—the most common method of sterilization used in the medical office; the steam is under pressure to achieve higher temperatures
  - Water temperature must be 212°F
  - Steam temperature must be 250°F to 254°F
  - Time required is between 20 and 40 minutes, depending on how tightly items are wrapped (the looser the wrap, the shorter the time required)
  - Sterilization bags or pouches, disposable paper wraps, or surgical towels are used for autoclaving surgical instruments, including those that will be placed on sterile fields; usually, double wrapping is required when using disposable paper wraps or surgical towels
  - Packages must be dry before removing them from the autoclave

- Procedure:
  1. Place cleaned and dried instruments in center of wrap (hinged instruments in open position) with sterilization indicator tape
  2. Position opened wrap on a flat surface in a diamond shape with a point toward you
  3. Fold the corner closest to you over the instrument
  4. Fold the first side corner toward the center, completely covering the instrument; fold extra material back to form a tab; repeat with the second side corner
  5. Fold the last corner toward the center and around the packet, ensuring the instrument is completely covered
  6. Fasten the packet with sterilization-sensitive tape

■ Standard or universal precautions

- Treat all blood and bodily fluids as contaminated
- Protect the patient from you (especially when patient's immune system is compromised)
- Protect yourself from the patient

■ Personal protective equipment (PPE)

- Gloves (nonsterile used for majority of patient procedures; sterile used only for procedures requiring sterile aseptic technique, e.g., surgery)
- Goggles or eye shields
- Masks
- Gowns
- Aprons

■ Other safety materials and actions

- Safety plan and policies and procedures
- Safety data sheets (SDS), these were formerly called material safety data sheets (MSDS); and labels for all hazardous agents
- Employee training
- "Sharps" (needles, scalpels, glass vials, etc.) containers
- Other biohazard receptacles for nonsharp material contaminated with body fluids
- Spill and eyewash stations
- Showers

TERMS

MICROORGANISMS AND ASEPSIS REVIEW

The following list reviews the terms discussed in this chapter and other important terms that you may see on the exam.

acquired immunodeficiency syndrome (AIDS) an often fatal condition caused by the human immunodeficiency virus (HIV)

alcohol hand disinfectant (AHD) an alcohol-based gel used to wash hands when water is not available

antibiotic a substance ingested, injected, or applied to a living being that has the power to inhibit the growth of or to destroy pathogens

antiseptic a chemical cleaning agent used on the skin to remove or to inhibit the growth of bacteria

asepsis the absence of or the control of microorganisms

bacteria (singular *bacterium*) one-celled microorganisms; may be found singularly or in chains

bactericide an agent or a process that kills bacteria

bacteriology the study of bacteria

bacteriostasis the process of inhibiting or controlling bacterial growth

blood-borne pathogen any type of disease-causing organism that lives in and is transmitted through blood

chain of infection elements necessary for disease to spread: reservoir, host, portal of exit, means of transmission, portal of entry, susceptible host

contagion the spread of disease by contact with a pathogen

disinfectant a bacteriostatic chemical agent used to clean and to decrease the number of pathogens on inanimate objects (such as surgical instruments, countertops); does not sterilize

emerging infections recently appearing infectious diseases in a population or diseases that are rapidly increasing or threatening to increase in the near future

endemic an increase in the normal number of a specific disease in a defined geographic area or locale

fomite contaminated food or drink and contaminated objects such as soiled hands; provide avenue for indirect transmission of microbes

general asepsis common techniques and procedures to reduce the number of pathogenic microorganisms in the normal environment and to decrease the opportunity for further spread

health-care–acquired infection (HAI) infection a patient acquires when in a health-care facility, typically a hospital setting; also known as nosocomial infection

human immunodeficiency virus (HIV) pathogen that causes AIDS

medical asepsis (clean technique) techniques and procedures that reduce the number of microorganisms in a health-care environment and decrease opportunities for further spread

methicillin-resistant staphylococcus aureus (MRSA) a bacterium responsible for a severe difficult-to-treat skin infection since it is resistant to methicillin and many other antibiotics

microorganisms microbes or germs; living organisms that are too small to see with the naked eye

mycology the study of fungi

OSHA (Occupational Safety and Health Administration) a federal agency that develops and monitors guidelines and mandates that address health and safety in the workplace

outbreak an excess of the normal number of occurrences of a specific disease

pandemic an epidemic that has spread over several countries or continents, usually affecting a large number of people

parasite an organism that lives at the expense of another organism

parasitology study of worms, protozoa, and other parasites

pathogens microorganisms that cause disease

portals of entry or means of entrance routes by which microorganisms enter the body

spores encapsulated bacteria in an inactive or resting state

sterilization process of destroying all living organisms

surgical asepsis (sterile technique) techniques and procedures intended to eliminate all microorganisms in an environment

virology study of virus

REVIEW QUESTIONS

All questions are relevant for all medical assisting certification exams. Questions 1 through 17 are relevant for all medical administrative certification exams.

1. The specific name used for any type of pathogen that lives in and is transmitted through blood is:
   A. anaerobic bacteria.
   B. parasitic amoeba.
   C. blood-borne pathogen.
   D. aerobic pathogen.

   Answer: **C**
   Why: A blood-borne pathogen is a microorganism that lives in and is transmitted through blood.
   Review: Yes ○   No ○

2. The chain of infection requires the microorganism to find a means of exit from the host. These means of exit include the following EXCEPT:
   A. sneezing.
   B. ingestion.
   C. coughing.
   D. blood.
   E. feces.

   Answer: **B**
   Why: Ingestion is the process of taking food or water into the body. This is a means by which a microorganism can enter the body but is not a means of exit.
   Review: Yes ○   No ○

3. An example of a viral disease is:
   A. ringworm.
   B. candidiasis.
   C. malaria.
   D. measles.

   Answer: **D**
   Why: Ringworm and candidiasis are examples of conditions caused by fungus. Malaria is caused by protozoal parasites.
   Review: Yes ○   No ○

4. A bacteria that lives without oxygen is:
   A. aerobic.
   B. aseptic.
   C. anemic.
   D. anoxic.
   E. anaerobic.

   Answer: **E**
   Why: An anaerobe is a microorganism that can live and grow in the absence of oxygen. The term anaerobic describes this type of bacteria. Aerobic means requiring oxygen for life and growth. Anoxic is a term used to describe the absence of oxygen in arterial blood. Anemic describes a condition in which the number of red blood cells or hemoglobin of the blood is below the normal level. Aseptic describes the absence or control of microorganisms.
   Review: Yes ○   No ○

5. The major reason for using proper aseptic procedures is to:
   A. follow office policies.
   B. destroy all bacteria on surfaces.
   C. control the patient's immune system.
   D. protect patients and health-care workers.

   Answer: **D**
   Why: Aseptic technique is practiced to protect patients, the public, and health-care workers from the transmission of disease-causing microorganisms. Asepsis is a condition in which living pathogenic organisms are absent: the environment is sterile.
   Review: Yes ○   No ○

6. The process that destroys all living organ-
   isms is:
   A. handwashing.
   B. sanitizing.
   C. autoclaving.
   D. cleansing.
   E. disinfecting.

   Answer: **C**
   Why: Autoclaving is the only process listed that ensures that all bacteria are destroyed and the items
   autoclaved are sterile.
   Review: Yes ○   No ○

7. Personal protective equipment includes
   the following EXCEPT:
   A. needles.
   B. gowns.
   C. gloves.
   D. masks.

   Answer: **A**
   Why: Personal protective equipment (PPE) includes
   any device or garment that protects the individual
   from contact with blood and body fluid that may
   contain blood-borne pathogens.
   Review: Yes ○   No ○

8. Ringworm or tinea corporis is an example
   of a:
   A. bacteria.
   B. fungus.
   C. protozoa.
   D. virus.
   E. parasite.

   Answer: **B**
   Why: Fungus is a simple parasitic plant. Ringworm
   is a type of fungal skin disease that forms a red,
   ringlike lesion on the skin.
   Review: Yes ○   No ○

9. The organization that develops and moni-
   tors guidelines and mandates health and
   safety practices in the workplace is:
   A. AMA.
   B. CDC.
   C. FDA.
   D. OSHA.

   Answer: **D**
   Why: The Occupational Safety and Health Administration (OSHA) is a federal agency that has
   developed policies for the workplace that include
   guidelines for health-care workers to prevent the
   transmission of blood-borne pathogens.
   Review: Yes ○   No ○

10. A chemical agent used to clean counter-
    tops to decrease the number of disease-
    causing organisms is a(n):
    A. antibiotic.
    B. disinfectant.
    C. antiseptic.
    D. sterile solution.
    E. germicidal soap.

    Answer: **B**
    Why: A disinfectant is used to clean surfaces to free
    them of pathogenic organisms. Antibiotics, anti-
    septics, and germicidal soaps are used on or in the
    body, not on inanimate objects. A sterile solution is
    any product that is free of microorganisms.
    Review: Yes ○   No ○

11. Characteristics of a susceptible host in-
    clude the following EXCEPT:
    A. lack of hygiene.
    B. poor nutrition.
    C. intact immune system.
    D. chronic illness.
    E. injury to the body.

    Answer: **C**
    Why: A susceptible host is a person who is more vul-
    nerable to a disease or disorder. Chronic illness, in-
    jury to the body, poor nutrition, and a lack of good
    hygiene contribute to the environment for microor-
    ganisms to cause infection or disease. A person with
    an intact immune system is more likely to be able to
    resist infections caused by pathogens.
    Review: Yes ○   No ○

12. One difference between a localized and a generalized infection is that a:
    A. localized infection is contained within a specific area.
    B. generalized infection has spread to one specific area of the body.
    C. localized infection is the same as a systemic infection.
    D. generalized infection is caused by non-specific microorganisms.

Answer: **A**
Why: A localized infection is confined to one area or part of the body, whereas a generalized infection has spread to many areas of the body or may be systemic.
Review: Yes ○   No ○

13. The most important guideline stated in the universal precautions is to:
    A. always wear gloves even if there is no risk for contact with blood-borne pathogens.
    B. treat all blood and bodily fluids as contaminated.
    C. label specimens from patients who are suspected of having a blood-borne pathogen such as HIV.
    D. conserve supplies by reusing gloves but changing them when visibly soiled with blood.

Answer: **B**
Why: All patients' blood and bodily fluids are considered contaminated, even if they are not. This practice will ensure you always use universal precautions with all patients, not just those suspected of having a blood-borne pathogen. It is not necessary to use gloves when performing procedures that will not put you at risk for contact with blood or body fluids. This includes most noninvasive procedures. Never reuse gloves on different patients.
Review: Yes ○   No ○

14. When a patient acquires an infection while in a medical facility, it is referred to as a:
    A. bacterial infection.
    B. causative infection.
    C. health-care–acquired infection.
    D. pathogenic infection.

Answer: **C**
Why: A health-care–acquired infection (HAI) is an infection separate from the patient's original condition that is acquired while the patient is being treated in a hospital or health-care facility.
Review: Yes ○   No ○

15. The chain of infection does not include:
    A. susceptible host.
    B. means of transmission.
    C. reservoir.
    D. asepsis.

Answer: **D**
Why: Asepsis is the absence or the control of microorganisms. The use of aseptic technique inhibits the spread of disease.
Review: Yes ○   No ○

16. Which of the following is a chemical cleaning agent used on the skin to remove bacteria?
    A. Disinfectant
    B. Antiseptic
    C. Immunization
    D. Cold sterilization solution
    E. Sterile water

Answer: **B**
Why: A disinfectant is a chemical agent used to clean inanimate objects. An immunization is a biologic or chemical agent that creates immunity to specific diseases. Immunizations are ingested or injected. Cold sterilization solution is used to soak instruments before autoclaving. Sterile water is not a chemical cleaning agent.
Review: Yes ○   No ○

17. Hepatitis B and rubella are examples of diseases caused by:
   A. yeasts.
   B. fungi.
   C. bacteria.
   D. protozoa.
   E. viruses.

Answer: **E**
Why: Viruses are the smallest form of microorganisms and are not susceptible to antibiotics. They are difficult to treat.
Review: Yes ○   No ○

18. Steps to follow for proper autoclaving include:
   A. keeping hinged instruments in an open position.
   B. wrapping instruments while they are wet.
   C. wearing sterile gloves to wrap autoclave packs for processing.
   D. storing autoclaved packs while they are damp.

Answer: **A**
Why: Instruments should be dry before they are wrapped for autoclaving. It is not necessary to wear sterile gloves to process wraps for autoclaving. After autoclaving, packs need to be dry before being placed in storage.
Review: Yes ○   No ○

19. Which of the following are bacteria normally found in the intestinal tract but that cause infection if introduced into the urinary tract or bloodstream?
   A. *Clostridium tetani*
   B. *Bacillus anthracis*
   C. *Escherichia coli*
   D. *Treponema pallidum*
   E. Coccidioidomycosis

Answer: **C**
Why: Escherichia coli is abbreviated to *E. coli*. It is a bacterium found in the intestinal tract and usually causes no problem except when it invades other body systems. *Clostridium tetani* causes tetanus, *Bacillus anthracis* causes anthrax, and *Treponema pallidum* causes syphilis.
Review: Yes ○   No ○

20. The process that kills spore-producing bacteria is:
   A. handwashing.
   B. chemical soaking.
   C. disinfecting.
   D. autoclaving.

Answer: **D**
Why: Autoclaving is the same as sterilizing. It is the use of steam under pressure. The autoclave is used at an average temperature of 250°F for an average time of 30 minutes. This process is used to ensure that spores will be killed.
Review: Yes ○   No ○

21. Which of the following is not part of proper surgical handwashing technique?
   A. Remove jewelry.
   B. Dry hands with sterile towel.
   C. Hold hands in a downward position while rinsing.
   D. Use foot- or knee-controlled faucet.
   E. Use a cuticle stick on nails.

Answer: **C**
Why: When performing a surgical handwash, hands should be held upward while rinsing so the water does not carry bacteria from the unscrubbed portion of the upper arm to the scrubbed portion of the arms and hands.
Review: Yes ○   No ○

22. The unique characteristic of spore-forming bacteria is that they:
    A. are easily destroyed with the use of chemical cleaners.
    B. are only found in cocci shapes or formation.
    C. account for most of the known viruses.
    D. are able to form a resistant capsule around themselves.

Answer: **D**
Why: Spore-forming bacteria are able to form a capsule or shell around themselves that is resistant to most means of asepsis, such as heat or chemicals. Autoclaving or sterilizing is the only method known to kill spores.
Review: Yes ○   No ○

---

23. Objects that provide an avenue for indirect transmission of microbes are called:
    A. spores.
    B. pathogens.
    C. PPE.
    D. fomites.

Answer: **D**
Why: Spores are bacteria that are able to form a capsule or shell around them that is resistant to most means of asepsis, such as heat or chemicals. Pathogens include any disease-causing microorganisms. PPE is personal protective equipment used for protection during procedures where there is a chance of contact with pathogens.
Review: Yes ○   No ○

---

24. A type of protozoa that causes vaginitis is:
    A. *Candida.*
    B. staphylococci.
    C. *Trichomonas.*
    D. tinea.

Answer: **C**
Why: Candida is an example of yeast, tinea is ringworm, and staphylococci are bacteria. *Trichomonas* are protozoa, single-celled parasites.
Review: Yes ○   No ○

---

25. The temperature setting and timing for proper autoclaving is:
    A. 175°F for 10 minutes.
    B. 212°F for 15 minutes.
    C. 250°F for 30 minutes.
    D. 275°F for 45 minutes.
    E. 300°F for 30 minutes.

Answer: **C**
Why: Most autoclave loads are processed at 250°F for 30 minutes. The timing or temperature may vary slightly because of the tightness of the wrap.
Review: Yes ○   No ○

---

26. Which of the following is an example of spherical or round bacteria?
    A. Staphylococci
    B. Tetanus
    C. *E. coli*
    D. *Shigella*

Answer: **A**
Why: Round or spherical-shaped bacteria are called *cocci*. Under the microscope, staphylococci appear as clusters or groups of round bacteria. Tetanus bacteria, *E. coli*, and *Shigella* are rod shaped.
Review: Yes ○   No ○

CRITICAL THINKING CASE REVIEW

It is cold and *influenza* (flu) season, and the staff in Dr. Grenger's office just received a training on asepsis.

1. The office policy is requiring all staff to receive a flu shot or:
   A. wear a mask during the flu season.
   B. wash hands more frequently.
   C. take an antibiotic.
   D. stay home during flu season.
   E. tender a resignation.

   Answer: **A**
   Why: Staff should always be washing hands appropriately and frequently. Therefore, it should not be necessary to do more during flu season. Antibiotics are not useful in preventing *influenza*, and due to emerging antibiotic resistant diseases, the use of antibiotics is decreasing, not increasing. It is not feasible to ask a staff member to stay home during the entire flu season, since it involves many months or to tender a resignation. Some offices do require any personnel who refuse a flu shot to wear a mask during the flu season. Masks should be worn by staff or patients who are coughing.
   Review: Yes ○   No ○

2. Influenza is a disease with the portal of entry of the:
   A. integumentary system.
   B. respiratory system.
   C. gastrointestinal system.
   D. vascular system.

   Answer: **B**
   Why: Influenza is a respiratory disease spread through droplets resulting from coughing and sneezing; contrary to some beliefs, influenza does not cause gastrointestinal problems but respiratory problems and even death in the more susceptible person.
   Review: Yes ○   No ○

3. The idea of coughing or sneezing into your elbow instead of your hands is to:
   A. avoid transmission of pathogens from your hands.
   B. cover your cough or sneeze more quickly.
   C. use your sleeve so as not to contaminate facial tissue.
   D. muffle your cough or sneeze to avoid disturbing people around you.
   E. encourage wearing long-sleeved clothing during the winter.

   Answer: **A**
   Why: When coughing or sneezing (**means of exit**) into the hand, the hand becomes contaminated and the pathogens are **transmitted** to the next person, for example, by handshake or a touched object, such as a pen; the pathogen eventually travels from there to the face, for example, by rubbing eyes, covering a yawn (**means or portal of entry**). Coughing or sneezing into your sleeve prevents your hand from becoming contaminated.
   Review: Yes ○   No ○

4. The recommendations and enforcement policies of which two organizations were probably used during the training in Dr. Grenger's office?
   A. CDC and OSHA
   B. CMC and OSHA
   C. CDC and CMC
   D. EEOC and OSHA

   Answer: **A**
   Why: The CDC establishes many of the standards and guidelines for asepsis in the health-care setting, and OSHA is the enforcement agency for these standards related to the workplace. The CMS is responsible for administering Medicare and Medicaid, and the EEOC is involved with ensuring that equal employment standards are observed.
   Review: Yes ○   No ○

5. It is necessary to practice asepsis:
- A. in the clinical portion of the medical practice.
- B. in all areas at all times.
- C. in all areas during cold and flu season.
- D. in the clinical and administrative areas.
- E. when you are aware of communicable diseases.

Answer: **B**

Why: All of the answers are correct. However, the best answer is in all areas at all times.

Review: Yes ⭕   No ⭕

CHAPTER

18

Patient Exams and Procedures

Review Tip:

The national exams often require you to identify instruments and equipment from a picture. Practice recognizing various instruments and their medical uses. Also, study the body positions described in this chapter, since they are always in the exams.

PROCEDURES

As previously cited, this is a review book, not a primary text. The material is not presented in detail as during initial learning but contains information that is likely to appear on the national exams. In addition to this chapter, procedure information is found in almost all chapters. Whether clinical or administrative, every procedure has the following commonalities:

■ always identify the patient using two metrics (usually name and birth date);

■ always utilize appropriate aseptic and safety practices;

■ always explain the procedure to the patient;

■ always assure the patient is provided with and understands any instructions.

The medical assistant, from the moment of contact, observes the patient for baseline behaviors, changes, and signs and symptoms. This first observation begins the patient exam, and observations continue throughout the patient visit. Specific medical record forms and drop-down screens are used to record the information. The medical assistant should note the data from previous visits as a comparison to the newly obtained information.

PATIENT INTERVIEW

The interview process discussed in this chapter incorporates the knowledge, techniques, and skills from previous chapters—including medical terminology, anatomy and physiology, communication, law and ethics, patient education, medical records, and microorganisms and asepsis. Professionalism and adherence to HIPAA are expected standards.

- Chief complaint—a summary in the **patient's words** explaining why he or she is seeking health care; best determined by asking an open-ended question such as "What brings you here today?"

- Symptoms—subjective descriptions of altered health indicators (e.g., nausea, headache); complaints that cannot be seen or measured

- Medical-related histories—accounts of past health status or practices and exposures that affect health status
  - Family history—medical history of the patient's close biologic relatives (e.g., grandparents, parents, siblings)
  - Patient medical history—the patient's past health status; usually conducted by a review of body systems
  - Social and environmental history—the patient's past and current personal habits and exposures and risks that influence health
  - Screen for abuse and domestic violence—a history-type questionnaire recommended by many professional organizations and mandated in some jurisdictions to assist in determining the presence of abuse in the patient's life
  - Preventive health maintenance status including recent
    - Immunization status (children and adults)
    - Bone density

    - Mammography, breast exam and self-breast exam
    - Pap smears
    - PSA, testicular exam and self-testicular exam
    - Colonoscopy
  - Condition-specific monitoring such as:
    - A1c hemoglobin for diabetics
    - TB risk assessment
    - Smoking and cessation
    - Weight control

COMMON ASSESSMENT MEASUREMENTS

Obtaining assessment measurements is also known as **anthropometry**. Anthropometry comprises signs, functions, and capacities that can be objectively determined by the senses (e.g., sight, hearing, smell, touch) or by specific equipment and tests. Medical asepsis is maintained in preparing, performing, and following all common assessment functions.

VITAL SIGNS

Vital signs are measurements of body temperature, pulse rate, respirations (TPR), and blood pressure (BP).

- Body temperature—measured by a thermometer using one of two scales, degrees Fahrenheit (F) or degrees Celsius (C), also referred to as centigrade; the normal range for infants, children, and adults is the same, but infants and small children are more sensitive to external temperature changes
  - Common anatomic locations to obtain temperature; refer to Table 18-1 for comparisons
    - Oral (temperature taken in the mouth) adult norm is 98.6°F or 37°C
    - Rectal (temperature taken in the rectum) norm is 1° higher than oral; adult norm is 99.6°F or 37.5°C
    - Axillary (temperature taken in the armpit) norm is 1° lower than oral; adult norm is 97.6°F or 36.4°C

TABLE 18-1 ▶ Normal body temperature comparisons by common sites

Route	Thermometer	Normal Temperature in Fahrenheit	Normal Temperature in Celsius (Centigrade)
Mouth	Oral	98.6°	37°
Rectum	Rectal	99.6°	37.5°
Armpit	Axillary	97.6°	36.4°
Ear	Otic, aural or tympanic	98.6°	37°

- Aural, otic, or tympanic (temperature taken in the ear) norm is the same as oral; adult norm is 98.6°F or 37°C
- Thermometer—instrument used to measure temperature
  - Mercury—a glass thermometer with a mercury column; no longer used due to mercury danger
  - Electronic—most common in the medical office; a thermometer with a power source, varieties are route-specific; the tympanic resembles an otoscope; displays the temperature digitally; converts from °F to °C or vice versa by flipping a small switch; stylus is covered by a disposable sheath
  - Disposable—one-time-use plastic thermometer strips, dots, or probes used on the skin or in the mouth; considered least reliable

- Pulse—"beat" caused by expansion and relaxation of the **artery wall**, expressed in beats per minute (bpm); the adult norm is 60 to 100 bpm in a regular rhythm, usually the same rate and rhythm as the heart; the infant norm is 100 to 160 bpm; and the norm of children to age 10 is 70 to 120 bpm
  - Anatomic sites—the pulse may be taken using any artery lying over bone; the most common follow in the order of frequency of use (refer to Fig. 18-1)
    - Radial—pulse located on the thumb side of the wrist; most common site used for adults
    - Brachial—pulse located medially on both arms anterior to the elbow; most common site used for children
    - Apical—pulse located at the fifth intercostal space midclavicular; common site used for infants; requires a stethoscope
    - Dorsalis pedis—pulse located medially on the top of both feet, often used to assess circulation to the extremities
    - Carotid—pulse located on both sides of the neck, lateral to the trachea
    - Femoral—pulse located bilaterally in groin
    - Popliteal—pulse located posterior to both knees, also used to assess circulation to the extremities
    - Temporal—pulse located bilaterally over temporal bone
  - Methods to obtain pulse
    - Manual—light compression of the artery with index and middle finger; count beats for 30 or 60 seconds, multiplying beats by 2 if 30-second count is used; for irregular pulses, a full-minute count is recommended
    - Doppler—ultrasonic device used to locate, audibly transmit, and sometimes record pulse

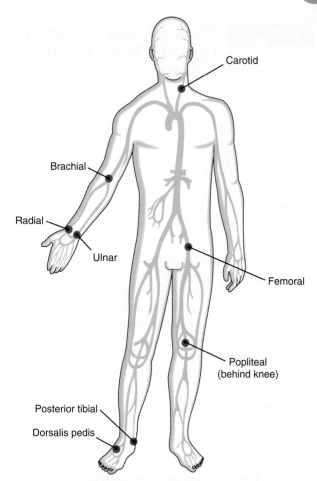

FIGURE 18-1 Location of common body pulses.

  - Electronic sphygmomanometer—device used to measure pulse and blood pressure simultaneously using a BP cuff
- Respiration—measurement of the number of respiratory cycles per minute, usually done by observation; a respiratory cycle consists of inspiration and expiration; the adult norm is 12 to 20 respiratory cycles per minute in a regular rhythm; the younger the infant or child, the more rapid the normal respiratory rate; refer to Table 18-2 for a comparison by age
- Blood pressure (BP)—measurement of the force of blood on the artery walls during contraction (systole)

TABLE 18-2	Comparison of normal respiration rates by age
Age	Respirations Rate
0–1 y	20–40
2–6 y	20–30
6 y through adult	12–20

TABLE 18-3 ▸ Blood pressure category designations from the National Heart, Lung and Blood Institute

Category	Systolic		Diastolic
Normal	<120	And	<80
Prehypertension	120–139	Or	80–89
High blood pressure (hypertension)			
Stage 1	140–159	Or	90–99
Stage 2	160 or higher	Or	100 or higher

and relaxation (diastole) of the heart; recorded as a fraction with systole as the numerator and diastole as the denominator; the adult norm has recently changed; refer to Table 18-3; above 130/89 is considered hypertension, but the diagnosis is not made on a single reading. BPs are not commonly taken in children younger than 4 years; the most accurate position for taking a BP is placing the arm at the level of the heart

- Korotkoff sounds—sounds heard through the stethoscope during the measurement of BP; there are five phases:
  1. Phase I—faint tapping sounds heard as the cuff deflates (systole)
  2. Phase II—soft swishing sounds
  3. Phase III—rhythmic, sharp, distinct tapping sounds
  4. Phase IV—soft tapping sounds that become faint
  5. Phase V—disappearance of sound (diastole)
- Pulse pressure—the difference between the systolic and diastolic pressures; the adult norm is 40; the difference should be approximately one-third of systole
- Orthostatic pressure—BP taken in all three positions (supine, sitting, and standing) at least 1 to 2 minutes apart
- Sphygmomanometer—the instrument used to measure BP; composed of a cuff for the arm, thigh, wrist, or finger, and a measurement device; the correct size and cuff fit influence the accuracy of the readings
  - Mercury sphygmomanometer—no longer in use because of mercury danger
  - Aneroid sphygmomanometer—a BP cuff with a numeric gauge to measure readings; stethoscope required
  - Electronic sphygmomanometer—BP cuff with an electronic device to measure BP and pulse readings; no stethoscope required
- Stethoscope—the instrument's diaphragm or bell is placed at the artery to be used to hear the sounds that compose the BP

OTHER MEASUREMENTS

Height
Height or length is commonly measured by a rod attached to a weight scale or fixed bar on a wall; a measuring tape is used for measuring the length of neonates and also the head circumference. Measurements are recorded in feet (ft) and inches (in), or centimeters (cm); the conversion is 2.5 cm per inch.

Weight
Weight is commonly measured in the medical office using a balance beam or an electronic scale. Measurements are recorded in pounds (lb) or kilograms (kg); the conversion is 2.2 lb per kg.

Comparisons of Height and Weight
Using the height and weight in formulas and charts provides the practitioner with an approximation of the patient's size related to normal standards. These methods are used to determine the patient's health risk for various diseases and conditions.

- **Body mass index (BMI)**—a health risk assessment tool for adults and children to estimate the percentage of body fat by using a formula based on the individual's height and weight; the calculations are somewhat complicated and can be calculated by going to the CDC website or downloading a specific BMI calculation application. For adults:
  - Normal range = 18.5 to 24.9
  - Underweight = <18.5
  - Overweight = 25 to 29.9
  - Obese = 30 and above
- **Pediatric growth chart**—supplied by the Centers for Disease Control and Prevention (CDC), this is considered a version of a BMI for infants and small children; the form is specific to the current age and sex of the child and contains the height, weight, and head circumference; the individual's measurements are compared by percentile to an established reference group (Fig. 18-2).

CDC Growth Charts: United States

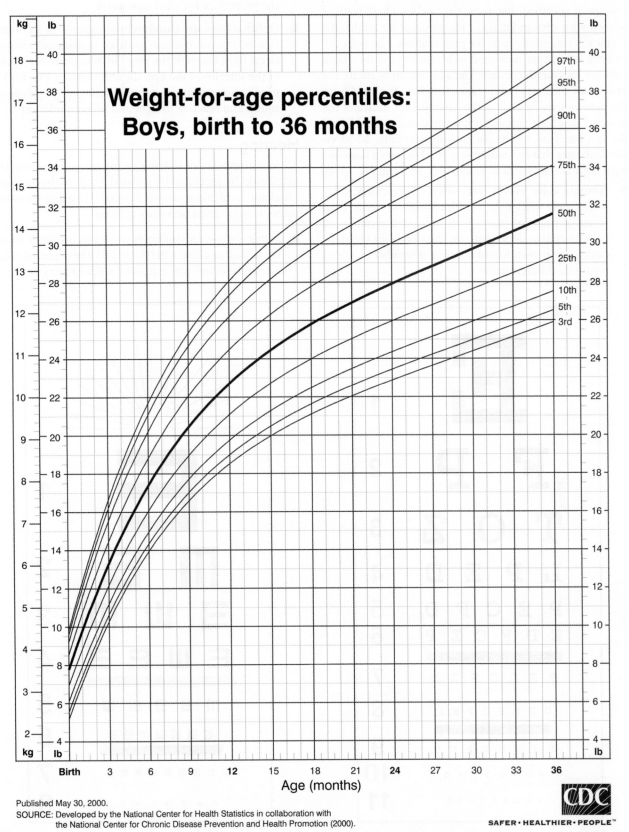

**Weight-for-age percentiles:
Boys, birth to 36 months**

Published May 30, 2000.
SOURCE: Developed by the National Center for Health Statistics in collaboration with
the National Center for Chronic Disease Prevention and Health Promotion (2000).

FIGURE 18-2 Centers for Disease Control and Prevention (CDC) growth chart for US males, birth to 36 months of age. (From the CDC.)

Vision

Visual acuity is the measurement of how well a person can see at specified distances; the **Snellen chart method** is used with various letters of the alphabet for adults; the E chart is commonly used for preschoolers. The right eye and the left eye are measured individually, and then both eyes are measured together. The adult norm is 20/20: the numerator indicates the distance the chart is placed from the patient, usually 20 feet; the denominator indicates the distance at which people with normal acuity could read the last line read by the patient—for example, 20/30 vision indicates that the patient sees at 20 feet what someone with normal vision sees at 30 feet (Fig. 18-3 and Fig. 18-4).

■ **Ishihara color vision test**—used to determine color vision deficiencies (color blindness); consists of a series of pages or plates with imbedded numbers of various colors; depending on the degree of the deficiency, the person would not see the number or would see it in a different color

■ **Tonometer**—an instrument used to measure the intraocular pressure of the eye to diagnose glaucoma; the procedure is called tonometry

■ **Ophthalmoscopy (funduscopy) exam**—an examination of the interior eye with an instrument that reflects light through the pupil to determine the health of the interior of the eye; the abbreviation **PERRLA** is used to document the normal finding of "pupils equal round and reactive to light and accommodation"

Hearing

All measurements of hearing or any action involving the ear should be preceded by a visual exam of the auditory canal and eardrum using an otoscope. Hearing measurements may be gross or highly defined.

■ Startle—gross measurement used with neonates; a loud noise such as a clap will be initiated; the expected result is that the infant will react with a jerk or a cry

FIGURE 18-3 Snellen eye chart for those who know the alphabet. (From Wikipedia.)

FIGURE 18-4 Snellen "E" eye chart for preschoolers. (From Wikipedia.)

- Whisper—screening measurement; the health-care provider will whisper to the patient and the patient repeats what is said; each ear is done separately
- Tuning fork—screening measurement for hearing and conduction; the instrument is activated by striking it with a hand; the placement is dependent on the test:
  - Weber test—the tuning fork is activated and usually placed on top of the patient's head equidistant from both ears; a normal test is when the patient hears the same in both ears
  - Rinne test—the tuning fork is activated and first placed and on each side of the patient's mastoid bone until the sound is no longer heard then immediately placed just outside the ear until the sound is no longer heard; a normal or positive test is when the sound outside the ear is louder than the sound with the mastoid placement
- Audiometry—a hearing test using an audiometer with earphones that measures the patient's response to tones; it is recorded in decibels (db) and frequencies
- Impedance audiometry—a hearing test using an audiometer and an ear probe that measures tympanic membrane mobility of the middle ear system and neural transmission
- Tympanometry—a test that uses a tympanometer (air pressure) to measure tympanic membrane mobility

Common Respiratory Tests

Part of the physical exam is to determine how well the lungs are functioning. The practitioner performs an initial evaluation by listening for normal breath sounds with a stethoscope. Other common respiratory tests are performed by the medical assistant.

- **Pulse oximetry**—a test using a pulse oximeter on the patient's digit to measure the percentage of oxygen (O_2) in the blood; this is a common test done with vital signs when visiting the medical office. The norm is 97% or higher.
- **Pulmonary function test (PFT)**—used to diagnose and measure the severity of lung problems by evaluating how well the lungs work: the amount of air the lungs can hold and how quickly the lungs move air in and out; measurements also include the efficiency of oxygenating the blood and removing carbon dioxide
  - **Spirometry**—the most common lung function test; measures how much and how quickly air is moved in and out of the lungs by breathing into a mouthpiece attached to a recording device (spirometer); a graph with the results (spirogram) is produced
  - **Peak flow meter**—a handheld device used to measure the **peak expiratory flow rate** (PEFR) to monitor asthmatics; the ranges are established by the practitioner, and usually three consecutive attempts are recorded

PHYSICAL EXAMINATION PREPARATION AND ASSISTANCE

The type of examination scheduled for the health-care provider to perform determines how the medical assistant prepares the patient and the supplies and tools used. Always explain the procedure to the patient. Ensure privacy is maintained, requesting that the patient undress to facilitate access to the body areas that will be examined; provide gowns and draping accordingly. Consideration for the patient's comfort includes room temperature, lighting, sound, and physical position while waiting and during the exam.

- Common supplies and instruments—the medical assistant is responsible for ensuring all supplies and equipment are readily available for the physical exam; Box 18-1 lists common supplies and tools for a routine patient exam; Figure 18-5 illustrates some of those tools
- Patient positions (Fig. 18-6)
  - **Supine**—patient lies on back with arms to the sides; commonly used for abdominal exams
  - **Dorsal recumbent**—patient lies on back with knees bent and feet flat on the exam table; commonly used to check progress of labor
  - **Lithotomy**—patient lies on back with buttocks on edge of exam table, legs elevated and resting in stirrups; commonly used for pelvic exams
  - **Sims'**—patient lies on left side with left leg slightly flexed and left arm behind body as comfortable;

BOX 18-1

Common supplies and tools for routine patient exam

4 × 4 gauze (nonsterile)	Slide and fixative or ThinPrep-type container and applicator (pelvic exam)
Exam gloves (nonsterile)	Sphygmomanometer
Laryngeal mirror	Stethoscope
Lubricant (pelvic and rectal exams)	Tape measure
Nasal speculum	Thermometer
Ophthalmoscope	Tissues
Otoscope	Tongue depressor
Penlight	Tuning fork
Percussion hammer	Vaginal speculum (pelvic exam)

A Sphygmomanometers

B Tuning forks

C Nasal specula

D Ophthalmoscope and otoscope

E Laryngeal mirror

F Vaginal specula

FIGURE 18-5 Select tools for routine physical exam. (Sklar Instruments, West Chester, PA.)

right leg is flexed toward chest and right arm is over the chest; commonly used for rectal exams and colonoscopies

- **Prone**—patient lies on stomach; commonly used for exam of posterior and administration of intramuscular injections on adults

- **Jackknife**—patient lies on stomach and the exam table is inverted with head lowered and with knees at a 90-degree angle; arms overhead; commonly used for sigmoidoscopic exams

- **Knee–chest position**—patient rests on knees with chest and arms on table and arms flexed over the head; commonly used for rectal and sigmoidoscopic exams when flexible exam table is not available

- **Fowler's**—patient lies face up on table with upper body elevated to a 45- to 90-degree angle; commonly used for patients short of breath and for head and neck exams

- **Semi-Fowler's**—the Fowler's position at a 45-degree angle

■ Examination techniques

- **Observation or inspection**—visual review of the body, inspecting for symmetry, abnormalities, and skin color and conditions

- **Palpation**—use of fingertips and hands to feel for sizes and positions of specific organs, masses, and other abnormalities; texture and firmness; skin temperature and moisture; and flexibility of joints

FIGURE 18-6 Patient positions for exams and procedures. (Reprinted with permission from Hosley JB, Jones SA, Molle-Matthews EA. *Lippincott's Textbook for Medical Assistants.* Philadelphia: Lippincott-Raven Publishers, 1997.)

- **Percussion**—process of determining density of specific internal structures by the sound (e.g., dull, hollow) produced by external tapping, usually with fingers or with a percussion hammer for testing neurologic reflexes

- **Auscultation**—use of an instrument, usually a stethoscope, to listen to internal body sounds for abnormalities

- **Manipulation**—passive movement of body joints to determine the extent of movement

- **Mensuration**—measurement of height or length and weight

COMMON MEDICAL IMAGING EXAMS AND SELECT PREPARATIONS

Medical assistants and certified medical administrative specialists do not perform radiology or medical imaging studies, except under a separate certification. Their job is to process the provider's orders; to assure authorization is obtained if required by the patient's insurance; and often, to coordinate and schedule the tests with an outside facility.

Radiology is the study and use of radioactive substances to visualize an internal structure and may be used for diagnostic purposes (e.g., to determine a fracture) or therapeutic purposes (e.g., as a treatment for cancer). Patient education and preparation is usually needed for these procedures, which is also the job of the medical assistant or the medical administrative specialist.

Not all medical imaging requires exposure to radiation. An example is ultrasound. Terminology and some patient preparations (preps) that may appear on the exams include:

- **X-ray (basic)**—radiation passing through a cassette or acquisition device that converts the image directly into a digital picture
  - When ordering an x-ray of a bone or bones of a body part that are bilateral, such as a foot, the provider frequently wants an x-ray of the same bone(s) of the opposite side as a comparison.

- **Angiography (angiogram)**—radiographic visualization of blood vessels and blood flow by injecting radiopaque material through a subcutaneous catheter
  - Instruct patient to consume nothing by mouth (NPO) for 8 hours before procedure
  - Determine whether the patient is on any blood-thinning medication, including aspirin and NSAIDs; these medications are usually stopped for a minimum of 24 hours prior to the procedure but is provider-specific

- **Arthrography (arthrogram)**—radiographic visualization of a joint by injection of contrast media

- **Barium enema (lower GI series)**—rectal administration of barium to radiographically visualize the lower portion of the gastrointestinal system
  - Instruct the patient to ingest only clear liquids the day before the test
  - Instruct NPO usually 8 hours before the procedure
  - Explain bowel cleansing per facility criteria
  - Instruct the patient to increase fluids after the exam and report if there is no bowel movement within 24 hours after the test

- **Barium swallow (upper GI series)**—oral administration of barium to radiographically visualize the upper portion of the gastrointestinal system
  - Instruct patient to have a light evening meal and NPO usually 8 hours before the procedure
  - Instruct the patient to increase fluids after the test; a laxative is usually recommended

- **Bone density scan**—radiographic exam to detect osteoporosis and osteopenia, which increase the patient's risk for fractures; the most common bone density scan is a called a **DEXA**

- **Cardiac catheterization**—passing a thin flexible tube (catheter) into the heart, using the femoral or radial artery under direct imaging for visualization to diagnose or treat certain heart ailments

- **Cholangiography (cholangiogram)**—radiographic visualization of the bile ducts by injection of contrast media; types include intravenous (IVC), percutaneous transhepatic (PTHC or PTC)
  - Instruct the patient to have a fat-free evening meal prior to the exam
  - Instruct the patient NPO after meal and prescribed tablets
  - Bowel cleansing may be ordered per facility criteria

- **Cholecystography (cholecystogram)**—radiographic visualization of the gallbladder structure and function

- **Computed tomography (CT)**—radiographic visualization of body structures in thin cross sections or layers; much more precise than traditional x-ray
  - Explain that contrast media will be ingested just prior to procedure; assure no iodine or other drug allergies
  - Other preparation may be specific to the part of the body being tested

- **HIDA scan**—imaging following injection of radioactive tracers to diagnose problems of the liver, gallbladder, and bile ducts

- **Intravenous pyelography (IVP)**—radiographic visualization of the kidneys, ureters, and bladder by injection of contrast media through a vein
  - Instruct the patient to ingest only clear liquids the day before the procedure
  - Instruct NPO usually 8 hours before the procedure
  - Explain bowel cleansing per facility criteria

- **Kidneys, ureters, and bladder (KUB)**—flat plate (x-ray) of the abdomen to visualize the kidneys, ureters, and bladder

- **Magnetic resonance imaging (MRI)**—visualization of internal structures, including soft tissue, by using a magnetic field in combination with radiation
  - Instruct patient to wear comfortable clothes without metal zippers or clasps and no metal hair clips or eye makeup

- **Mammography**—radiographic examination of breasts (usually female) with specialized x-ray equipment
  - Instruct the patient not to apply lotion, deodorant, or powder from the neck to the waist
  - Instruct the patient to avoid caffeine one week before the test if this is a facility criterion

- **Myelography (myelogram)**—radiographic visualization of the spinal cord and nerve roots by injection of contrast media into the subarachnoid space

- **Nuclear medicine**—area of medicine using radioisotopes to diagnose and treat specific pathology; used in some cancer therapies

- Positron emission tomography (PET)—process of producing color images by injecting radioisotopes that combine with particles in the body; used to assess physiology and metabolic activity, not just structures; especially useful in detecting malignancies.
  - Explain to the patient the necessity for a low-carbohydrate diet and no sugars the day prior to the scan
  - Instruct the patient to fast with only water allowed six hours prior to the scan
  - Avoid exercise 48 hours prior to the scan per criteria of facility
- Radiation therapy—using radiation to treat diseases, typically cancer, by shrinking the tumor; may be performed in medical imaging department or outpatient facility
- Retrograde pyelography—radiographic visualization of the kidneys, ureters, and bladder by administration of contrast media through a urinary catheter
- Ultrasonography (ultrasound)—use of high-frequency ultrasonic waves to produce an image and identify and measure deep body structures and abnormalities
  - Echocardiography (echocardiogram)—ultrasound waves used to diagnose or monitor heart disease
  - Fetal ultrasound—ultrasound waves used during various stages of fetal development to discover fetal abnormalities or, in some cases, the size or sex of the baby

---

TERMS

PATIENT EXAMS REVIEW

The following list reviews the terms discussed in this chapter and other important terms that you may see on the exam.

angiography radiographic visualization of blood vessels and blood flow by injecting radiopaque material through a subcutaneous catheter

anthropometry obtaining assessment measurements; comprises signs, functions, and capacities that can be objectively determined by the senses (e.g., sight, hearing, smell) or by specific equipment or tests

arthrography radiographic visualization of a joint by injection of contrast media

audiometry a hearing test using an audiometer with earphones that measures the patient's response to tones; it is recorded in decibels (db) and frequencies

auscultation use of an instrument, usually a stethoscope, to listen to internal body sounds for abnormalities

body mass index (BMI) a health risk assessment tool for adults and children to estimate the percentage of body fat by using a formula based on the individual's height and weight

cardiac catheterization passing a thin flexible tube (catheter) into the heart, using the femoral or radial artery and direct x-ray for visualization to diagnose or treat certain heart ailments

chief complaint a summary of the patient's words explaining why he or she is seeking health care

cholangiography radiographic visualization of the bile ducts using contrast media

cholecystography radiographic visualization of the gallbladder structure and function

computed tomography (CT) radiographic visualization of body structures in thin cross sections or layers

Doppler an ultrasonic device used to locate, audibly transmit, and sometimes record pulses

impedance audiometry a hearing test using an audiometer and an ear probe that measures tympanic membrane mobility of the middle ear system and neural transmission

intravenous pyelography (IVP) radiographic visualization of the kidney, ureters, and bladder by injection of contrast media through a vein

Ishihara color vision test used to determine color vision deficiencies (color blindness); consists of a series of pages or plates with imbedded numbers of various colors; depending on the degree of the deficiency, the person would not see the number or would see it in a different color

kidney, ureter, and bladder (KUB) flat plate (x-ray) of the abdomen

Korotkoff sounds sounds heard through the stethoscope during the measurement of blood pressure; there are five phases

magnetic resonance imaging (MRI) film visualization of internal structures, including soft tissue, by using a magnetic field with radiation

mammography radiographic examination of breasts (usually female) with specialized x-ray

manipulation passive movement of body joints to determine the extent of movement

mensuration measurement of height or length and weight

myelography radiographic visualization of the spinal cord and nerve roots by injection of contrast media into the subarachnoid space

observation visual review of the body, inspecting for symmetry, abnormalities, and skin color and conditions

ophthalmoscope (funduscope) an instrument that reflects light throughout the pupil to determine the health of the interior of the eye

orthostatic pressure comparative blood pressures taken in the supine, sitting, and standing positions

otoscope an instrument to examine the auditory canal and eardrum

palpation use of fingertips and hands to feel for sizes and positions of specific organs, masses, or other abnormalities; texture and firmness; skin temperature and moisture; and flexibility of joints

peak flow meter a handheld device used to measure the peak expiratory flow rate (PEFR) to monitor asthmatics

percussion process of determining density of specific internal structures by the sound produced by external tapping, usually with fingers or with a percussion hammer for testing neurologic reflexes

PERRLA pupils equal, round, reactive to light and accommodation; abbreviation used to describe the normal pupil of the eye

positron emission tomography (PET) process of producing color images by injecting radioisotopes that combine with particles in the body; used to assess physiology and metabolic activities such as malignancies

pulmonary function test (PFT) used to diagnose and measure the severity of lung problems by evaluating how well the lungs work: the amount of air the lungs can hold and how quickly the lungs move air in and out; measurements also include the efficiency of oxygenating the blood and removing carbon dioxide

pulse oximetry a test using a pulse oximeter to measure the percentage of oxygen in the blood

radiology the study and use of radioactive substances to visualize an internal structure

radiolucent a substance or structure that x-rays will penetrate

radiopaque substance or structure that is not penetrated by x-rays

retrograde pyelography radiographic visualization of the kidney, ureters, and bladder by administration of contrast media through a urinary catheter

Snellen chart poster with letters in rows of graduated sizes used to measure how well a person can see at specified distances

sphygmomanometer instrument used to measure blood pressure; the instrument is composed of a cuff for the arm, thigh, wrist, or finger and a measurement device

spirometry the most common lung function test; measures how much and how quickly air is moved in and out of the lungs by breathing into a mouthpiece attached to a recording device (spirometer); a graph with the results (spirogram) is produced

stethoscope an instrument used to listen (auscultate) the action of a person's heart or lungs, and to take an apical pulse or blood pressure; typically having a small disk-shaped device to place against the chest and two tubes connected to earpieces

symptoms subjective descriptions of altered health indicators (e.g., nausea, headache); complaints that cannot be seen or measured

tonometry a test using an instrument (tonometer) to measure the intraocular pressure of the eye to diagnose glaucoma

tuning fork used for gross measurement for hearing and sound conduction; the instrument is activated by striking it with the hand and is then placed on top of a patient's head, beside each ear, and on each side of the patient's mastoid bone

tympanometry a test that uses a tympanometer, which uses air pressure to measure tympanic membrane mobility

ultrasonography (ultrasound) use of high-frequency ultrasonic waves to produce an image and identify and measure deep body structures and abnormalities

vital signs measurements of body temperature, pulse rate, respirations (TPR), and blood pressure (BP)

x-ray an image produced on a radiosensitive surface or a radiation beam passed through an object

REVIEW QUESTIONS

All questions are relevant for all medical assisting and medical administrative assisting certification exams.

1. The main reason why an ill patient is seeking medical care is referred to as the:
   A. assessment.
   B. symptoms.
   C. chief complaint.
   D. observation.

   Answer: **C**
   Why: When a patient seeks medical care, the medical assistant should summarize the patient's words explaining why the patient has come to see the doctor. The abbreviation of "chief complaint" is CC. Assessment means to evaluate or measure. Symptoms are subjective health indicators such as nausea and headache. Observation is a visual inspection of the body.
   Review: Yes ○   No ○

2. What is the normal adult pulse range in beats per minute?
   A. 50 to 120
   B. 60 to 100
   C. 70 to 130
   D. 80 to 140
   E. 90 to 140

   Answer: **B**
   Why: The normal adult pulse should be between 60 and 100 beats per minute (bpm) and should have a regular rhythm.
   Review: Yes ○   No ○

3. The pulse point located behind the knee is the:
   A. femoral.
   B. dorsalis pedis.
   C. temporal.
   D. popliteal.

   Answer: **D**
   Why: The popliteal pulse, located behind the knee, is used to assess circulation to the extremities. The temporal pulse is located on the side of the head above the eye, the dorsalis pedis on the top of the foot, and the femoral in the groin.
   Review: Yes ○   No ○

4. The instrument used to measure the blood pressure is a(n):
   A. pulse oximeter.
   B. Doppler.
   C. sphygmomanometer.
   D. tympanometer.
   E. audiometer.

   Answer: **C**
   Why: The medical terminology root *sphygm* means "pulse," and *meter* means "an instrument for measuring." A pulse oximeter measures the amount of oxygen in the blood. A Doppler is an ultrasonic device used to locate and audibly transmit a pulse. A tympanometer uses air pressure to measure tympanic membrane mobility. An audiometer measures the patient's hearing based on his or her response to tones.
   Review: Yes ○   No ○

5. The instrument used in the physical exam to determine hearing and conduction is a:
   A. reflex hammer.
   B. stethoscope.
   C. tuning fork.
   D. speculum.

   Answer: **C**
   Why: A tuning fork is a metal device that vibrates and produces a humming sound. It is used to determine whether a patient can hear. After striking the tuning fork, it is placed on the patient's head or mastoid bone to examine conductive and sensorineural hearing loss.
   Review: Yes ○   No ○

6. The formula used to change pounds to kilograms is:
A. 22 lb = 1 kg
B. 2.2 kg = 1 lb
C. 100 lb = 1 kg
D. 1 lb = 100 kg
E. 2.2 lb = 1 kg

Answer: **E**
Why: Remember, it takes approximately twice the number of pounds to equal a kilogram.
Review: Yes ○   No ○

7. The examination technique used to listen to internal body sounds is:
A. palpation.
B. percussion.
C. mensuration.
D. auscultation.

Answer: **D**
Why: Auscultation is performed with the use of a stethoscope. The physician can listen to the sounds made as air moves in and out of the lungs. Bowel sounds are also heard when the stethoscope is placed over the abdomen.
Review: Yes ○   No ○

8. Which of the following items is not considered necessary for a routine patient exam?
A. Ophthalmoscope
B. Percussion hammer
C. Sterile gloves
D. Tongue depressor
E. Otoscope

Answer: **C**
Why: Nonsterile exam gloves are used during a routine patient exam. Sterile gloves are only used when performing a procedure that requires sterile aseptic technique.
Review: Yes ○   No ○

9. A Snellen chart is used to:
A. record a child's growth.
B. measure a patient's vision.
C. determine normal values in spirometry.
D. monitor vital signs.

Answer: **B**
Why: The Snellen chart is a poster with rows of letters in graduated sizes and is used to measure vision at specific distances. A person with 20/20 vision can see the letters at 20 feet away from the chart the same as a person with normal vision can at 20 feet.
Review: Yes ○   No ○

10. The average adult respiration rate is:
A. 20 to 24 per minute.
B. 10 to 12 per minute.
C. 12 to 20 per minute.
D. 25 to 30 per minute.
E. 30 to 35 per minute.

Answer: **C**
Why: Respiration ranges vary by age. Infants have a respiration rate of at least 20 per minute or greater, children's respiratory rate is 18 to 20 per minute, and the average adult breathes in and out (one respiration) 14 to 20 times a minute.
Review: Yes ○   No ○

11. The patient exam position used for a patient who is having difficulty breathing is:
A. dorsal recumbent.
B. lithotomy.
C. prone.
D. Fowler's.

Answer: **D**
Why: In Fowler's position, the patient lies face up on the exam table with the upper body elevated at a 45- to 90-degree angle.
Review: Yes ○   No ○

12. The pulse point located on the thumb side of the wrist is the:
    A. apical.
    B. brachial.
    C. carotid.
    D. radial.
    E. popliteal.

Answer: **D**
Why: The radial pulse is palpated at the wrist on the thumb side over the radial bone—the bone in the lower arm on the lateral side.
Review: Yes ○   No ○

13. The systolic pressure is described as:
    A. soft tapping sounds that become faint, or phase IV.
    B. faint tapping sounds heard as the cuff deflates, or phase I.
    C. rhythmic, sharp, distinct tapping sounds, or phase III.
    D. a soft swishing sound, or phase II.

Answer: **B**
Why: The Korotkoff sounds are those sounds heard through the stethoscope during the measurement of blood pressure. There are five phases; phase I is the determination of the systolic pressure. This is the sound made when arterial blood starts flowing back through the blood vessels as the cuff is deflated.
Review: Yes ○   No ○

14. A percussion hammer is used for which kind of examination?
    A. Orthopedic
    B. Neurologic
    C. Gynecologic
    D. Urologic
    E. Otologic

Answer: **B**
Why: A percussion hammer is used to test neurologic reflexes. Neurologic refers to the nerves. If a patient has diminished reflexes, this may indicate some nerve involvement. Orthopedic refers to the skeletal and muscular system. Otologic refers to the ear. Gynecologic refers to women, and urologic refers to the urinary system.
Review: Yes ○   No ○

15. The instrument used to visualize the ear canal and tympanic membrane is the:
    A. otoscope.
    B. audiometer.
    C. nasoscope.
    D. ophthalmoscope.

Answer: **A**
Why: The root *oto* refers to the ear. A scope is an instrument used to examine a body part. Sometimes, a scope has a light source attached. An otoscope is a lighted instrument used to look into the ear canal and examine the eardrum (tympanic membrane). An audiometer is used to measure hearing (*audio* means hearing or sound). A nasoscope is an instrument used to examine the nose, and an ophthalmoscope is used to examine the eyes.
Review: Yes ○   No ○

16. The exam method used to check for conjunctivitis (pinkeye) is:
    A. auscultation.
    B. palpation.
    C. percussion.
    D. inspection.
    E. mensuration.

Answer: **D**
Why: Conjunctivitis, or pinkeye, is an inflammation of the conjunctiva of the eye. The physician visually inspects the eyes for the signs of infection and inflammation.
Review: Yes ○   No ○

17. The exam method used when a physician is determining a patient's range of motion is:
A. auscultation.
B. palpation.
C. manipulation.
D. mensuration.

Answer: **C**
Why: Manipulation is the passive movement of the joints of the body to determine the extent of movement. Mensuration refers to the measurement of height, weight, and length. Auscultation is the act of listening to internal body sounds, usually using a stethoscope. Palpation is using the fingertips and hands to feel for sizes and positions of specific organs, masses, and abnormalities.
Review: Yes ○   No ○

18. An oral temperature registers 99.4°F, which equates to a(n):
A. rectal reading of 101.4°F.
B. axillary reading of 98.4°F.
C. otic reading of 100.4°F.
D. rectal reading of 99.4°F.
E. axillary reading of 99.4°F.

Answer: **B**
Why: The temperature reading taken rectally is 1° higher than oral. An axillary temperature, under the arm, is 1° lower, and a temperature taken in the ear is the same as an oral temperature.
Review: Yes ○   No ○

19. If the blood pressure is 130/90, the pulse pressure is:
A. 40
B. 60
C. 90
D. 130

Answer: **A**
Why: The pulse pressure is the difference between the systolic and diastolic readings. Therefore, 130 minus 90 equals 40.
Review: Yes ○   No ○

20. What position would be used to examine the back or spine?
A. Fowler's
B. Supine
C. Knee–chest
D. Dorsal recumbent
E. Prone

Answer: **E**
Why: In the prone position, the patient is lying face down on the exam table. Supine is face up, and dorsal recumbent is face up with knees bent and feet flat on the table. The knee–chest position requires the patient to kneel on the table and lower the chest to the table. The knee–chest position is used to perform rectal exams.
Review: Yes ○   No ○

21. Which of the following pulse sites requires a stethoscope to take the pulse?
A. Brachial
B. Carotid
C. Apical
D. Femoral

Answer: **C**
Why: The apical pulse is located at the fifth intercostal space midclavicular. A stethoscope is placed on the chest at this location to listen to the pulse.
Review: Yes ○   No ○

22. When performing a physical exam, the abbreviation PERRLA is used to describe what part(s) of the body?
A. Abdomen
B. Nose and sinuses
C. Ears
D. Eyes
E. Heart

Answer: **D**
Why: PERRLA means pupils equal, round, and reactive to light and accommodation. This abbreviation is used to describe normal pupils in the eye.
Review: Yes ○   No ○

23. Which of the following instrument or supply item is not included for a pelvic exam?
    A. Lubricant
    B. Cytology slide
    C. Sterile gloves
    D. Vaginal speculum

Answer: **C**
Why: It is not necessary to include sterile gloves with a pelvic exam tray setup; only regular nonsterile exam gloves are used.
Review: Yes ◯   No ◯

24. When measuring the blood pressure, the medical assistant will normally place the stethoscope over which artery?
    A. Apical
    B. Brachial
    C. Carotid
    D. Radial
    E. Aorta

Answer: **B**
Why: The term **brachial** means "relating to the arm." The brachial artery is located on the inner aspect of the anterior of the arm, and the pulse is felt at the elbow region.
Review: Yes ◯   No ◯

25. Blood pressure readings taken 1 to 2 minutes apart in the supine, sitting, and then standing position are the:
    A. pulse pressure.
    B. metastatic pressure.
    C. orthostatic pressure.
    D. orthopedic pressure.

Answer: **C**
Why: The term **orthostatic** refers to "erect posture or position." A patient's blood pressure can fluctuate when changing positions from lying down to standing up.
Review: Yes ◯   No ◯

CRITICAL THINKING REVIEW QUESTIONS

Ms. Nashtos presented to Dr. Ricardo's office for her annual well-woman's physical exam. After obtaining her height and weight, you calculated her BMI which was 32.

1. The 32 BMI is:
    A. normal.
    B. underweight.
    C. overweight.
    D. obese.
    E. not accurate with only the height and weight.

Answer: **D**
Why: The normal range for the BMI is 18.5 to 24.9; below that range is considered underweight. Between 25 to 29.9 is considered overweight, and anything above 30 is considered obese; 32 is considered obese. BMI is calculated using the height and weight.
Review: Yes ◯   No ◯

2. You also checked her blood oxygen saturation and her blood pressure using a(n):
    A. spirometer and sphygmomanometer.
    B. glucometer and spirometer.
    C. pulse oximeter and sphygmomanometer.
    D. audiometer and pulse oximeter.

Answer: **C**
Why: The pulse oximeter is used to determine the oxygen saturation in the blood, and the sphygmomanometer is used to determine blood pressure. The spirometer is used to determine movement of air out of the lungs and the glucometer to measure blood sugar. The audiometer measures hearing.
Review: Yes ◯   No ◯

3. Ms. Nashtos's blood pressure is 160/86.
A. The systolic is prehypertensive, and the diastolic is hypertensive.
B. The systolic is hypertensive, and the diastolic is normal.
C. The systolic is hypertensive, and the diastolic is prehypertensive.
D. The systolic and the diastolic are normal.
E. The systolic is normal, and the diastolic is hypertensive.

Answer: **C**
Why: According to the table published by the NHLBI, Stage 2 hypertension is a systolic of 160 and higher; a diastolic of 80 to 89 is pre-hypertensive. A diagnosis is not made on one reading, and the physician would probably have the patient monitor her blood pressure and conduct other tests before diagnosing hypertension.
Review: Yes ○   No ○

4. The remainder of the vital signs were taken, and Ms. Nashtos's temperature was normal which is:
A. rectally 36.4°C.
B. tympanic 97.8°F.
C. oral 37°C.
D. axillary 99.6°F.

Answer: **C**
Why: The normal rectal temperature is 99.6°F or 37.5°C; the normal tympanic temperature is 98.6° or 37°C; the normal oral temperature is 98.6°F or 37°C; the normal axillary temperature is 97.6°F or 36.4°C.
Review: Yes ○   No ○

5. You are preparing the patient for the physician's portion of the well-woman's exam. The exam will begin in the sitting position for eyes, ears, neck, heart, and lungs. The next position for the patient will be:
A. lithotomy.
B. Fowler's.
C. semi-Fowler's.
D. prone.
E. supine.

Answer: **E**
Why: The physician will next examine the patient's breasts and abdomen requiring the supine position, which is the patient lying on her back with arms to her sides. Lithotomy requires the patient to lie on her back with buttocks at the end of the table and feet in stirrups positioned for the pelvic exam, which will follow the breast and abdominal exams. Fowler's is sitting on the exam table with the head at a 45 to 90 degree. Prone is lying flat on one's stomach.
Review: Yes ○   No ○

CHAPTER

19

Medical Office Surgery

Review Tip:

Chapter 17, "Microorganisms and Asepsis," has direct application to surgical procedures—be sure you understand those concepts before reviewing this chapter. Minor surgery is another area of the national exams that contains questions requiring identification (sometimes by picture), care, and usage of surgical instruments.

Most states define and regulate types of surgery that are considered appropriate for the medical office. Medical malpractice insurance carriers also play a role. Refer to Chapter 4, "Law and Ethics," for issues concerning licensure, scope of practice, patient rights, informed consent, malpractice, confidentiality, quality improvement, and safety. As in all areas of medical assisting and medical administrative specialists, patient education is an important component (see Chapter 8).

General anesthesia is not usually administered for surgery in the medical office and is not covered in this book.

OVERVIEW OF THE MEDICAL ASSISTANT'S ROLE

Surgical asepsis must be maintained throughout the preparation and performance of surgical procedures. In general, the medical assistant's role is to assure that:

- All needed instruments and materials, including personal protective equipment (PPE), are present and sterile

- The patient is appropriately prepared, including signed consents

- The trays are opened maintaining sterile technique and materials are opened and placed on the sterile field

- The surgical prep is performed (the physician may prefer to do this)

- Assistance is provided to the physician per physician preference such as cutting sutures as he or she ties them

- Postoperatively, the wound is cleaned and appropriately dressed

- All sharps and contaminated materials are properly disposed

- Dirty instruments are placed in the recommended soak solution for cleaning and wrapping

- The specimen, if any, is labeled, prepared for transport and appropriately stored

- Postoperative instructions are given and understand along with follow-up appointments

- The patient is rested; able to ambulate and assisted to his home transport; the patient should not drive himself or herself home.

PREPARATION

- Surgical handwashing (scrub)—remove all jewelry; use foot- or knee-controlled faucet; wash hands, wrists, and forearms for 10 minutes (first surgical scrub of day); hold hands in upward position while rinsing; use brush and cuticle stick on nails; do not apply lotion; dry with sterile towel; apply sterile gloves

- PPE for surgery
  - Gloves—sterile
  - Goggles or eye shields—nonsterile
  - Masks—nonsterile
  - Gowns—sterile
  - Aprons—sterile if worn over surgical gown

- Sterile field—a pathogen-free area containing sterile instruments, solutions, sponges, and other items that will come in direct contact with another sterile item or the surgical field; this includes the hands and anterior neck to waist of the surgical team
  - Ensure sterile indicators and dates on instruments and solutions are intact and current before opening and placing on a sterile field
  - Examine sterile items for signs of break in packaging or presence of moisture (discard item if either is noted)
  - Open the sterile package(s) (Fig. 19-1)

FIGURE 19-1 Opening a sterile pack.

  - Open the top flap first; open away from you to avoid reaching over sterile field
  - Open the right and left flaps to the sides
  - Open the last flap toward you
- Allow only sterile items to come into contact with other sterile items
- Keep all sterile items and hands above the waists of the surgical team
- Maintain a border of 1 inch between nonsterile and sterile areas
- Do not turn your back to a sterile field or leave it unattended
- Do not lean or reach over sterile field
- Do not pass contaminated or nonsterile items over a sterile field
- Pour liquids such as sterile saline or an antiseptic into a sterile waterproof container on the sterile field
  - Do not touch the container with the nonsterile bottle
  - Do not drip or spill liquid on the sterile field
- Do not talk, cough, or sneeze over a sterile field

- Surgical site preparation
  - Hair removal—shave or cut hair at surgical site only with physician order (usually in procedure file); use only disposable blades; sterile instruments should be covered during hair removal; all loose hair should be removed before application of antiseptic
  - Skin cleansing—using an antiseptic cleansing solution (check for patient allergies) such as Betadine® or Hibiclens®, cleanse the surgical site using a circular motion from the point of the incision outward; use a clean sponge to repeat
  - "Painting" and draping—after performing the previous steps, a sterile member of the surgical team

will use a sterile sponge stick and sterile sponges to apply, or "paint," an antiseptic solution on the surgical site, using circular motions beginning with the incision site and working outward (one sponge per layer of antiseptic); fenestrated drapes (a drape with a hole or opening) or sterile towels, held in place by sterile towel clips, are applied, as well as any other drapes (sterile coverings) required by the size of the sterile field

- When local anesthetic is required, the physician will hold the sterile syringe with sterile-gloved hands; the medical assistant shows the physician the label on the bottle, ensures the bottle top is not contaminated (may use alcohol swab), and holds the bottle upside down for the physician to draw out the required amount of medication then shows the physician the label, again

INSTRUMENTATION

All instruments or parts of instruments (such as transfer forceps) that enter the sterile field must be sterile. Chapter 17 covered the two common procedures for sterilization: autoclaving and cold or chemical sterilization. Biosafety (e.g., the use of sharps containers and other biohazard receptacles) was also addressed in Chapter 17.

COMMON INSTRUMENTS (FIG. 19-2)

- **Curette**—sharp or smooth spoon-shaped instrument used to scrape tissue or other substances from a body orifice or organ; the most common types are ear and uterine
- **Dilator**—solid instrument used to stretch or widen the opening to an anatomic structure
- **Forceps**—a two-handled instrument used to grasp, move, or crimp tissue; or sterile objects may be with or without "teeth"
  - **Splinter forceps**—fine-pointed, tweezer-like forceps without teeth used to remove splinters and other foreign objects
  - **Thumb forceps**—smooth (without teeth) forceps; the general-use forceps
  - **Adson forceps**—tweezer-like forceps, with or without teeth, with a smaller tip for smaller areas
  - **Bayonet forceps**—tweezer-like forceps shaped like a bayonet used for placing packing in areas (e.g., the nostrils)
  - **Ring (sponge) forceps**—long, two-handled forceps with open ovals on the ends to grasp tissue, hold sponges, or transfer sterile instruments
  - **Hemostat**—sometimes referred to as a forceps; straight or curved instrument used to compress or

crimp capillaries and other blood vessels to stop bleeding; also referred to as a clamp or a Crile; common types are given below:
  - ○ Kelly hemostat—a medium-size hemostat; may be curved or straight
  - ○ Mosquito hemostat—a small hemostat used for pediatric, plastic, or microsurgery; may be curved or straight

- **Needle holder**—a two-handled instrument that clasps a suture needle, allowing the physician to push and pull the needle with suture material through various anatomic structures
- **Probe**—a straight instrument with ends of various shapes, used primarily to explore ducts, canals, and other anatomic structures
- **Retractors**—instruments of various shapes and sizes used to hold back tissue and organs to facilitate exposure to the operative site
- **Scalpels**—knives of various blade shapes and sizes, used to make surgical incisions; the blade is always disposable; the knife handle may or may not be disposable
- **Scissors**—two-bladed instrument used to cut tissue and materials during surgical procedures
  - **Surgical/operating scissors**—scissors used during surgery to cut and dissect tissue; may be curved or straight, blunt or sharp (e.g., Mayo scissors)
  - **Suture scissors**—straight-bladed scissors used to cut suture material during the suturing procedure; **they are sometimes also used for suture removal.**
  - **Suture-removal scissors**—specific scissors with a hook toward the distal end of one blade to get under sutures and safely snip during suture removal; sometimes referred to as suture scissors, although suture removal is their only use.
  - **Bandage scissors**—angled scissors with a blunt knobbed end to insert under dressings to remove them without injuring tissue
- **Sound**—a straight or curved instrument used to explore body cavities for measurement of depth and presence of masses or foreign bodies
- **Tenaculum**—a long, two-handled instrument with pointed ends used to grasp tissue during surgery; a cervical tenaculum is commonly used in well-woman exams
- **Towel clamps** (clips)—small instruments of various shapes used to keep sterile towels, used as drapes, in place during surgery

COMMON SURGICAL TRAY INSTRUMENTS

Each office maintains a file card of all instruments, supplies, and equipment needed for each surgical procedure. The following are select surgical trays and their instruments.

A Hemostats   **B** Tenaculum   **C** Needle holder   **D** Ring (sponge) forceps   **E** Splinter forceps

F Surgical scissors   **G** Suture removal scissors   **H** Bandage scissors   **I** Towel clip

J Retractors (rake)   **K** Probe   **L** Sounds   **M** Curettes   **N** Bayonet forceps

FIGURE 19-2 Common surgical instruments. (Sklar Instruments, West Chester, PA.)

- General minor surgery tray used for procedures such as removal of lesions—towel clips (four), scalpel and blade, curved and straight hemostats (two each), surgical scissors, thumb forceps, forceps with teeth, suture scissors, needle holder (retractors and other instruments may be added as needed), specified type of surgical sponge; sutures and sizes may be on the file card or requested by the physician during the procedure

- Suture tray—towel clips (four), curved hemostat, forceps with teeth, thumb forceps, suture scissors, needle holder, sterile 4 × 4 gauze; sutures identified by the physician and added to the setup

- Suture- or staple-removal tray—suture-removal scissors or staple remover, thumb forceps, sterile 4 × 4 gauze

ENDOSCOPE

An **endoscope** is a special instrument used to examine the interior of canals and hollow viscus; the specific design and name is dependent on the organ (e.g., arthroscope, gastroscope, bronchoscope). The instrument usually contains fiber-optic technology that allows lighting, video transmission, and other technologic procedures; biopsies and select surgical procedures may be performed through the endoscope, eliminating or minimizing a surgical incision. These instruments are usually sterilized using the cold chemical process after thoroughly cleaning.

Other Common Instrumentation with Power Sources

- Electrosurgery—a method of dissection and cauterization using an electric current directed to a specific anatomic area to cut, destroy, or coagulate; the power source is initiated and controlled through a boxlike unit that transmits to a hand piece with sterile removable tips that come in direct contact with the surgical site; the patient must be grounded and safety precautions enforced

- Cryosurgery—a method of destroying tissue by freezing (cryogenics) using liquid nitrogen applied from a tank with a gauge and removable hand pieces (e.g., for removal of cervical lesions), or other cryo materials requiring simple spray canisters (e.g., for removal of skin lesions)

- Laser surgery—a method using high concentrations of electromagnetic radiation in narrow beams for surgical and diagnostic applications (e.g., coagulation of retinal hemorrhage); uses vary and are dependent on the color spectrum; common terms associated with laser surgery are *argon*, *continuous wave*, *pulsed wave*, *excimer*, *krypton*, *KTP*, *YAG*, and *Q-switched*; goggles should be worn and special training provided before assisting in laser surgery

- **Mohs procedure or surgery**—removal of skin tissue which is then prepared and examined while the patient waits to determine the presence of carcinoma and, if present, more tissue may be removed for cancer-free edges; specially trained medical assistants may prepare the specimen for microscopic examination

CLOSURE MATERIALS

The type of material used for closure is dependent on several factors. Is the closure on an internal anatomic structure or on the skin? What are the depth, thickness, and length of the closure site? What are the healing capacity factors of the patient (e.g., nutritional status, diabetes, recent history of steroid administration, smoking)?

- Suture—derived from Latin, meaning "a sewing"; threadlike materials (ligature) and needle used to close a wound; the needle and ligature used in the medical office are usually mechanically attached (swaged) by the manufacturer

- Ligature
  - Absorbable—material that dissolves in the body (e.g., catgut); used for internal suturing
  - Nonabsorbable—material that does not dissolve (e.g., silk, nylon and other synthetics, wires); generally for external use, although some wires may be used internally; most nonabsorbable sutures are removed after healing takes place
  - Size—determined by the thickness of the diameter; the range is approximately from 7, the largest, to 11-0, the smallest (Box 19-1)

BOX 19-1

Range of common suture material sizes

Larger to smaller

7	6	5	4	3	2	1	0	1-0	2-0	3-0	4-0	5-0	6-0	7-0	8-0	9-0	10-0	11-0

Large ← → Small

- Needle
  - Cutting—needle with sharp, flat edge used on tough tissue (e.g., skin)
  - Noncutting—needle with sharp, smooth, rounded edge used on finer tissue, such as peritoneum
  - Curved—the shape of the needle; may have cutting or noncutting edge; needle holder used
  - Straight (Keith)—the shape of the needle; may have cutting or noncutting edge; no needle holder required; rarely used
  - Size—determined by the size of the ligature to be used; physician will ask for ligature size on a cutting or noncutting, curved or straight needle
- Staples—metal clips used to approximate skin edges during healing or occlude internal structures; materials vary per use (e.g., stainless steel used on skin, silver used for neurosurgery); external staples must be removed with a staple remover (not to be confused with the type used for office staples)
- Steri-Strips—adhesive strips of material used in minor lacerations or as a follow-up to sutures to hold wound edges together during healing
- Glue—bonding material used externally to approximate skin edges or internally to affix structures; often used in neurologic or orthopedic surgeries

WOUNDS

Wounds are traumas to body tissues caused by physical means. The trauma may be unintentional, such as a fall, or intentional, such as surgery. The type of wound determines the treatment and the potential for healing. Surgical wounds are considered clean wounds because they are initiated under sterile conditions. Dirty wounds are those sustained under contaminated conditions (e.g., a knife wound while preparing a meal).

- Abrasion—outer layers of skin scraped off, resulting in a small amount of sanguineous or serosanguineous drainage, such as a "skinned" knee
- Contusion—bleeding below unbroken skin caused by blunt trauma; a bruise
- Incision—a smooth cut as in surgery or as made with a razor; the amount of bleeding depends on the location and depth
- Laceration—a jagged traumatic cut resulting in irregular wound edges
- Puncture—a hole in the skin made by a sharp pointed object
- Healing—physiologic process of wound closure; there are two predominant types

- First intention (primary)—wound edges are approximated and healing process occurs in all layers (e.g., incision, laceration)
- Secondary intention (granulation)—wound edges do not approximate and healing begins at wound bottom, forming granular projections on the wound surface (e.g., a wound from a drain)
- Dressings—defined as sterile coverings placed over a wound but often used synonymously with bandaging; types of dressing include gauze, occlusives (e.g., Vaseline gauze), nonstick (e.g., Telfa), nonopaque (e.g., BioDerm), and commercial gauze impregnated with medication (e.g., NuGauze); dressings should be applied using sterile technique
- Bandages—sterile or nonsterile materials that splint or protect injured tissue (e.g., Kerlix, Ace bandages, triangular slings, tube gauze [frequently used on digits]), maintain pressure over an area (such as abdominal pads, Coban), and hold sterile dressings in place (e.g., Montgomery straps, rolled gauze)

THE JOINT COMMISSION AND SURGICAL SAFETY

Disposal of biohazard waste such as needles and grounding of patients for electrosurgery instrumentation are two examples of patient surgical safety. The Joint Commission's Patient Safety Goals also include **the time out**. This is a practice or standard recommended at the beginning of each surgical procedure. The team members pause to ensure the:

- Correct patient identity (use two identifiers such as name and birthday)
- Correct surgical site
- Correct procedure

The documentation of the time out is often the job of the medical assistant.

SURGICAL SPECIMENS

Common medical office surgical specimens include the following:

- Moles, nevi, skin tabs, and other skin lesions
- Toenails, fingernails
- Vas deferens (vasectomies)
- Tissue biopsies from endoscopic procedures or excisions
- Cultures from body fluids and drainage
- Foreign bodies

Sometimes a specimen is disposed of as biohazard waste and other times a specimen may be sent to a laboratory to determine if it is malignant or for identification. The medical assistant should always ask the physician if a specimen should be sent to the laboratory. Do not assume.

Additional safety standards include placing the specimen in an appropriate container and labeling the specimen with the patient's name, birthday, the date and the time the specimen was obtained, and the source (such as lesion of left forearm). The patient should be asked to read the label for the correct name and birthdate then the specimen should be placed in a plastic bag and sealed for transport. Further discussion on handling specimens is discussed in Chapter 21: Laboratory Procedures.

TERMS

MINOR SURGICAL PROCEDURES REVIEW

The following list reviews the terms discussed in this chapter and other important terms that you may see on the exam.

abrasion outer layers of skin scraped off, resulting in a small amount of sanguineous or serosanguineous drainage, such as a "skinned" knee

contusion bleeding below unbroken skin caused by blunt trauma; a bruise

cryosurgery a method of destroying tissue by freezing (cryogenics) using liquid nitrogen applied from a tank with a gauge and removable hand pieces, or other cryo materials requiring simple spray canisters

curettes sharp or smooth spoon-shaped instruments used to scrape tissue or other substances from a body orifice or organ; most common are ear and uterine

dilators solid instruments used to stretch or widen the opening to an anatomic structure (e.g., uterine, urethral sounds)

electrosurgery a method of dissection or cauterization using an electric current directed to a specific anatomic area to cut, destroy, or coagulate

endoscope special instrument used to examine the interior of canals and hollow viscus; design and name are dependent on the organ; it usually contains fiber-optic technology allowing lighting, video transmission, and other technologic procedures

forceps a two-handled instrument used to grasp, move, or crimp tissue

hemostat sometimes referred to as a *forceps*; straight or curved instrument used to compress capillaries and other blood vessels to stop bleeding; (hemostasis) also referred to as a *clamp* or a *Crile*

incision a smooth cut as in surgery or as made with a razor

laceration a jagged traumatic cut resulting in irregular wound edges

laser surgery a method using high concentrations of electromagnetic radiation in narrow beams for surgical and diagnostic applications

needle holder a two-handled instrument that clasps a needle, allowing the physician to push and pull the needle with suture material through various anatomic structures

probe a straight instrument with ends of various shapes; used primarily to explore patency of ducts, canals, and other anatomic structures

puncture a hole in the skin made by a sharp pointed object

retractors instruments of various shapes used to hold back tissue and organs to facilitate exposure to the operative site

scalpels knives with various blade shapes and sizes, used to make surgical incisions

sound a straight or curved instrument used to explore body cavities for measurement of depth and presence of masses or foreign bodies

suture-removal scissors scissors with a hook toward the distal end of one blade to get under sutures and safely snip during suture removal

suture scissors straight-bladed scissors used to cut suture material during the suturing procedure and sometimes for suture removal

tenaculum a long, two-handled instrument with pointed ends used to grasp tissue during surgery; a cervical tenaculum is commonly used in well-woman exams

time out patient safety practice recommended by TJC; at the beginning of each surgical procedure, the team members pause to ensure the correct patient identity, correct surgical site, and correct procedure

towel clamps (clips) small instruments of various shapes used to keep sterile towels used as drapes in place during surgery

REVIEW QUESTIONS

All questions are relevant for all medical assisting certification exams.

1. An instrument used to grasp tissue is a:
   A. probe.
   B. curette.
   C. dilator.
   D. forceps.

   Answer: **D**
   Why: There are many types of forceps, such as splinter forceps, thumb forceps, Adson forceps, and sponge forceps. These are used to grasp tissue or supplies.
   Review: Yes ○   No ○

2. The instrument used to remove stitches is:
   A. operating scissors.
   B. Kelly hemostat.
   C. suture scissors.
   D. Mayo scissors.
   E. needle holder.

   Answer: **C**
   Why: Sutures and stitches are the same. Suture scissors and suture-removal scissors are often used synonymously; and is the best choice here those designed solely for suture stitch removal have a hook on the end of one of the blades. This hook is slipped under the stitch/suture, and the stitch is cut for removal.
   Review: Yes ○   No ○

3. A procedure that uses liquid nitrogen to freeze and destroy tissue is:
   A. electrosurgery.
   B. laser surgery.
   C. endoscopic surgery.
   D. cryosurgery.

   Answer: **D**
   Why: The root *cryo* means "cold." Liquid nitrogen produces a freezing effect that destroys tissue. This method is frequently used to destroy cervical lesions.
   Review: Yes ○   No ○

4. Which of the following statements is true regarding the sizing of suture, or ligature?
   A. 2-0 suture is finer than 6-0 suture.
   B. 3 suture is thicker than 6 suture.
   C. 4-0 suture is finer than 2-0 suture.
   D. 5-0 suture is finer than 6-0 suture.
   E. 4 suture is finer than 2 suture.

   Answer: **C**
   Why: Suture is available in different sizes or gauges. When the size ends in a zero, suture sizes become smaller as the number gets larger. A 2-0 suture is thicker than a 10-0 suture. The opposite is true when the suture size is a whole number. The higher the whole number, the larger or thicker the suture. For example, size 7 suture is thicker than size 2.
   Review: Yes ○   No ○

5. Which of the following sutures does not require removal from the body?
   A. Catgut
   B. Silk
   C. Nylon
   D. Cotton

   Answer: **A**
   Why: Catgut suture is an absorbable suture made from the intestines of sheep or cattle. It is readily broken down by the body and usually does not require removal.
   Review: Yes ○   No ○

6. The type of wound caused by scraping off the outer layers of skin is a(n):
   A. incision.
   B. abrasion.
   C. contusion.
   D. laceration.
   E. bruise.

Answer: **B**
Why: An example of an abrasion is a skinned knee, in which the top layers of skin are scraped off.
Review: Yes ◯   No ◯

7. Which of the following instruments is used to scrape foreign substance from an ear?
   A. Dilator
   B. Hemostat
   C. Retractor
   D. Curette

Answer: **D**
Why: A curette is a sharp or smooth, spoon-shaped instrument used to scrape tissue or other substances from a body orifice or organ. A dilator is a solid instrument used to stretch or widen the opening to an anatomic structure. A hemostat is used to compress or crimp capillaries and other blood vessels to stop bleeding. A retractor is used to hold and separate tissue.
Review: Yes ◯   No ◯

8. The type of bandage material that is not intended to apply pressure but to hold a dressing in place on the forearm is:
   A. elastic bandage.
   B. rolled gauze.
   C. triangular bandage.
   D. tubular gauze.
   E. 4 × 4 gauze.

Answer: **B**
Why: Rolled gauze is available in different widths from 1 inch to 6 inches and in various lengths. It is used to wrap around a body part such as an arm or a leg. Elastic bandage is made from a stretchy material and is used to apply pressure. Triangular bandages are used to make a sling for the arm. Tubular gauze is used to bandage toes and fingers. Gauze squares are used to cover wounds and are available in 1-inch to 4-inch squares.
Review: Yes ◯   No ◯

9. A type of wound caused by a blunt trauma to the body that results in bleeding below unbroken skin is a(n):
   A. puncture.
   B. laceration.
   C. contusion.
   D. abrasion.

Answer: **C**
Why: A contusion causes a bruise. A bruise forms from bleeding beneath the skin. The skin is not broken, but the injury is visible through the surface of the skin.
Review: Yes ◯   No ◯

10. Items that are placed on the sterile field of a biopsy surgical tray setup include the following EXCEPT:
    A. scalpel.
    B. needle holder.
    C. bandage scissors.
    D. hemostat.
    E. curette.

Answer: **C**
Why: Bandage scissors are used to cut through and remove bandages and have a blunt end so they do not injure the patient during use. They are not included on the tray for a biopsy.
Review: Yes ◯   No ◯

11. The type of material preferred to bandage a digit is:
  A. 4 × 4 gauze.
  B. tube gauze.
  C. Ace bandage.
  D. 2 × 2 gauze.

Answer: **B**
Why: Tube gauze is gauze manufactured into a tube shape. It stretches and conforms to body parts such as fingers and toes (digits).
Review: Yes ◯   No ◯

12. Which of the following statements is true regarding the sterile tray setup?
  A. All bandage materials are added to the sterile tray for easy access after the procedure.
  B. You should pour solutions into the basin on the sterile tray holding the bottle label down so you can see the liquid in the container.
  C. Surgical handwashing is not required.
  D. You should reach over the sterile field, not around it, to access something on the other side of the tray.
  E. A 1-inch border around the sterile field is considered contaminated.

Answer: **E**
Why: Bandage materials are not placed on the sterile field. Only those items that are sterile are on the tray. For example, adhesive and surgical tape are not sterile. When pouring solutions from a bottle, pour the liquid from the container with the label face up, so that if liquid drips down the bottle, the label will not be destroyed or damaged. Before setting up a sterile tray, it is essential to perform a surgical handwash. You should never reach over a sterile tray.
Review: Yes ◯   No ◯

13. A fenestrated sterile drape:
  A. is used to cover the sterile tray after it is set up to protect it from becoming contaminated.
  B. has an opening in the middle and is placed over the area of the patient where a surgical incision will be made.
  C. is a type of bandaging material used to cover a large area of the body.
  D. is a sterile drape impregnated with an anesthetic medication.

Answer: **B**
Why: The word *fenestra* is a Latin term for "window" or "opening." This sterile drape is approximately 18 × 24 inches and has a 2-inch square opening in the middle. The drape is placed over the patient, with the opening over the area where the surgical procedure will be performed.
Review: Yes ◯   No ◯

14. To ensure package sterility, the medical assistant should:
  A. use a torn sterile package only if the tear is small.
  B. use sterile packages up to 30 days after the expiration date to conserve the need to re-autoclave.
  C. use only dry, undamaged sterile packages.
  D. only transport sterile packages with sterile gloves.
  E. perform a surgical handwash before wrapping packs for sterilization.

Answer: **C**
Why: You should not use a sterile package if it is wet or damp or has become damaged. Packs sterilized in-house expire 30 days from the preparation date. The outside of the sterile package is not considered sterile, only the contents within the pack. Therefore, sterile gloves are not required to transport the pack. It is not necessary to perform a surgical handwash before wrapping packs.
Review: Yes ◯   No ◯

15. Electrosurgery is used to:
   A. retract tissues.
   B. dilate openings in the body.
   C. dissect and coagulate tissue.
   D. freeze tissue.

Answer: **C**
Why: Electrosurgery is a method of cauterization using an electric current to dissect or coagulate tissue. Surgical instruments are used to retract or to hold back structures of the body during surgery. Dilation is the process of making an opening larger. Cryosurgery is the method used to freeze tissue.
Review: Yes ◯   No ◯

16. The first step performed to set up a sterile field is to:
   A. open the sterile package.
   B. pour solutions that will be used during the procedure.
   C. wash your hands.
   D. don sterile gloves.
   E. prepare the local anesthetic in a syringe and place it on the sterile field.

Answer: **C**
Why: Handwashing is performed before any procedure. When setting up a sterile field, a surgical handwashing is performed for 10 minutes.
Review: Yes ◯   No ◯

17. After a surgical procedure, the guidelines for discarding materials include:
   A. placing all sharps in a biohazard sharps container.
   B. placing only visibly soiled materials in a biohazard sharps container.
   C. discarding all paper materials in the trash can.
   D. pouring unused solutions back into their proper containers.

Answer: **A**
Why: All items that are disposable and considered sharp are discarded in the biohazard sharps container. This includes suture materials with needles attached, syringes and needles, and scalpel blades. All other materials soiled with body fluids should be placed in a biohazard container, but not in one specifically designed for sharps. Red trash bags are most commonly used for these items.
Review: Yes ◯   No ◯

18. An instrument used to explore anatomic structures is a:
   A. hemostat.
   B. curette.
   C. forceps.
   D. dilator.
   E. probe.

Answer: **E**
Why: A probe is a straight instrument with various shaped ends that are usually blunt, used primarily to explore the patency of ducts, canals, and other anatomic structures.
Review: Yes ◯   No ◯

19. Instruments used to hold back tissue and organs are:
   A. thumb forceps.
   B. Kelly forceps.
   C. retractors.
   D. curettes.

Answer: **C**
Why: Retractors may be plain or toothed and may be sharp or blunt. They are designed to be either held by an assistant or screwed open to be self-retaining.
Review: Yes ◯   No ◯

20. A common antiseptic solution used to prep the surgical site is:
  A. Betadine⁻.
  B. alcohol.
  C. hydrogen peroxide.
  D. formaldehyde.
  E. sterile saline.

Answer: **A**
Why: Formaldehyde is not intended for use on the skin. Alcohol is used for surface cleansing of the skin for minor invasive procedures and to wipe items such as stethoscopes. Hydrogen peroxide does not have the antiseptic qualities necessary for prepping the skin before surgery. Sterile saline is a salt solution that is free from all microorganisms.
Review: Yes ◯   No ◯

21. A jagged traumatic cut resulting in irregular wound edges is a(n):
  A. contusion.
  B. laceration.
  C. incision.
  D. abrasion.

Answer: **B**
Why: A contusion does not break the skin but bleeding occurs beneath the skin, resulting in a visible bruise. An incision is a smooth cut, as made with a razor or a scalpel. An abrasion is a wound caused from scraping away the top layers of skin.
Review: Yes ◯   No ◯

22. An instrument used to examine the interior of canals or of hollow organs is a(n):
  A. retractor.
  B. catheter.
  C. dilator.
  D. curette.
  E. endoscope.

Answer: **E**
Why: An endoscope is an illuminated optic instrument used for visualizing the interior of a body cavity or of an organ. Scopes include a gastroscope, which is used to examine the stomach; a bronchoscope, which is used to examine the bronchi of the lungs; and a sigmoidoscope, which is used to examine the sigmoid colon.
Review: Yes ◯   No ◯

23. The procedure for delivering local anesthetic to the sterile field is to:
  A. fill the syringe with the proper amount of solution before the procedure and place it on the sterile field.
  B. place the vial of solution on the sterile field so the physician can have access to it.
  C. remove the syringe from the sterile field, fill the syringe with the amount of solution required, and return the syringe to the sterile field for the physician to use.
  D. while the physician holds the syringe with sterile-gloved hands, the medical assistant holds the vial of solution for the physician, and the physician draws out the required amount of solution.

Answer: **D**
Why: The vial of medication is not sterile and should not be placed on the sterile field. Using sterile technique, a syringe is placed on the sterile field. The physician holds the syringe and directs the needle into the rubber stopper of the vial and withdraws the required amount of solution. The medical assistant must remember to wipe the top of the vial with alcohol before offering the vial to the physician. Also, it is usually required that the medical assistant either show the physician the vial label or read the label out loud before using the solution to ensure the solution is the correct one.
Review: Yes ◯   No ◯

24. The bandage material preferred when pressure is required over the injured area is:
    A. 4 × 4 gauze.
    B. elastic bandage.
    C. roller gauze.
    D. triangular bandage.
    E. Telfa pad.

Answer: **B**

Why: The elastic (Ace) bandage is form-fitting and used as a pressure bandage. It is important to check the patient's extremities for proper blood return into toes and fingers. If the bandage is too tight, it can restrict blood flow to the body part.

Review: Yes ○   No ○

25. A wrapped, autoclaved, sterile package is opened on the Mayo stand by opening the top flap of the wrapper:
    A. toward the right side of the table.
    B. toward the left side of the table.
    C. away from you.
    D. toward you.

Answer: **C**

Why: The top flap is opened away from you so that as the other flaps are opened you will not have to reach over the sterile contents of the package. After the top flap is open, the right and left flaps are opened to the sides. The last flap, closest to you, is opened by lifting it toward you.

Review: Yes ○   No ○

CRITICAL THINKING CASE REVIEW QUESTIONS

The minor surgeries performed in a medical office integrate many previously learned topics included in the national exams. The following questions are related to the surgical patient and will test your recall.

1. Prior to any type of surgery it is important to obtain:
   A. implied consent.
   B. informed consent.
   C. second opinion.
   D. insurance information.
   E. advance directive.

Answer: **B**

Why: Informed consent is a patient's permission for a procedure given after receiving all the information necessary to make an educated decision. Implied consent is an action that probably indicates consent. Implied consent should not be used for an invasive procedure. Obtaining a second opinion is not always necessary, especially when a minor surgery is involved. Insurance information is correct but not the best answer. Advance directives should be encouraged but not necessary for an office surgery.

Review: Yes ○   No ○

2. The agent used to prepare the patient's skin prior to an incision is a(n):
   A. disinfectant.
   B. cold sterilization.
   C. antiseptic.
   D. antibiotic.

Answer: **C**

Why: A disinfectant is used to clean and decrease pathogens on inanimate objects; cold sterilization is used for heat-sensitive equipment. An antiseptic is a cleaning agent for the skin. An antibiotic is not used to prepare skin prior to surgery.

Review: Yes ○   No ○

3. For reimbursement of a surgical procedure, the insurance company usually requires:
   A. coordination of benefits.
   B. capitation.
   C. assignment of benefits.
   D. prior authorization.
   E. coinsurance.

Answer: **D**

Why: Coordination of benefits is when a person is covered by more than one insurance company and they work together to determine who will pay for what. Capitation is a fixed amount paid to a health-care provider for each patient regardless of the amount or type of care. Assignment of benefits is authorization by the patient for the insurance company to pay the physician directly. Prior authorization is approval by the insurance company for the surgery to be performed. Coinsurance is an established cost of the insurance that the patient must pay; not all insurance plans require a coinsurance.

Review: Yes ◯   No ◯

4. Prior to the surgery, the medical assistant takes the adult patient's vital signs which are normal. What group of vitals is normal?
   A. T 37 C orally, P 68, R 14
   B. T 98.6 F axillary, P 72, R 10
   C. T 36.4 C axillary, P 22, R 62
   D. T 98.6 F tympanic, P 98, R 40

Answer: **A**

Why: This group of vital signs is the only one with the three measurements in the normal range for an adult: oral temperature 37°C or 98.6°F, pulse 60 to 100, respirations 12 to 20.

Review: Yes ◯   No ◯

5. Before the surgery was performed, the team conducted a time out which included:
   A. a few minutes to take a break.
   B. time to check the patient's insurance coverage.
   C. an opportunity for the patient to ask questions.
   D. patient education
   E. the correct patient identification.

Answer: **E**

Why: Time out is The Joint Commission standard when, prior to surgery, the team pauses to determine and concur that it is the correct patient, the correct surgical site, and the correct procedure.

Review: Yes ◯   No ◯

CHAPTER

20

Electrocardiography

Review Tip:

Refer to Chapter 6, "Anatomy and Physiology," and review the cardiovascular system, including the functions, components, cardiac cycle, and cardiac conduction. Exam questions may involve identifying a cardiac rhythm or PQRST waves from a picture of an electrocardiogram strip or identifying cardiac leads.

The **electrocardiogram** (**ECG or EKG**) is the graphic representation of the **electrical** activity that passes through the heart. It is monitored at the skin surface with sensors called **electrodes** that produce specific **leads** or views of the heart, which is a three-dimensional organ. The ECG is a painless and noninvasive tool used to collect baseline information (e.g., during a routine physical exam) and to diagnose and monitor various heart diseases such as myocardial infarctions and other ischemia, heart blocks and other conduction defects, benign and life-threatening arrhythmias, and the effects of cardiac drugs.

OVERVIEW

The electrical activity of the heart begins at the cellular level. It then follows the conductive pathway bringing about the cardiac cycle, which results in the heart pumping blood throughout the body (see Chapter 6, Figs. 6-19 and 6-21).

■ Cardiac polarity—electrical status of cardiac muscle cells; an attempt to maintain electronegativity (ability to attract electrons) inside these cells to ensure an appropriate distribution of ions or electrolytes (e.g., potassium, sodium, chloride, calcium)

- Polarization—resting cardiac muscle cells
- Depolarization—charged and contracting cardiac muscle cells
- Repolarization—recovering cardiac muscle cells; returning to equilibrium

■ Cardiac cycle—the pumping of the heart in a rhythmic cycle of contraction and relaxation (the sound through a stethoscope is often described as "lub dub")

- Normally 60 to 100 cycles or beats per minute (normal adult heart rate)
- Phases of atrial and ventricle contractions (systole) and relaxation (diastole)
  - Atrial systole—contraction of atria, forcing blood into ventricles through tricuspid and mitral valves
  - Ventricle diastole—relaxation of ventricles, allowing them to fill with blood from atria
  - Ventricle systole—contraction of the ventricles, forcing blood through the aortic and pulmonic valves to the aorta and pulmonary artery
  - Atrial diastole—relaxation of atria, allowing them to fill with blood from the vena cava and pulmonary veins

■ ECG complex—a full cardiac electrical cycle (one heartbeat) represented by PQRST waves (and sometimes U wave) working together as a complex (Fig. 20-1)

- P wave—an upward curve representing atrial contraction; used to measure the atrial rate
- Q wave—a downward deflection after the P wave

- R wave—a large upward spike after the Q wave
- S wave—a downward deflection after the R wave
- T wave—an upward curve after the S wave, representing the repolarization and resting of the ventricles
- U wave—a small upward curve sometimes following the T wave, representing slow repolarization or return to resting
- QRS complex—the QRS waves representing contraction of the ventricles
- PR interval—the P wave and the line connecting it to the QRS complex, representing the time the electrical impulse travels from the sinoatrial (SA) node to the atrioventricular (AV) node
- QT interval—the QRST waves representing a full cardiac electrical cycle
- ST segment—a slight upward line connecting the QRS waves to the T wave and representing the time between contraction of the ventricles and relaxation or recovery

■ Types of ECGs

- Single-lead ECG—information recorded from one view of the heart; a lead is a specific view of the heart, which is a three-dimensional organ; usually, lead II is selected
- 12-lead (multichannel) ECG—information recorded from 10 electrodes, representing 12 views of the heart from 12 different angles
- Six-lead ECG—information generally recorded from three electrodes representing Einthoven triangle and producing six views of the heart; commonly used for cardiac monitoring or a screening ECG
- Telemetry—single-lead or 12-lead ECGs transmitted via radio, electronic, or telephone waves to another site for monitoring or interpretation
- Interpretive ECG—a computerized ECG machine that is programmed to analyze data and produce a printed interpretation with the graph

FIGURE 20-1 Normal cardiac electrical cycle recorded on standard ECG paper. (Reprinted with permission from Pillitteri A. *Maternal and Child Nursing.* 4th Ed. Philadelphia: Lippincott Williams & Wilkins, 2003)

ELECTRODES, PLACEMENT, AND LEADS

The terms "electrodes" and "leads" are sometimes used synonymously. *This is not correct.* An **electrode** is the sensor attached to the ECG machine that adheres to the skin. A **lead** is the view of the heart produced by a standard combination of electrode placements. The *12-lead ECG* is the "gold standard" for diagnosing cardiac problems and is produced using *10 electrodes* (Fig. 20-2). The correct placement of these electrodes influences the quality and accuracy of the rhythm strip. The right leg (RL) is

FIGURE 20-2 Twelve-lead electrocardiogram electrode placement. (Reprinted with permission from Hosley JB, Molle-Matthews E. *Lippincott's Pocket Guide to Medical Assisting.* Philadelphia: Lippincott Williams & Wilkins, 1999)

the grounding electrode and not used as part of any lead. Electrodes should never be placed over a bony prominence or clothing.

PLACEMENT OF ELECTRODES (10 SENSORS)

■ Chest electrodes (six)
  • V1—fourth intercostal space at right margin of sternum
  • V2—fourth intercostal space at left margin of sternum
  • V3—midway between V2 and V4
  • V4—fifth intercostal space at left midclavicular line
  • V5—placed midway between V4 and V6
  • V6—fifth intercostal space at the left midaxillary line
■ Limb electrodes (four)
  • RA—right arm
  • LA—left arm
  • RL—right leg (ground)
  • LL—left leg

ECG LEADS (12 VIEWS OF THE HEART)

■ Limb leads or **six views** produced by **four electrodes**
  • Bipolar limb leads—record cardiac electrical activity between two electrodes
    ○ Lead I—heart view between LA and RA electrodes
    ○ Lead II—heart view between LL and RA electrodes
    ○ Lead III—heart view between LL and LA electrodes
    ○ Lead I, lead II, and lead III with RL (ground) form **Einthoven triangle** (Fig. 20-3)
  • Unipolar (augmented voltage) limb leads
    ○ aVR (RA electrode)
    ○ aVL (LA electrode)
    ○ aVF (LL electrode)
■ Chest (precordial) leads (six)—all chest leads are unipolar and equate to the six chest electrodes
  • V1
  • V2
  • V3
  • V4
  • V5
  • V6

FIGURE 20-3 Einthoven triangle representing views of the heart in leads I, II, and III.

The national certification examinations frequently ask questions about identification of ECG leads.

ECG PAPER

ECG paper is standardized paper designed for ECG machines. It has a combination of small and large blocks to measure the cardiac electrical activity demonstrated in Figure 20-4.

- Horizontal line = time
  - Small block is 1 × 1 mm, representing 0.04 second on the horizontal axis

- Large block is 5 × 5 mm or five times larger than the small block representing 0.20 second on the horizontal axis (Box 20-1)
- Vertical line = voltage or amplitude
  - Small block is 1 × 1 mm, representing 0.1 mV on the vertical axis
  - Large block is 5 × 5 mm or five times larger than the small block representing 0.5 mV on the vertical line
- Vertical slashes above the graph—mark 3-second intervals (15 large blocks); used to calculate heart rate

Time used to estimate heart rate (horizontal axis)	
Small block	Represents 0.04 second
Large block (5 small squares)	Represents 0.20 second
Calculation	0.04 × 5 = 0.20 second
Voltage or amplitude (vertical line)	
Small block	Represents 0.1 mV
Large block (5 small squares)	Represents 0.5 mV
Calculation	0.1 × 5 = 0.5 mV

FIGURE 20-4 Calculating ECG time and voltage using ECG paper.

BOX 20-1

Criteria for identifying Normal Sinus Rhythm (NSR)

Rhythm (Regular)	Rate (Adult 60–100 bpm)	P Wave (Present)	Normal PR Interval (0.12–0.20 s)	Normal QRS Interval (between 0.06 and 0.10 s)

- Paper speed—25 mm/second is the usual speed for adults; 50 mm/second is usual speed for children
- Calibration—10-mm (two large blocks) vertical mark is the normal standard; it is sometimes referred to as the *standardization mark*; the calibration is changed to 5 mm (one-half standard) in situations where the R wave is too large and the ECG machine amplitude must be decreased to allow the tracing to fit on the paper

STYLUS

A **stylus** is a heated penlike instrument of the ECG machine. It receives impulses via electrodes and moves on heat-sensitive paper recording the electrical activity of the heart.

CRITERIA TO IDENTIFY NORMAL SINUS RHYTHM

Normal sinus rhythm (NSR) is a standard cardiac cycle that begins in the SA node (Fig. 6-21). The role of the medical assistant is not to interpret an ECG. The expectation is that the medical assistant can differentiate NSR from abnormal cardiac rhythms and notify the physician of irregularities. The physician may order a rhythm strip, a long tracing of lead II, as opposed to a complete ECG. The purpose is to evaluate a longer interval of complexes that may be compared to a previous ECG. Five criteria for NSR are (Box 20-1):

1. **Rhythm must be regular**; the same number of spaces must be between all R waves
2. **Heart rate must be normal**—normal adult heart rate is 60 to 100 beats per minute
   a. Calculation method 1—count the number of large blocks between two R waves and divide into 300 (e.g., five large blocks between two R waves = 300/5 = 60 beats per minute)
   b. Calculation method 2—count the number of R waves between 6-second marks (30 large blocks) and multiply by 10 (e.g., 6 R waves in 6 seconds = 6 × 10 = 60 beats per minute)

3. P waves must be present before each QRS complex
4. PR interval must be normal, 0.12 to 0.20 second (three to five small blocks)
5. QRS complex must be normal, 0.06- to 0.10-second duration (1.5 to 2.5 small blocks)

CARDIAC ARRHYTHMIAS

Cardiac **arrhythmias** or dysrhythmias are irregular heart activities resulting in loss of a regular rhythm. If all the criteria for NSR, as stated previously, are not met, the beat is considered abnormal. You will have to name select arrhythmias for the exams. Figure 20-5 illustrates a NSR and some examples of arrhythmias.

- Bradycardia—a heart rate slower than 60 beats per minute
- Tachycardia—a heart rate faster than 100 beats per minute
- Asystole—absence of a heart rate, no complexes; flat line; cardiac arrest
- Ectopic beat—a beat originating outside the SA node, the pacemaker of the heart
- Ventricular arrhythmias—irregularities in the ventricular activity (usually widened or odd-shaped QRS)
  - Premature ventricular contraction (PVC)—a contraction of the ventricles occurring early; may be life-threatening, depending on the ratio of PVCs to normal ventricular contractions; report to physician
  - Ventricular tachycardia—ventricular rate of more than 100 to 150 beats per minute, a wide QRS complex; considered a life-threatening arrhythmia and should be reported to the physician immediately; do not leave the patient and prepare for CPR
  - Ventricular flutter—ventricular rate of 150 to 300 beats per minute; considered a life-threatening arrhythmia and should be reported to the physician immediately; do not leave the patient and prepare for CPR
  - Bigeminy—every other beat is ectopic and/or premature (PVC); considered life-threatening and should be reported to the physician immediately; do not leave the patient and prepare for CPR

A Normal sinus rhythm

B Premature ventricular contractions (PVCs)

C Ventricle tachycardia

D Atrial fibrillation

E Atrial flutter (sawtooth)

FIGURE 20-5 Select electrocardiogram strips. (Reprinted with permission from Smeltzer SC, Bare BG. *Textbook of Medical-Surgical Nursing*. 9th Ed. Philadelphia: Lippincott Williams & Wilkins, 2000.)

WANDERING BASELINE

SOMATIC MUSCLE TREMOR

AC INTERFERENCE

FIGURE 20-6 Electrocardiogram artifacts. (Reprinted with permission from Hosley JB, Jones SA, Molle-Matthews EA. *Lippincott's Textbook for Medical Assistants*. Philadelphia: Lippincott-Raven Publishers, 1997.)

- Ventricular fibrillation—uncoordinated, ineffective ventricular contractions, "quivering of the heart"; displayed on the ECG as coarse or fine trembles with no identifiable waves or complexes; a life-threatening arrhythmia and should be reported to the physician immediately; begin CPR

■ Atrial arrhythmias—irregularities in the atrial activity

- Premature atrial contraction (PAC)—a contraction of the atria that occurs early

- Atrial tachycardia—also called AT; atrial rate of 150 to 250 beats per minute; P waves are often unidentifiable or hidden in previous T wave

- Paroxysmal atrial tachycardia (PAT)—atrial tachycardia that starts, and often stops, suddenly

- Atrial flutter—atrial rate of 250 to 350 beats per minute; "sawtooth" pattern on ECG; the ventricular rate is dependent on the number of nonconducted beats

- Atrial fibrillation—atrial rate of 350 to 500 beats per minute; P waves not distinct because of rapid rate; R to R waves are usually irregular; often with a rapid ventricular rate

Use Box 20-1 and Figure 20-5 to practice identifying NSR versus an arrhythmia.

ARTIFACTS

Artifacts are interruptions or disturbances in the ECG strip resulting from activity outside the heart. Figure 20-6 demonstrates examples of some of the following artifacts;

- Somatic tremors or movement—involuntary or voluntary muscle or other movement by the patient

- Alternating current (AC) interference—caused by other sources of electricity in the room, such as other equipment including some cell phones, crossed wires, improper grounding

- Wandering baseline—movement of the stylus from the center of the ECG paper in a "roaming" or "wandering" manner; causes may be electrodes that are too loose or too tight, corroded or dirty electrodes, oil or lotion on the patient's skin

- Interrupted baseline—a break between complexes, usually resulting from a wire becoming disconnected from an electrode or a broken wire

OTHER COMMON CARDIAC TESTS

- Holter monitor—a portable ECG device worn by a patient for 24 hours; monitors heart activity during normal activities of daily living and requires a patient to keep a diary of activities to help physician with diagnosis; electrodes are placed in the following locations:
  - Fourth intercostal space, right sternal margin
  - Right clavicle, lateral to sternal notch
  - Left clavicle, lateral to sternal notch
  - Fifth intercostal space, left axillary line
  - Lower right chest wall

- Stress test—ECG recordings taken while the patient exercises using a treadmill, stationary bicycle, or stair climber; monitors the response of the heart to increased demand

- Echocardiogram—ultrasound (sound waves) transmitted through the heart producing a picture on a screen; used to test the heart for structural or functional abnormalities

- Angiogram—an X-ray visualization with contrast material injected into a blood vessel to determine the presence of structural or functional abnormalities

- Cardiac catheterization—insertion of a catheter into a major blood vessel to visualize the heart's activity, to measure pressures, and to identify abnormalities, especially blockages

TERMS

ELECTROCARDIOGRAM REVIEW

The following list reviews the terms discussed in this chapter and other important terms you may see on the exam.

arrhythmia irregular heart activity resulting in loss of a rhythm

artifacts interruptions or disturbances in the ECG strip resulting from activity outside the heart

asystole absence of a heart rate, no complexes; represented by a flat line; cardiac arrest

atrial fibrillation atrial rate of 350 to 500 beats per minute; P waves not distinct because of rapid rate; R to R waves usually irregular, often with a rapid ventricular rate

atrial flutter atrial rate of 250 to 350 beats per minute; a "sawtooth" pattern on ECG; the ventricular rate is dependent on the number of nonconducted beats

atrial tachycardia (AT) atrial rate of 150 to 250 beats per minute; P waves are often unidentifiable or hidden in previous T wave

bigeminy every other beat is ectopic or premature

bradycardia a heart rate slower than 60 beats per minute

depolarization charged and contracting cardiac muscle cells; systole

ECG complex a full cardiac electrical cycle (one heartbeat) represented by the PQRST (and sometimes U) waves

echocardiogram reflected sound waves used to test the heart for structural or functional abnormalities

ectopic beat a beat originating outside the sinoatrial (SA) node, the pacemaker of the heart

Einthoven triangle the views of the heart from the placement of lead I, lead II, and lead III, which form a triangular shape

electrocardiogram (ECG or EKG) the graphic representation of the heart's electrical activity monitored at the skin surface with sensors called electrodes

electrodes skin sensors used to capture or monitor electrical activity of various organs (e.g., the heart, the brain)

Holter monitor a portable ECG device worn by a patient for 24 hours; heart activity is monitored during normal activities of daily living

lead a standard combination of electrode placements that designates a specific view of the heart

normal sinus rhythm (NSR) a standard cardiac cycle that begins in the SA node

paroxysmal atrial tachycardia (PAT) atrial tachycardia that starts, and often stops, suddenly

polarization resting cardiac muscle cells

premature atrial contraction (PAC) a contraction of the atria occurring early

premature ventricular contraction (PVC) a contraction of the ventricles occurring early; may be life-threatening, depending on the ratio of PVCs to normal ventricular contractions

repolarization recovering cardiac muscle cells; diastole; returning to equilibrium

sinoatrial (SA) node pacemaker of the heart

stress test ECG recordings taken while the patient exercises on a treadmill, stationary bicycle, or stair climber

stylus a heated penlike instrument of the ECG machine that receives impulses via electrodes and moves on ECG paper, recording the electrical activity of the heart

tachycardia a heart rate faster than 100 beats per minute

ventricular fibrillation uncoordinated and ineffective ventricular contractions, "quivering of the heart"; displayed on the ECG as coarse or fine trembles with no identifiable waves or complexes; considered a life-threatening arrhythmia

ventricular flutter ventricular rate of 150 to 300 beats per minute; considered a life-threatening arrhythmia

ventricular tachycardia ventricular rate of more than 100 to 150 beats per minute, wide QRS complex; considered a life-threatening arrhythmia

REVIEW QUESTIONS

All questions are relevant for all medical assisting certification exams.

1. The measurements of the smallest blocks on standard ECG graph paper are:
   A. 1 mm wide by 5 mm high.
   B. 1 cm high by 1 cm wide.
   C. 5 mm wide by 1 mm high.
   D. 1 mm wide by 1 mm high.

   Answer: **D**
   Why: The small blocks are 1 mm by 1 mm, and the large blocks are 5 mm by 5 mm. Five small blocks equal one large block.
   Review: Yes ◯   No ◯

2. Lead I of the ECG tracing is the heart view between the:
   A. right arm (RA) and the left arm (LA).
   B. right arm (RA) and the left leg (LL).
   C. left arm (LA) and the left leg (LL).
   D. right leg (RL) and the left leg (LL).
   E. left arm (LA) and the right leg (RL).

   Answer: **A**
   Why: Leads I, II, and III are the standard limb leads; they are also known as bipolar leads. Lead I is designated as the first lead, starting at the top of the body with both arms.
   Review: Yes ◯   No ◯

3. In a standard ECG, lead V3 is located:
   A. at the midaxillary line at the horizontal level of position V4 and position V5.
   B. at the fifth intercostal space and left mid-clavicular line.
   C. midway between position V2 and position V4.
   D. at the fourth intercostal space at the right margin of the sternum.

   Answer: **C**
   Why: After the location of V2 and V4 have been determined, V3 is located on an imaginary line midway between V2 and V4.
   Review: Yes ◯   No ◯

4. Proper preparation of the patient includes the following *except*:
   A. nylon hose should be removed to expose the area of the legs where the sensors will be placed.
   B. place the electrodes or sensors over bony prominences of the arms and legs where the electrical activity is more easily conducted.
   C. position the power cord away from the patient to lessen the chance of artifacts in the ECG tracing.
   D. make the patient comfortable and reassure patient that the procedure is not painful and that there is no transfer of electricity.
   E. place the ground sensor on the right leg.

   Answer: **B**
   Why: Electrodes or sensors should be placed over fleshy, muscular parts of the upper arms and lower legs. Conduction will be impaired if placed on bony prominences.
   Review: Yes ◯   No ◯

5. The height of a normal standardization mark on an ECG tracing is:
   A. 5 mm.
   B. 10 mm.
   C. 20 mm.
   D. 25 mm.

Answer: **B**
Why: A normal standardization mark that marks the accuracy of the ECG machine should be 10 mm high. The mark should have a square top. Most ECG machines automatically place a standardization mark at the beginning of the tracing. To manually insert a standardization mark, you need to push the Standard button on the machine.
Review: Yes ◯   No ◯

6. AC interference is an artifact in an ECG tracing that means:
   A. the patient is having a muscle tremor.
   B. there is a loose electrode connection.
   C. there is electrical interference in the room.
   D. the electrodes are too tight on the patient.
   E. the patient may be cold and shivering.

Answer: **C**
Why: There may be electrical machines, computers, or other devices causing interference with the function of the ECG machine. It may be necessary to unplug other appliances or equipment in the room, or the patient may need to be moved to another room to properly complete the ECG.
Review: Yes ◯   No ◯

7. The cardiac testing procedure that requires the patient to keep a diary of daily activities is a(n):
   A. cardiac stress test.
   B. echocardiogram.
   C. 12-lead electrocardiogram.
   D. Holter monitor.

Answer: **D**
Why: The Holter monitor is a small, portable ECG device that a patient wears while continuing with daily activities. Usually a 24-hour period is adequate to record and monitor the heart's activity. The patient maintains a written diary or log of activities and events during this time. The physician can determine if there is any correlation between abnormal heart function and the daily activity that took place during that period.
Review: Yes ◯   No ◯

8. The ECG grounding lead is the lead attached to the:
   A. right arm.
   B. left arm.
   C. right leg.
   D. chest, midway between V2 and V4.
   E. left leg.

Answer: **C**
Why: The grounding lead helps to reduce alternating current (AC) interference. It keeps the average voltage of the patient the same as the instrument.
Review: Yes ◯   No ◯

9. The ECG tracing is printed on graph paper at a standard speed for an adult of:
   A. 25 mm/sec.
   B. 50 mm/sec.
   C. 10 cm/sec.
   D. 20 cm/sec.

Answer: **A**
Why: Each block on the ECG graph paper represents 1 mm. When an ECG tracing is moving at a standard speed, the paper is advancing at 25 mm (25 small squares) each second.
Review: Yes ◯   No ◯

10. Lead II of the ECG tracing records the electrical activity through the heart from the:
   A. right arm to left arm.
   B. right arm to left leg.
   C. right leg to left leg.
   D. right arm to right leg.
   E. left arm to left leg.

Answer: **B**
Why: The standard limb leads—lead I, lead II, and lead III—form an imaginary triangle when lines connect the reference points. Lead I is the top horizontal line of the triangle, the left side of the triangle is lead II, and the right side of the triangle is lead III.
Review: Yes ○   No ○

11. During the electrical heart cycle, **repolarization** refers to the:
   A. recovering phase.
   B. discharging phase.
   C. resting phase.
   D. contracting phase.

Answer: **A**
Why: During the heart cycle, cardiac cells are exchanging positive and negative charges within the cell membranes. During repolarization, negative ions are transferred to the inside of the cell, and the positive ions return to the outside. Repolarization is a recovery time for the cells and is a necessary process for another heartbeat to take place.
Review: Yes ○   No ○

12. The chest lead V1 is located at which intercostal space?
   A. Fourth
   B. Fifth
   C. Between fourth and fifth
   D. Sixth
   E. Third

Answer: **A**
Why: V1 is located at the fourth intercostal space at the right margin of the sternum.
Review: Yes ○   No ○

13. The image traced on the ECG paper is a(n):
   A. image created by an echocardiogram of the heart.
   B. needle scratching the image on the paper.
   C. graph representing the electrical activity of the heart.
   D. measurement of the blood volume going through the heart at a specific speed.

Answer: **C**
Why: The ECG paper is a graph representing the electrical activity of the heart, hence the term electrocardiogram. An echocardiogram is a study done with sound waves to determine the functioning of the heart. ECG machines work digitally, and no needles are involved. Blood volume cannot be measured by an ECG, but excessive or decreased blood volume can affect the ECG.
Review: Yes ○   No ○

14. The purpose of adjusting the normal standard to one-half standard is to:
   A. conserve paper.
   B. enlarge the height of the patient's ECG tracing.
   C. decrease the size of the patient's ECG tracing.
   D. eliminate artifacts in the tracing.
   E. ensure proper lead placement.

Answer: **C**
Why: When the ECG machine setting is changed from the normal 10-mm-high standard mark to one-half standard, 5 mm high, it decreases the size of the patient's ECG tracing. This is necessary when the tracing is so large it goes off the paper. The physician cannot properly measure the complex unless the entire complex is on the paper.
Review: Yes ○   No ○

15. When a patient has trouble relaxing or cannot remain still for the ECG, the artifact that may occur is:
    A. somatic muscle tremor.
    B. wandering baseline.
    C. AC interference.
    D. electrode interference.

Answer: **A**
Why: A somatic muscle tremor appears as a static line in between the complexes on the ECG paper. To avoid this artifact, make sure the patient is comfortable and not cold. Pillows may be placed under the knees to help the patient relax.
Review: Yes ◯   No ◯

16. The type of cardiac procedure that requires the use of a treadmill is:
    A. echocardiography.
    B. cardiac stress test.
    C. cardiac angiography.
    D. 12-lead ECG.
    E. Holter monitoring.

Answer: **B**
Why: A cardiac stress test is a procedure that measures the body's response to increased demands made on the heart muscle. The patient walks on a treadmill while the ECG tracing is recorded. Some cardiac abnormalities may be exhibited on exertion rather than at rest.
Review: Yes ◯   No ◯

17. The medical assistant should gather all the appropriate patient data before the ECG procedure *except*:
    A. patient's height and weight.
    B. date of the patient's first ECG procedure.
    C. patient's current medications.
    D. time and date of the recording.

Answer: **B**
Why: It is not important to know when the patient had his or her first ECG procedure. However, it may be important to know when the patient had his or her last ECG. Some patients have had many electrocardiograms performed. If the patient had a prior ECG with the same physician, the record will be in the patient's file, and the physician can do a comparison.
Review: Yes ◯   No ◯

18. The leads aVR, aVL, and aVF are the:
    A. standard leads.
    B. bipolar leads.
    C. limb leads.
    D. chest leads.
    E. augmented voltage leads.

Answer: **E**
Why: Augmented voltage leads provide additional information about the electrical activity of the heart. They use the electrical midpoint of the three limb sensors as the negative pole, and each limb sensor is considered the positive pole. Lead aVR, augmented voltage right, uses a midpoint between the left leg and left arm as the negative pole and the right arm as the positive pole. Lead aVL uses a midpoint between the left leg and right arm as the negative pole and the left arm as the positive pole. Lead aVF uses a midpoint between the right arm and left arm as the negative pole and the left leg as the positive pole.
Review: Yes ◯   No ◯

19. The QRS complex of the ECG tracing represents:
    A. atrial depolarization.
    B. atrial repolarization.
    C. ventricular depolarization.
    D. ventricular repolarization.

Answer: **C**
Why: The QRS complex represents the contraction of the ventricles as positive ions enter the cells and negative ions leave them. Depolarization is the electrical activity that causes the heart to contract.
Review: Yes ◯   No ◯

20. The atrial arrhythmia that is sometimes re-
ferred to as sawtoothed is:
   A. ventricular fibrillation.
   B. ventricular tachycardia.
   C. atrial fibrillation.
   D. atrial flutter.
   E. asystole.

Answer: **D**
Why: The atrial rate of 250 to 350 creates a sawtoothed appearance (Fig. 20-5E). Ventricular
fibrillation and ventricular tachycardia refer to
the QRS complex. Atrial fibrillation is a faster
atrial response, and P waves are not distinguish-
able; the rhythm is also very irregular. Asystole is
"flatline."
Review: Yes ○   No ○

21. A long strip of QRS complexes of a certain
lead used to define certain cardiac arrhyth-
mias is a(n):
   A. monitor strip.
   B. stress strip.
   C. rhythm strip.
   D. artifact strip.

Answer: **C**
Why: A rhythm strip is run to give the physician
a tracing longer than the typical lead length. This
allows the physician to determine whether the
patient has an abnormality that only shows up occasionally and not with each beat.
Review: Yes ○   No ○

22. If the electrodes are too loose on the patient,
what artifact might you find on the ECG
tracing?
   A. Wandering baseline
   B. Somatic tremor
   C. AC interference
   D. Electrical interference
   E. Muscle tremor

Answer: **A**
Why: A wandering baseline appears as a tracing
that wanders back and forth from the bottom to
the top of the paper. The normal baseline should
stay within the middle of the paper. Check all
electrodes for proper connection. If electrodes are
too loose, the baseline may wander on the tracing
paper.
Review: Yes ○   No ○

23. The purpose of setting the ECG paper speed
at 50 mm/sec is to:
   A. help record rapid heartbeats.
   B. increase the size of the complex on the
      paper.
   C. help record slow heartbeats.
   D. decrease the size of the complex on the
      paper.

Answer: **A**
Why: When a patient has a rapid heartbeat, the
faster speed allows the complexes to space farther
apart on the paper. It is easier to determine the
quality of the complexes when they are not plot-
ted close together. Rapid heartbeats are normal for
infants and young children.
Review: Yes ○   No ○

24. The P wave represents the:
   A. last waveform of the ECG complex.
   B. activity of the ventricles.
   C. resting phase of the heart muscle.
   D. atrial depolarization.
   E. ventricle repolarization.

Answer: **D**
Why: The P wave is the first waveform of the ECG
complex and represents the electrical activity that
spreads from the SA node through the atria, causing atrial contraction. During this time, the cells
are depolarizing.
Review: Yes ○   No ○

25. What should the medical assistant tell a patient if the patient asks if he or she will feel any discomfort from the ECG procedure?
    A. If you feel any shocks or electrical tingling, please let me know.
    B. Don't worry, we do lots of these exams every day.
    C. The ECG procedure does not hurt and does not send electricity through you.
    D. The electrodes are cold and may feel too tight, but we need to get a good connection.

Answer: **C**
Why: Reassure the patient that the ECG machine does not send out any electricity and that it does not hurt to have the procedure performed. The medical assistant should ask the patient if there is anything that would make him or her more comfortable during the exam, especially if the patient has a problem that could cause discomfort when lying down. Pillows used as support for the arms or legs could help relax the patient.
Review: Yes ○   No ○

CRITICAL THINKING CASE REVIEW QUESTIONS

Ms. Jarvis is a patient of Dr. Celaya. She was diagnosed with gallstones and scheduled for surgery. Prior to her surgery, the physician has asked you to perform a 12-lead ECG. This is Ms. Jarvis' first ECG.

1. The primary purpose of this ECG is to:
    A. monitor any potential heart condition.
    B. treat any potential heart problem prior to surgery.
    C. conform with the standard of care for diagnostic studies prior to surgery.
    D. establish a baseline ECG and determine if the patient's heart is fit for surgery.
    E. allow you an opportunity to hone your ECG skills and to perform patient teaching since this the patient's first ECG.

Answer: **D**
Why: Since this is the patient's first ECG, it establishes her baseline; it also gives an indication if her heart is fit for surgery. You are not monitoring or treating the heart. While C and E may be true, they are not the best answers.
Review: Yes ○ No ○

2. The electrode placed on the right leg is usually used as the ground which:
    A. prevents the patient from becoming shocked.
    B. reduces electrical interference.
    C. completes the Einthoven triangle from the left arm to the right leg for lead IV.
    D. shuts off the machine if there is a power failure.

Answer: **B**
Why: The purpose of the ground electrode is to reduce interference. Electrical shock is virtually impossible for the patient during an ECG, and the ground electrode will not shut off the machine in a power failure. The right leg does not make up any part of the Einthoven triangle. It is the right arm to the left arm, the left arm to the left leg, and the left leg to the right arm.
Review: Yes ○ No ○

3. In order to obtain an accurate ECG, you instruct Ms. Jarvis to:
    A. breathe normally and remain still.
    B. hold her breath and remain still.
    C. maintain comfort during the procedure and move as necessary.
    D. ask for a blanket if she becomes cold.
    E. leave on her shoes and stockings.

Answer: **A**
Why: The patient should be instructed to breathe normally and remain still. Holding one's breath could affect the bpm, since the body is not circulating oxygen, and movement causes artifacts. A blanket could also cause artifacts and not necessary, since the procedure is quite rapid. Stockings must be removed in order for the leg electrodes to have contact with the skin. Shoes are optional.
Review: Yes ○ No ○

4. During the ECG, you notice two PVCs, one at the beginning of the strip and one at the end. The appropriate thing for you to do is to:
   A. run and notify Dr. Celaya.
   B. tell Ms. Jarvis that you are seeing an abnormality and call for Dr. Celaya.
   C. repeat the ECG to assure that you did it correctly
   D. complete the test normally and show it to Dr. Celaya.

Answer: **D**

Why: Although two PVCs are not normal, they are not life-threatening. You would not run to tell the doctor nor say anything to the patient regarding the arrhythmia. It is not appropriate to repeat the ECG at this time, since it is the baseline test. You would complete the test as you normally would and show the strip to the doctor.

Review: Yes ○ No ○

5. As the test prints out, Ms. Jarvis notices that different portions of the graph look different and she becomes upset. You would:
   A. inform her that she does have some abnormalities but nothing serious.
   B. tell her that most people feel this way after they see the graph and she is normal.
   C. explain to her that there are different views of the heart and they should not look the same.
   D. do not say anything but stay with her until the doctor comes into the room.
   E. explain to her that you are not able to read an ECG and you could not tell her why the different lines look different.

Answer: **C**

Why: A, you would be diagnosing and that is not in your scope of practice. B is not true, and it is never appropriate to be untruthful with a patient. C is correct and the truth that there are different views of the heart created by the placement of the electrodes producing varying visualizations. D, there is no reason not to give the patient the explanation expressed in C relieving unnecessary anxiety. E, you can tell the patient that you are not able to read the ECG, but you should know why the lines look different and be able to articulate the reason to the patient.

Review: Yes ○ No ○

CHAPTER 21

Laboratory Procedures

ReviewTip:

Review Chapter 17, "Microorganisms and Asepsis," which contains information that is needed for laboratory procedures. Understand the concepts in that chapter before beginning this chapter. Study the laboratory norms and other information contained in the tables, boxes, and review terms in this chapter. If you know the normal values of laboratory tests you will recognize what is abnormal in exam questions.

Laboratory procedures, whether for diagnosis or treatment, are an integral part of health care provided in the medical office. The medical assistant plays a major role and is often the one to obtain, prepare, and process the laboratory specimen. The integrity of the specimen and adherence to the processing procedure can determine the correctness of the test results, the accuracy of the patient's diagnosis, and even the efficacy of the treatment. The medical administrative assistant also plays an integral role, often, as the person who follows up to assure that results were received by the practice, reviewed by the provider, and reported to the patient.

LABORATORY DIVISIONS

Laboratory procedures are divided into areas or divisions of expertise. The divisions are named according to the types of tissues or organisms to be studied and require different equipment, reagents, and staff training. Although many of the laboratory procedures are not performed in the medical office, the specimens are collected there and general knowledge of divisions is needed.

- Clinical chemistry/metabolic testing—analysis that identifies and measures chemical components in blood, urine, spinal fluid, tissue, and other body fluids as indicators of health status and to help to identify pathology; common examples include laboratory tests for glucose, cholesterol, calcium, globulin, blood urea nitrogen (BUN), chloride, sodium, potassium, bilirubin, triglycerides, cardiac, and liver enzymes

- Cytology—analysis of cells to determine abnormalities; examples include Papanicolaou (Pap) smears to detect cervical cancer and chromosomal studies

- Hematology—study of blood and blood-forming tissue; analysis of blood to determine abnormalities in the blood cells, number of cells or the clotting; examples include tests for hemoglobin, hematocrit, prothrombin time (PT) for blood clotting, international normalized ratio (INR) with PT for blood clotting, partial thromboplastin time (PTT) also for blood clotting, platelet count, red blood cell (RBC) count, and differential white blood cell (WBC or diff) count (Table 21-1 lists common blood tests and their normal ranges)

- Histology—microscopic study of cells, tissues, and organs in association with their functions; examples of tests include biopsy and tissue analysis

- Immunology (serology and blood banking)—study of immunity, sensitivity, and induced sensitivity; the presence of antibodies/antigens and pathology; examples include tests for Rh typing, ABO blood typing, Rh antibody titer, rapid plasma reagent (RPR), erythrocyte sedimentation rate (ESR) and C-reactive protein (CRP) for inflammation and autoimmune diseases such as lupus and rheumatoid arthritis, mononucleosis, helicobacter pylori (H. pylori) antibodies, and human gonadotropin (HCG) for pregnancy

- Microbiology—study of microorganisms; in the laboratory, this division usually determines the presence and identity of microorganisms found in specimens; examples are tests for tuberculosis, meningitis, pertussis, streptococcal infections, and salmonella; often requires collection of a specimen for culture such as a nasopharyngeal, wound drainage, or throat swab

- Parasitology—study of human parasites and ova (eggs); examples include tests for hookworm, scabies, pinworms, tapeworms, toxoplasmosis, malaria, and amebiasis

- Urinalysis—physical, chemical, and microscopic analysis of urine; Table 21-2 lists normal ranges for urinalysis; examples include tests for:

TABLE 21-1 ▶ Common blood tests: normal ranges

Test	Adult Normal Range
Bleeding time	2–7 min
Blood urea nitrogen (BUN)	10–20 mg/dL
Chloride	98–110 mEq/L
Cholesterol: total	140–200 mg/dL
High-density lipoprotein	30–90 mg/dL
Low-density lipoprotein	30–100 mg/dL
Creatinine	0.6–1.3 mg/dL
Erythrocyte sedimentation rate (ESR, sed rate)	(Results are age- and method-dependent) Male: 0–20 mm/h Female: 0–30 mm/h
Glucose (fasting blood glucose, FBS)	70–110 mg/dL
Hematocrit (HCT or "crit")	Male: 39%–49% packed RBCs Female: 35%–45% packed RBCs
Hemoglobin (Hb, Hgb)	Male: 13.2–17.3 g/dL Female: 11.7–16.0 g/dL
Hemoglobin A1c	4.5%–6% (5.7%–6.4% prediabetic)
*International normalized ratio (INR) (may be reported as PT/INR)	*0.9–1.1
Platelets	$150–400 \times 10^3$ cells/µL
Potassium	3.5–5.0 mEq/L
Prostate-specific antigen (PSA)	0–6.5 ng/mL (age-specific ranges)
*Prothrombin time (PT)	*11–13.5 s
*Partial thromboplastin time (PTT)	*25–35 s
Red blood cells (RBCs)	Male: $4.3–5.7 \times 10^3$ cells/µL Female: $3.8–5.1 \times 10^3$ cells/µL
Rheumatoid factor (RF)	<30 U/mL
Sodium	135–148 mEq/L
Triglycerides	Male: 40–163 mg/dL Female: 35–128 mg/dL
White blood cells (WBCs)	$4.5–11.0 \times 10^3$ cells/µL

µL = mm^3 (sometimes used to measure WBCs).
*indicates normal values for patients not on anticoagulants (blood thinners).

- Color, clarity, specific gravity (physical)
- pH, glucose, ketones, nitrites, HCG for pregnancy (chemical)
- RBCs, WBCs, crystals (microscopic)

TABLE 21-2 Components of reagent strip urinalysis and results

Test	Norm
pH	4.5–8
Protein	Negative
Glucose	Negative
Ketone	Negative
Bilirubin	Negative
Blood	Negative
Leukocytes	Negative
Nitrites	Negative
Urobilinogen	Negative
Specific gravity	1.020–1.030
Color	Pale–dark yellow
Clarity	Clear
Odor	Distinct

CLINICAL LABORATORY IMPROVEMENT AMENDMENTS

Enacted in 1988 by Congress, the Clinical Laboratory Improvement Amendments (CLIA) placed all laboratories involved with testing human laboratory specimens under the regulation of the Health Care Finance Administration (now called the Centers for Medicare and Medicaid Services) and the Centers for Disease Control and Prevention (CDC). The standards developed were divided into three areas: personnel, testing, and quality assurance.

The CDC also identifies and publishes a list of CLIA-waived laboratory tests. These are tests generally permitted in a medical office without the stringent standards associated with non–CLIA-waived tests performed in laboratories. The waived tests specify the names of approved commercial products including instrumentation for conducting these tests. The medical assistant may perform the CLIA-waived tests for:

- Blood
  - Blood count; spun microhematocrit
  - Blood chemistry (whole blood) analysis
  - Blood glucose by FDA-approved monitoring devices
  - CPR protein in the body that rises when inflammation such as rheumatoid arthritis and lupus are present
  - ESR, nonautomated
  - Hemoglobin by copper sulfate, nonautomated
  - Hemoglobin by single-analyte instruments
  - INR
  - Lipid panel
- Urine
  - Dipstick or tablet reagent urinalysis for the following:
    - Glucose
    - Hemoglobin (blood)
    - Ketone
    - Leukocytes
    - Nitrite
    - pH
    - Protein
    - Specific gravity
    - Urobilinogen
  - HCG by visual color comparison (pregnancy test)
  - Ovulation tests by visual color for human luteinizing hormone (HLH)
  - Rapid drug tests for the following:
    - Amphetamine
    - Cocaine
    - Marijuana (THC) test
    - Methadone
    - Morphine
    - Opiates
    - Oxycodone
    - PCP
- Fecal occult blood/guaiac testing
- *Helicobacter pylori* antibodies breath test (blood and feces specimens are not CLIA-waived)
- Rapid tests from nasal aspirate or wash or nasal pharyngeal (NP) specimen
  - *Influenza* antibodies
  - Respiratory syncytial virus (RSV) antigen
- Sperm check for male fertility
- *Streptococcus* A (throat swab)

LABORATORY QUALITY ASSURANCE

To ensure the accuracy of CLIA-waived testing and the integrity of collected specimens, the following are quality assurance measures:

- Know the protocol for the collection, processing, and storage for each test before performing
- Monitor and record daily temperatures of refrigerators and incubators

- Be aware of room temperature for equipment function and storage of materials used in testing that do not require refrigeration
- Adhere to equipment maintenance schedules as recommended by the manufacturer
- Perform and record daily calibration of instrumentation
- Perform daily control testing
- Store reagents and other supplies per the manufacturers' directions
- Use appropriate aseptic technique, PPE, and biohazard waste disposal to avoid contamination
- Label each specimen with the patient's name, second identifier, date, time of collection, and source
- Have patient verify labeling
- Preserve specimens for transport appropriately (check protocol if refrigeration is needed)
- Maintain logs of tests performed and specimens collected/transported

COMMON SPECIMENS COLLECTED FOR TRANSPORT

Although only CLIA-waived tests are performed in the medical office, many specimens are collected there and sent to reference laboratories for processing. Correct specimen collection is vital to test results and is often the responsibility of the medical assistant.

- **Biopsies**—removing tissue from patients for microscopic examination to determine cancer or other abnormalities; may be done surgically or with endoscopes, biopsy punches, or other instruments
- **Phlebotomy**—incision or needle puncture into a vein to draw blood (see Box 21-1)
  - Blood components (see Fig. 21-1)
    - Plasma—relatively clear yellow liquid portion of blood; composes 55% of whole blood; upper layer in specimen tube
    - Buffy coat—light grayish liquid portion of blood containing WBCs; composes 1% of whole blood; middle layer in specimen tube
    - RBCs—dark red opaque portion of blood containing RBCs; composes 44% of whole blood; bottom layer of specimen tube
    - Serum—liquid portion of blood after clotting factors are removed; composition includes portions of plasma and buffy coat
  - Collection tubes—glass and plastic; Box 21-2 lists the order of collection for glass and for plastic tubes
    - Yellow top—used to collect serum for bacteriologic tests; does not contain an additive
    - Red top—used to collect serum for chemistry and serology; a "clot tube"; does not contain an additive
    - Speckled top (red and black)—used to collect serum for chemistry and serology; different from red top in that it contains a gel that separates serum and RBCs during centrifugation

---

BOX 21-1

Venous blood collection reminders

- Identify the patient using two pieces of information, usually name and birthday.
- Ask the patient about latex and tape allergies.
- Use appropriate PPE.
- Choose the site; the antecubital fossa medial cubital vein is the preferred site for blood draw.
- The vein of choice is the median cubital.
- The tourniquet should be placed 3 to 4 inches above the point of puncture.
- The tourniquet should not be left on for more than 1 minute.
- Cleanse the site using a circular pattern beginning at the point of puncture and moving to the outside.
- Allow the antiseptic to dry before inserting safety needle.
- Always anchor the vein.
- Safety needle is attached to the tube collection holder (use a butterfly only for difficult draws).
- During insertion, the bevel of the needle should be face up at a 15° to 30° angle.
- Release the tourniquet when filling the last tube.
- Gently invert the collection tubes 8 to 10 times to mix tube additives.
- Using a sterile dressing, apply direct pressure to the site.
- Do not tape until bleeding has stopped.
- Label specimen and have patient verify information.

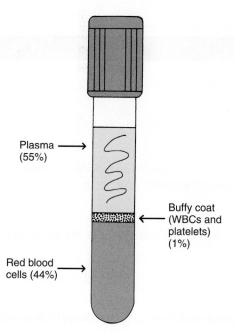

Plasma (55%)

Buffy coat (WBCs and platelets) (1%)

Red blood cells (44%)

FIGURE 21-1 Centrifuged blood specimen. (Reprinted with permission from McCall RE, Tankersly CM. *Phlebotomy Essentials*. 3rd Ed. Philadelphia: Lippincott Williams & Williams, 2003.)

- ○ Lavender top—used to collect plasma for hematology testing; contains an anticoagulant additive
- ○ Blue top—used to collect plasma for coagulation studies; contains anticoagulant sodium citrate additive
- ○ Green top—used to collect plasma for urgent chemistry studies; contains anticoagulant additive
- ○ Gray top—used to collect blood for glucose and alcohol testing; contains anticoagulant additive
- • **Capillary puncture**—dermal puncture of finger, earlobe, or heel (in infants) to obtain a blood specimen; examples include tests for blood glucose and hemoglobin; also used for mandated neonatal specimen collection in the United States for the following:

BOX 21-2

Order of draw to avoid cross-contamination of additives

Order of Draw Using Plastic or Glass Tubes

1. Yellow-top tubes requiring sterility (for blood cultures)
2. Light-blue top
3. Red or speckled top
4. Green top
5. Lavender top

- ○ **Phenylketonuria (PKU)**—capillary specimen from the infant's heel used to detect phenylalanine
- ○ Hypothyroidism—capillary specimen from infant's heel used to detect thyroid hormone levels
- • Capillary puncture technique
  - ○ Avoid squeezing tip of finger
  - ○ May gently "milk" hand and finger
  - ○ Discard first drop of blood
  - ○ Avoid scraping collection tube over puncture
  - ○ Avoid air bubbles or spaces in the collection area of the tube

- ■ **Cerebral spinal fluid**—clear, colorless fluid that covers the spinal cord and brain, obtained for testing by a lumbar puncture performed by a physician or mid-level provider

- ■ **Cervical scrapings/brushings**—specimens obtained during a pelvic exam; used to test for cancer of the cervix and other diseases

- ■ **Nasal pharyngeal swab**—specimen collected with a fine Dacron or other soft applicator inserted up the nares to the pharyngeal passageway (Box 21.3 and Fig. 21-2); used to test for pertussis, RSV by culture, or **polymerase chain reaction (PCR)** to identify DNA presence of a pathogen

- ■ **Sputum**—secretions from the respiratory system obtained by deep coughing; used to culture for presence of tuberculosis (*Mycobacterium tuberculosis*) and other disease-causing microorganisms

- ■ **Stool**—fecal specimen used to test for ova and parasites, pathologic bacteria, and occult blood (e.g., hemoccult), which may indicate cancer

- ■ **Throat swabbing** (with sterile cotton applicator)—specimen collected for culture and sensitivity (C&S) to detect disease-causing microorganisms in the throat and to test for the appropriate antibiotic to combat them

- ■ **Urethral brushings**—specimen collected with a fine brushlike applicator inserted in the urethra; used to test for sexually transmitted infections

- ■ **Urine**

  - • Random sample—urine specimen collected at any time

  - • Clean-catch sample—urine specimen collected after cleaning the urinary meatus from front to back using three antibacterial pads, one per side and the third down the middle for the female; for the male use a circular motion from the urethra outward; the patient then begins to void, stops, collects a portion of urine in the provided container, and finishes voiding in the toilet; referred to as a "midstream" urine; used for tests to determine the presence of bacteria in the urine

BOX 21-3

Specimen collection using a nasopharyngeal swab

- Identify the patient using two pieces of information, usually name and birthday.
- Ask the patient about latex and tape allergies.
- Use appropriate PPE.
- Position patient with head straight.
- Determine correct swab material for test, for example, Dacron.
- Insert straight back into one nostril along the floor of the nasal passage for several centimeters until resistance is met which should be the nasopharynx (approximately distance from nose to ear); *never* force.
- If blockage is felt; use the other nostril.
- Rotate the swab 5 to 10 seconds to obtain adequate specimen.
- Place immediately into transport media at least ½ inch below top of media material; stick should be broken or folded to allow secure attachment of top of carrier.
- Label specimen appropriately and keep at refrigerator temperature.

FIGURE 21-2 Collecting nasopharyngeal specimen.

- 24-hour sample—all urine voided in a 24-hour period is collected directly into a specified container; used to determine the presence of substances released only sporadically and to measure the amount of urinary output
- First-voided sample—urine collected in the morning after a night's sleep; used to obtain more concentrated substances for pregnancy testing and microscopic exams
- Catheterized or sterile sample—urine collected by insertion of a sterile tube into the urinary bladder; used to measure the amount of residual urine in the bladder or to obtain a sterile urinary specimen for culturing to determine the presence of pathogens in the bladder, not the external urinary structures that would contaminate the specimen
- **Postprandial urine or blood**—collected after patient has consumed a meal

- **Wound swabbings** (with sterile applicator)—drainage from wounds; used to culture for pathogens

---

PREPARATION FOR SPECIMEN EXAMINATION

- **Centrifuge**—a machine that separates whole blood or urine into various components for additional testing
- **Smear**—using a swab-type applicator, a small amount of the specimen is applied to a glass slide and allowed to dry or a **fixative** which is substance to preserve the specimen is applied
- **Wet mount**—a drop of normal saline (0.9% sodium chloride) is placed on a slide that has been smeared with the specimen; a cover slide is placed on top, and the specimen is ready for examination with a microscope
- **Potassium hydroxide (KOH) mount**—primarily used to identify fungal infections; the specimen is prepared as a wet mount, substituting KOH for the saline; the specimen is allowed to sit at room temperature until examination under the microscope
- **Stains**—a smear of the specimen is prepared; when dry, the slide is heated and stain material applied; specific bacteria hold certain color stains, allowing identification
  - Purple stain—identifies gram-positive bacteria
  - Red stain—identifies gram-negative bacteria
  - Acid–fast—certain bacteria are not susceptible to color staining; these bacteria are called acid–fast (e.g., *Mycobacterium tuberculosis*)

■ **Culture**—the process of growing pathogens from specimens **inoculated** into a culture media and **incubated** to grow; the purpose is to identify the microorganisms contained in the specimen to target treatment

- **Common culture media**—substances used to promote growth of bacteria by providing a nutrition source; may be a liquid or gel-like state

  ○ Transport media—usually a tube structure with a substance used to keep the bacteria alive until they can be plated on an appropriate culture media; specific tubes may be used for specific specimens

  ○ **Petri dish**—a round plastic dish that contains **agar**, a gelatin-like culture material made from algae or other media appropriate to grow suspected organisms, and has a cover to minimize contamination of the specimen with environmental bacteria; the covered petri dish should be placed in the incubator upside down, with the patient identification and other information placed on the bottom of the, *not* the top of the, plate. This assures the correct specimen belongs to the correct patient

  ○ **Plating or inoculating**—process of inoculating agar with the specimen swab and sometimes with a sterile inoculating loop

  ○ **Incubate**—maintaining a culture in a special device (incubator) that provides an optimal temperature (approximately 36°C for 3 to 7 days for most bacteria), humidity, and other conditions such as carbon dioxide or oxygen to grow microorganisms

- **Sensitivity**—testing to determine a pathogen's susceptibility to specific antibiotics

---

THE MICROSCOPE

The microscope (scope) is an instrument used to magnify very small objects, usually objects not visible to the naked eye. Anton van Leeuwenhoek (17th century) is attributed with being the first to use an instrument with lenses to visualize "germs." Many different types and strengths of microscopes are used in clinical and research laboratories. The most common one found in the medical office is the binocular, or two-eyepiece, scope. It is used to identify microorganisms placed on slides from various body specimens using the processes previously mentioned. The main portions of the microscope are described below and illustrated in Figure 21-3.

■ Ocular lens(es)—eyepiece(s)

■ Frame—structure that supports the scope

FIGURE 21-3 Basic parts of the microscope.

- Base—bottom portion of the frame that holds entire structure
- Arm—extension of the frame that holds upper portion of the scope
- Head—portion of the frame below the eyepiece(s)

■ Stage—platform that holds the slide during observation

■ Condenser—lens beneath the stage that focuses light on the slide; it may be raised or lowered

■ Light source—located on base; provides light to the condenser

■ Diaphragm—controls the amount of light on the condenser

■ Nosepiece—portion below the head that holds the objective lenses

■ Objective lenses—lenses below the nosepiece marked with specified magnifications; these are summarized in Table 21-3

- Low power—magnification 10×; used for initial focus
- High-power dry—magnification 40×; used to locate and focus on the specimen
- Oil immersion—magnification 100×; used with oil to perform differential count of blood smear

■ Coarse adjustment—outside knob used with low-power objective lens

TABLE 21-3 ▶ Objective lens magnification		
Ocular Lens	Lens Magnification	Total Lens Magnification
Low power	10 × 10×	100×
High-power dry	10 × 40×	400×
Oil immersion	10 × 100×	1000×

■ Fine adjustment—inside knob used with both high-power and oil-immersion objective lenses

TERMS

LABORATORY PROCEDURES REVIEW

The following list reviews the terms discussed in this chapter and other important terms you may see on the exam.

anticoagulant substance that prevents blood from clotting

biopsy removing tissue from patients for microscopic examination to determine the presence of cancer or other abnormalities; may be done surgically or with endoscopes, biopsy punches, or other instruments

calibration a measurement compared with a standard; a method for testing the accuracy of equipment; a quality assurance procedure

capillary puncture dermal puncture of finger, earlobe, or heel in infants to obtain a blood specimen

centrifuge laboratory instrument that spins at high speeds, separating particles in specimens such as blood and urine

clinical chemistry analysis to identify and to measure chemical components in blood, urine, spinal fluid, tissue, and other body fluids

complete blood count (CBC) panel of blood tests that includes hematocrit, hemoglobin, red blood cells, white blood cells, and differential white blood cells (diff)

control a specimen with known values that serves as a check of test accuracy

C-reactive protein (CPR) protein in the body that rises when inflammation such as rheumatoid arthritis and lupus are present

crossmatching laboratory testing process to determine compatibility of blood donated by one person with the blood of a potential recipient

culture the process of growing pathogens from specimens inoculated into a culture medium and maintained at a designated temperature; the purpose is to identify the microorganisms contained in the specimen

cytology analysis of cells to determine abnormalities

evacuated tube (ET) a tube, sealed to maintain the vacuum, that is used for obtaining blood specimens; it may have additives, depending on the type of blood specimen to be obtained

fasting sample blood collected after the patient has not eaten or drank (except water) for 6 to 8 hours

fibrinogen a protein in blood plasma that assists clotting

hematocrit percentage of red blood cells in the total blood volume

hematology study of blood and blood-forming tissue; analysis of blood to determine abnormalities

hemoglobin oxygen-carrying portion of red blood cells

hemoglobin A1C blood test to help diagnose type 1 and type 2 diabetes and to measure the average blood glucose over a 2- to 3-month period

histology microscopic study of cells, tissues, and organs in association with their functions

human chorionic gonadotropin (HCG) hormone present in blood and urine during pregnancy; urine or blood tests are used to determine pregnancy by the presence of HCG

immunohematology specialized immunology dealing with blood, the presence of antibodies/antigens, and pathology

immunology study of immunity, sensitivity, and induced sensitivity; the presence of antibodies/antigens and pathology

incubation maintaining a controlled environment to promote growth of microbial or tissue cultures

international normalizing ratio (INR) ratio derived from the prothrombin time to help determine blood clotting; often reported as **PT/INR**

lancet a sharp, sterile, disposable instrument used to puncture skin for collecting capillary blood

microbiology study of microorganisms; in the laboratory, this division usually determines the presence and the identity of microorganisms found in specimens; examples include tests for tuberculosis, meningitis, and diphtheria

microscope (scope) an instrument used to magnify very small objects usually not visible to the naked eye

Mohs procedure or surgery removal of skin tissue which is then prepared and examined while the patient waits to determine the presence of basal cell or squamous cell carcinoma and, if present, the amount of tissue to remove for cancer-free edges

Papanicolaou (Pap) smear to detect cervical cancer

parasitology study of human parasites and ova (eggs)

partial thromboplastin time (PTT) blood test to determine abnormal clotting or to monitor anticoagulation medication

phenylketonuria (PKU) a disease resulting in mental retardation caused by a deficiency in the metabolic process; tested for by using a capillary specimen from an infant's heel, a test required by law in the United States

phlebotomy incision or needle puncture into a vein to draw blood

plasma relatively clear yellow liquid portion of blood; composes 55% of whole blood; upper layer in specimen tube

plating process of inoculating agar with a specimen swab and sometimes a sterile inoculating loop

point-of-care testing (POCT) laboratory testing performed at the location where the patient is receiving his or her health care (usually the medical office) using small, rapid instruments and methods; these tests are Clinical Laboratory Improvement Amendments (CLIA)-waived

polymerase chain reaction (PCR) laboratory test to identify DNA presence of a pathogen

prothrombin time (PT) blood test to determine abnormal clotting or to monitor anticoagulation medication

qualitative analysis the identification of a type of pathogen by its appearance in the specimen

quantitative analysis the method used to determine the number of bacteria present in a specimen

reagent a substance that, when added to a solution of another substance, participates in a chemical reaction; it may be used to identify or to quantify the presence of another substance

sensitivity testing to determine a pathogen's susceptibility to specific antibiotics

serum liquid portion of the blood that remains after clotting factors are removed

universal donor a person who has O-negative blood, which is theoretically able to be transfused into a person with another blood type in an emergency situation

urinalysis the physical, chemical, and microscopic analysis of urine

urinometer a sealed glass float placed in approximately 15 mL of urine and that measures specific gravity

REVIEW QUESTIONS

All questions are relevant for all medical assisting certification exams.

1. The process of removing tissue from a patient for microscopic examination is called:
   A. cytology.
   B. microbiology.
   C. biopsy.
   D. histology.

Answer: **C**
Why: The process of removing tissue from the body for examination is called a biopsy. Cytology and histology are both a process of analysis or examination of cells. Microbiology is the study of all microscopic organisms.
Review: Yes ◯   No ◯

2. The following blood collection tubes contain an anticoagulant EXCEPT:
   A. blue.
   B. lavender.
   C. gray.
   D. green.
   E. red.

Answer: **E**
Why: A red-stoppered collection tube is used to collect serum for chemistry and serology tests. The tube does not contain any additive, enabling the blood to form a clot and the serum to be separated from the clot or clotted cells.
Review: Yes ◯   No ◯

3. A urine specimen that is collected at any time of the day is referred to as:
   A. clean catch.
   B. random.
   C. 24-hour.
   D. postprandial.

Answer: **B**
Why: Random means at any time. Clean catch is a method of collection of urine in which the patient cleans the area of the urinary meatus and collects the urine in midstream. A 24-hour urine is a collection of all urine in a 24-hour period. Postprandial means after a meal.
Review: Yes ◯   No ◯

4. The clear liquid portion of blood that composes 55% of whole blood is:
   A. serum.
   B. plasma.
   C. hemoglobin.
   D. fibrinogen.
   E. thrombin.

Answer: **B**
Why: Serum is the fluid portion of blood that remains after coagulation. It contains no fibrinogen, a plasma protein essential to the blood clotting process. Hemoglobin is a protein–iron compound found in the blood; it carries oxygen to the cells from the lungs and carries carbon dioxide away from the cells to the lungs. Fibrinogen, a globulin, and thrombin, an enzyme, are products found in the blood that are required for proper clotting.
Review: Yes ◯   No ◯

5. Appropriate locations for collecting capillary blood include the following EXCEPT:
   A. fingertip.
   B. earlobe.
   C. antecubital space.
   D. heel.

Answer: **C**
Why: The antecubital space, in the inner surface of the bend of the elbow, is where the veins are located that are used for phlebotomy. Capillary punctures are not performed here.
Review: Yes ◯   No ◯

6. When multiple tubes of blood are to be drawn, which is drawn first?
   A. Tubes with anticoagulant additive
   B. Blood culture tubes
   C. Tubes with no additive
   D. Tubes containing heparin
   E. Tubes containing sodium citrate

Answer: **B**
Why: Any time a sterile specimen is required, such as blood cultures, special care is taken not to contaminate the specimen—therefore, these specimens are drawn first. After that, tubes containing no additive are drawn and then tubes with additive. This order of draw prevents contamination of tubes with the additives.
Review: Yes ○   No ○

---

7. The specimen used to perform a culture test for the presence of tuberculosis is:
   A. sputum.
   B. capillary blood.
   C. venous blood.
   D. swab from throat.

Answer: **A**
Why: Tuberculosis typically infects the lungs. Sputum is the material coughed up from the lungs. A culture of this material will grow the acid–fast bacillus *Mycobacterium tuberculosis*.
Review: Yes ○   No ○

---

8. A blood test used to indicate the level of kidney function is:
   A. sedimentation rate.
   B. complete blood count.
   C. blood urea nitrogen.
   D. human chorionic gonadotropin.
   E. hematocrit.

Answer: **C**
Why: Blood urea nitrogen (BUN) is a measurement of the amount of nitrogenous substance present in the blood as urea. Urea is a major end product of protein and amino acid metabolism. The kidneys are responsible for excreting this product. If the levels are elevated, it may indicate kidney failure. A sedimentation rate is used to monitor the course of inflammation in rheumatoid arthritis. A complete blood count (CBC) will provide information about the formed white and red cells in the body, both quantity and quality. Human chorionic gonadotropin is a hormone present in blood or urine during pregnancy. This test is used to determine pregnancy. A hematocrit is a blood test that determines the percentage of packed cells in a volume of blood.
Review: Yes ○   No ○

---

9. The solution used to identify fungal infections is:
   A. 0.9% sodium chloride.
   B. sodium citrate.
   C. PSA.
   D. KOH.

Answer: **D**
Why: Potassium hydroxide (KOH) is mixed with skin scrapings, and the mixture is placed on a microscope slide for analysis. Sodium chloride 0.9% is the solution used for a wet mount. Sodium citrate is an additive in a blue-top evacuated tube used for coagulation studies. PSA is an abbreviation for prostate-specific antigen, which is used in the detection of cancer of the prostate.
Review: Yes ○   No ○

---

10. A urine test that compares the weight of urine with that of distilled water is:
   A. sedimentation rate.
   B. clarity.
   C. specific gravity.
   D. pH.
   E. ketone analysis.

Answer: **C**
Why: Distilled water is used as a measure of density against other liquids such as urine. Distilled water with a specific gravity of 1.000 is compared with urine, which has particles dissolved in it. The normal specific gravity of urine is 1.005 to 1.030.
Review: Yes ○   No ○

11. Which of the following is proper technique when performing venipuncture?
    A. The bevel of the needle is face up, and the insertion angle is 15° to 30°.
    B. The bevel of the needle is face down, and the insertion angle is 30°.
    C. The bevel of the needle is face up, and the insertion angle is 45° to 60°.
    D. The placement of the bevel is not critical, but the insertion angle should be at least 45°.

Answer: **A**
Why: The bevel of the needle should always be face up when performing venipuncture. If it is face down during insertion, the bevel may lodge against the back wall of the vein and no blood would be obtained. Insertion should be at a slight angle, no greater than 30°.
Review: Yes ◯ No ◯

12. Proper sites for a capillary puncture include the following EXCEPT the:
    A. tip of ring finger.
    B. heel of infant.
    C. tip of index finger.
    D. earlobe.
    E. tip of middle finger.

Answer: **C**
Why: The index finger tends to be more calloused and may not provide proper blood flow from a lancet puncture.
Review: Yes ◯ No ◯

13. The normal range of urine pH is:
    A. 3.0 to 5.0
    B. 5.0 to 8.0
    C. 5.0 to 10.0
    D. 8.0 to 10.0

Answer: **B**
Why: On the pH scale, 7.0 represents a neutral reading. Readings lower than 7.0 are acidic and higher than 7.0 are basic. The normal range of urine is from slightly acid to slightly basic.
Review: Yes ◯ No ◯

14. Which of the following is a normal adult WBC count?
    A. 1,000 cells/mm^3
    B. 7,000 cells/mm^3
    C. 20,000 cells/mm^3
    D. 50,000 cells/mm^3

Answer: **B**
Why: The normal range for a white blood cell count is 4.5 to 11.0 × 10^3 cells/mm^3. This means there are 4,500 to 11,000 white blood cells in a cubic millimeter. A white blood cell count range is also reported as 4.5 to 11.0 × 10^3 cells/µL.
Review: Yes ◯ No ◯

15. A urine pregnancy test measures:
    A. RPR.
    B. VDRL.
    C. HCG.
    D. HDL.

Answer: **C**
Why: HCG is the human chorionic gonadotropin hormone present in blood and urine during pregnancy.
Review: Yes ◯ No ◯

16. Which of the following is an incorrect technique to use when performing phlebotomy?
    A. Check the expiration dates printed on vacuum collection tubes to make sure they are not expired.
    B. Put on sterile gloves to ensure use of universal standard precautions.
    C. Apply the tourniquet snugly, but not too tightly.
    D. After the puncture site is determined and cleansed, do not touch the site.
    E. Release the tourniquet before removing the needle from the patient's vein.

Answer: **B**
Why: It is not required that you wear sterile gloves for routine venipuncture; however, clean gloves must be used with each patient.
Review: Yes ◯ No ◯

17. The color of the stopper of the vacuum collection tube used to collect plasma for coagulation studies is:
    A. yellow.
    B. red.
    C. red and black.
    D. blue

Answer: **D**
Why: The yellow-, red-, and red-and-black-top tubes do not contain any anticoagulant additive. Blood collected in these tubes will clot and cannot be used for clotting or coagulation blood tests.
Review: Yes ○   No ○

---

18. The term used to describe cloudy urine is:
    A. pale.
    B. straw.
    C. transparent.
    D. amber.
    E. turbid.

Answer: **E**
Why: Pale, straw, and amber are used to describe the color of urine; transparent is the term to describe clear urine. Turbid or cloudy urine indicates the presence of some particles in the urine, such as chemicals, blood cells, bacteria, or mucus.
Review: Yes ○   No ○

---

19. Which department of the laboratory performs hemoglobin and hematocrit tests?
    A. Cytology
    B. Bacteriology
    C. Immunology
    D. Hematology

Answer: **D**
Why: Cytology is the department that analyzes cells to determine abnormalities. Immunology is the study of immunity and antibodies/antigens. Bacteriology is the study of bacteria, culture, and sensitivity. Hematology includes the study of the blood for any abnormalities of the blood-forming tissue and the quality of the blood cells.
Review: Yes ○   No ○

---

20. Which of the following is part of proper capillary blood collection technique?
    A. Use the index finger as the preferred site for capillary puncture.
    B. Squeeze the tip of the finger for at least 30 seconds before a puncture of the skin.
    C. Scrape the tip of the collection tube over the tip of the finger to get every drop of blood in the tube.
    D. After performing the skin puncture, use the first drop of blood that comes to the surface of the skin.
    E. When collecting blood, avoid air bubbles in the microhematocrit collection tube.

Answer: **E**
Why: When using a microhematocrit collection tube, the test will be inaccurate if there are air pockets in the tube. Proper technique requires that the index finger not be used but that the ring or middle finger be used instead. You should not scrape the skin during the collection process, because this encourages platelet activation, which can cause the blood to clot and alter the test results. To encourage blood flow, make sure the site chosen is warm. Gently massage from the base to the top of the site but do not squeeze the finger. Squeezing or milking the site will dilute the specimen with tissue fluid. Always wipe away the first drop of blood before starting to collect the specimen. The first drop of blood contains a higher concentration of tissue fluid, which may alter the test results.
Review: Yes ○   No ○

---

21. A hematocrit reading of 40 means that:
    A. 40% of the total blood volume consists of RBCs.
    B. 60% of the total blood volume consists of RBCs.
    C. 40% of the total blood volume is plasma.
    D. 60% of the total blood volume is WBCs.

Answer: **A**
Why: A hematocrit is the percentage of red blood cells contained in whole blood. A reading of 40 means that of 100% total blood volume, 40% is red blood cells, and 60% is plasma, WBCs, and platelets.
Review: Yes ○   No ○

22. When whole blood is allowed to clot, the clear portion visible after centrifugation is the:

A. plasma.
B. buffy coat.
C. serum.
D. hemoglobin.
E. fibrinogen.

Answer: **C**

Why: Serum is the clear liquid portion of the blood that contains no blood cells, platelets, or fibrinogen. Plasma is the clear portion of blood that still contains clotting agents. The buffy coat is the light grayish liquid portion of blood containing WBCs; it composes 1% of whole blood and is the middle layer in the specimen tube. Hemoglobin is the oxygen-carrying portion of RBCs. The platelets and fibrinogen are clotting agents that form the clot.

Review: Yes ○   No ○

23. Which of the following would be considered a normal finding for urine?

A. Protein—positive, 4+
B. Clarity—cloudy
C. Color—straw
D. Specific gravity—1.055

Answer: **C**

Why: The color of normal urine is yellow and is typically described as straw-colored. The protein content in urine should be negative. A positive reading could indicate a kidney disorder. The clarity or characteristic of urine should be clear, not cloudy or turbid. The specific gravity of urine is 1.003 to 1.035. The higher the reading, the more dense the urine is because of dissolved particles in the urine. These could be blood cells, chemicals, or bacteria.

Review: Yes ○   No ○

24. Parasitology includes the study of:

A. worms.
B. fungi.
C. cells.
D. bacteria.
E. antibodies.

Answer: **A**

Why: Parasitology is the study of human parasites (worms and scabies) and ova (eggs).

Review: Yes ○   No ○

25. Which of the following represents an error in performing venipuncture?

A. Using the proper size needle to avoid hemolysis of the specimen
B. Vigorously shaking the anticoagulated blood specimens to completely mix the anticoagulant with the blood
C. Labeling the tube with the date, time of draw, patient's name, and your initials
D. Allowing the venipuncture site to completely dry before insertion of the needle

Answer: **B**

Why: If a blood specimen is vigorously shaken, the blood cells will rupture (hemolyze) and release hemoglobin into the plasma. This can result in erroneous readings. Blood drawn in anticoagulant tubes should be well mixed by gently tilting the tube back and forth several times.

Review: Yes ○   No ○

CRITICAL THINKING CASE REVIEW QUESTIONS

Dr. Celaya ordered preoperative lab work for his cholecystectomy patient, Ms. Jarvis.

1. Her hemoglobin is 15.0 g/dL and her hematocrit is 44% which is:
   A. normal.
   B. slightly below normal.
   C. slightly above normal.
   D. above normal and concerning.
   E. below normal and concerning.

   Answer: **A**
   Why: The normal female hemoglobin range is 11.7 to 16.0 g/dL; the normal female hematocrit range is 35% to 45%. Her numbers fall within the normal range.
   Review: Yes ◯   No ◯

2. Dr. Celaya also ordered electrolytes. The normal potassium range should be:
   A. 2% to 6%
   B. 2.0 to 6.0 mEq/L
   C. 32% to 45%
   D. 3.5 to 5.0 mEq/L

   Answer: **D**
   Why: The normal potassium range is the same for males and females at 3.5 to 5.0 mEq/L.
   Review: Yes ◯   No ◯

3. The patient's WBC is 15×10^3 cells/μL which is:
   A. normal.
   B. slightly below normal.
   C. slightly above normal.
   D. above normal and concerning.
   E. below normal and concerning.

   Answer: **D**
   Why: The normal white blood count (WBC) range is 4.5 to 11.0×10^3 cells/μL; 15.5×10^3 cells/μL is above normal and concerning, since it most likely indicates an infection.
   Review: Yes ◯   No ◯

4. Ms. Jarvis also had a urine analysis done. Since she was scheduled for a cholecystectomy for gallbladder problems, it would not be a surprise if _____ was detected in her urine:
   A. glucose
   B. bilirubin
   C. nitrites
   D. blood

   Answer: **B**
   Why: Bilirubin in the urine may indicate liver damage or the flow of bile from the gallbladder is blocked. Since Ms. Jarvis is having gallbladder problems, if the bile flow was blocked, bilirubin would most likely appear in her urine.
   Review: Yes ◯   No ◯

5. The urine test could be conducted in the medical office by the medical assistant, since it is:
   A. approved by the FDA.
   B. sanctioned by the CDC.
   C. CLIA-waived.
   D. performed by dipstick.
   E. not a sterile procedure.

   Answer: **C**
   Why: A and D are also correct, but C is the best answer. All laboratory tests performed in the medical office must be CLIA-waived even if they are approved by the FDA. The dipstick urine is a CLIA-waived test.
   Review: Yes ◯   No ◯

CHAPTER

22

Physical Modalities

Review Tip:

Your medical practice may not provide services for physical modalities or fitting of ambulation devices; however, it is important that the medical assistant recognize improper fitting and use when patients present with crutches, walkers, or canes. Information may be obtained from durable medical equipment vendors or retailers.

Physical modalities are noninvasive therapeutic agents, procedures, and preventive measures used in:

- Physical medicine (physiatry)—diagnosis and treatment of disease and disability using physical means, such as diathermy
- Rehabilitative medicine—restores and improves function impaired by disease or injury
- Sports medicine—prevents and treats injuries and impairments that are sports-related
- Preventive health—applies techniques and uses devices to prevent injury and impairment (e.g., body mechanics)

MOBILITY TESTING

- Goniometry—measurement of degrees of joint motion using a goniometer
- Range-of-motion (ROM) test—exam requiring the patient to perform various joint motions to

determine the extent of movement; may be active or passive

- Strength tests—exams requiring the patient to perform select muscle or muscle group actions to determine the strength of function
- Gait tests—exams observing and evaluating the person's way of walking
- Posture tests—exams assessing the patient's posture related to the spinal curve, symmetry of shoulders, hips, and knees
- Activities-of-daily-living (ADL) tests—exams that determine the patient's ability to perform common tasks (e.g., opening doors, brushing hair)

THERAPIES

THERMOTHERAPY

Thermotherapy uses heat to reduce swelling and to decrease pain by dilating blood vessels (vasodilation), increasing circulation to the affected area; it is not used in the initial phase of injury treatment.

- Dry heat—heat without moisture
  - Heating pads—electrically or microwave-heated packs for thermotherapy use; should always be covered with fabric before placing on skin; check cords for safety and frequently monitor temperature to avoid burns
  - Chemical hot packs—heating pads filled with a chemical compound that produces heat when activated (usually by applying pressure); follow same precautions as for heating pads
  - Infrared—heat produced by wavelengths in various lamp-like structures; position a safe distance from skin and monitor frequently to avoid burns
  - Ultraviolet—sunlamps used to treat specific conditions (e.g., psoriasis, newborn jaundice); patient's eyes should be covered and length of exposure timed and monitored to avoid burns
- Moist heat—heat with moisture sources
  - Hot soaks—water or water with antiseptic or other solution is warmed between 100°F and 105°F; affected area requiring treatment is submerged for a specific period
  - Hot compresses—fabric is wet with water or antiseptic or other solutions and placed on affected area; plastic-type wrap may be used to cover compress and conserve heat
- Paraffin—hand or foot is immersed in melted wax with additive such as mineral oil; plastic bags or "mittens" are worn after wax is applied to retain heat;

when cool, the wax is peeled off; used for relief of arthritis pain

- Diathermy—deep heat therapy using a mechanical energy source
  - Ultrasound—heat therapy using high-frequency sound waves; a special gel substance is placed on the head of the ultrasound attachment to improve conductivity
  - Microwave—heat therapy using electromagnetic radiation for tissues; should not be used with moisture or on patients with pacemakers

CRYOTHERAPY

Cryotherapy uses cold to prevent or minimize swelling and to reduce pain by causing blood vessels to constrict (vasoconstriction); it is used in the initial treatment of an injury.

- Dry cold—cold therapy without moisture
  - Ice pack—waterproof bag filled with ice; air should be removed and bag covered with fabric before placing on skin; monitor to prevent skin damage
  - Chemical ice bag—pack filled with a chemical compound that produces cold when activated (usually by applying pressure); follow same precautions as with ice pack
- Moist cold—cold therapy using moisture
  - Cold soaks—water or water with antiseptic or other solution is cooled with ice and affected area is submerged for a given period
  - Cold compresses—fabric is wet with cold water or antiseptic or other solution and placed on affected area

HYDROTHERAPY

Hydrotherapy uses hot- or cold-water regimens for therapy; not used in the initial treatment of an injury.

- Whirlpool—a bath or other container in which water is continually circulated to provide massage and heat therapy
- Hot to cold (alternating)—the affected area is alternately plunged between hot and cold baths or packs to contract and dilate vessels

EXERCISES

Exercise is an action to strengthen, develop, or maintain muscle.

- Active exercise—an action to strengthen, develop, or maintain muscle that is performed directly by the patient
  - Isometric exercises—exercises that contract opposing muscles without the muscles shortening

Flexion/extension

Pronation/supination

Abduction/adduction

Circumduction

Dorsiflexion/plantar flexion

Eversion/Inversion

Rotation

FIGURE 22-1 Range of motion of selected joints.

- Resistance exercise—exercises performed with counter pressure applied to increase the effectiveness and determine improvement
- Water exercises—exercises performed in water
- ■ Passive exercise—exercises performed on the patient by another person or by a mechanical device
  - Electrical stimulation—electrical device used to stimulate muscles or nerves
  - Passive motion device—a mechanical apparatus placed on a patient to passively exercise the affected area; frequently used on knees after surgery; speed and flexion may be increased or decreased according to the patient's pain tolerance
  - Massage—rubbing, stroking, kneading, and tapping tissue with hands or devices to alleviate pain and improve function

RANGE OF MOTION AS A THERAPY

A method of testing joints, **ROM** can also be a therapy using passive or active exercises; the patient or caregiver performs standard joint motions (Fig. 22-1) to maintain or improve the extent of movement.

OTHER COMMON PHYSICAL THERAPIES

- ■ Manipulation—maneuvers to realign affected area; frequently used on joint dislocations or spinal injuries
- ■ Immobilization—prevention of movement, usually of joint or bone, through the use of splints, casts, and other devices to reduce pain and allow healing to

occur; do not confuse "immobilization" with "mobilization," which is movement

- Traction—application of a slow pulling force; commonly used to realign fractured bones

COMMON ASSISTIVE DEVICES

- Cane—a rod-type device used for minimal standing or walking support as a result of weakness on one side or balance problems; the handle may be candy cane–shaped or straight and perpendicular to the rod
  - Types—single-pronged, tripod, or four-pronged (quad); the length may be adjustable or nonadjustable
  - Fit—the patient's elbow should be at a 30-degree angle when standing to obtain proper cane length
  - Gait—cane is held on patient's strongest side, tip 4 to 6 inches lateral to the foot, tip flat on the ground; cane moves forward approximately 12 inches followed by the affected limb, which stops at the cane; the stronger limb moves forward to the cane, and steps are repeated
  - Caution—stronger limb is first going up stairs, weaker limb first going down

- Crutches—assistive walking devices, used singly or as a pair, which transfer weight bearing to upper extremities
  - Common types—standard or axillary crutches usually used for temporary conditions; Lofstrand or forearm crutches usually used for long-term disability
  - Fit—measure with the shoes the patient will be wearing; patient standing; normally crutch tips are placed 4 to 6 inches lateral to each foot and 2 inches in front of feet; allow two- to three-finger widths between the axilla and the axillary support on crutches; adjust crutch height to accommodate; adjust handgrips to 30 degree of elbow flexion
  - Common crutch gaits (Fig. 22-2)—crutches placed on ground 4 to 6 inches lateral and 2 inches in front of feet; this is referred to as the tripod
    - Swing-to gait—bilateral weight bearing required; patient moves both crutches forward simultaneously, plants them, and lifts body to crutches; repeat steps
    - Swing-through gait—bilateral weight bearing required; patient moves both crutches forward simultaneously, plants them, and lifts body past crutches; repeat steps
    - Two-point gait—bilateral weight bearing required; the patient moves one crutch forward and the opposite foot at the same time, followed by the other crutch and other foot; repeat steps
    - Three-point gait (most commonly taught in medical office)—for weight bearing on one leg; patient moves both crutches and affected leg forward simultaneously and follows with unaffected leg; repeat steps
    - Four-point gait—bilateral weight bearing required; the patient moves right crutch forward, followed by the left crutch, and then the left leg forward parallel to the left crutch, followed by the right leg forward parallel to the right crutch; repeat steps
  - Caution—shoes should be flat and nonskid; avoid throw rugs, wet areas, and other hazards; to avoid axilla nerve damage, support weight using handgrips, not crutch underarm pads

- Gait or transfer belt—a wide-woven belt used to assist in lifting or steadying the patient during ambulation or transfer (e.g., car or wheelchair)
  - Placement—buckled over patient's clothes around waist at midabdominal area; allow room for two fingers to fit between the waist and the belt
  - Caution—the belt should not be used if patient has no use of lower extremities; check for abdominal, back, or rib conditions and ostomy or feeding devices

- Walker—waist-high assistive walking device with four legs, used when a cane is not enough support; may be folded when not in use
  - Types—standard (fixed) with rubber-tipped legs; or can roll on wheels
  - Fit—client's elbows flexed at 30-degree angle; hand rests should be approximately at top of patient's femur
  - Gait—patient steps into the walker and grasps handgrips, moves walker forward 6 to 12 inches then moves one foot at a time back into walker; repeat steps
  - Caution—walkers should not be used on stairs or narrow passages

- Wheelchair—a mobile chair with adjustable or nonadjustable footrests and brakes, used when a patient cannot ambulate
  - Types—nonmechanical or mechanical, standard size or custom-fitted to patient
  - Caution—always lock brakes when patient is getting into or out of chair; do not allow patient to place arms around your neck

ERGONOMICS

The Merriam Webster dictionary defines ergonomics as *a science that deals with designing and arranging things so that people can use them easily and safely.* The intent is to:

- Reduce work-related musculoskeletal injuries
- Lessen muscle fatigue
- Increase productivity

2-POINT GAIT	3-POINT GAIT	4-POINT GAIT	SWING THROUGH/ TRIPOD
Partial weight bearing both feet Provides less support Faster than a 4-point gait	Non-weight bearing (left foot) Requires good balance Requires arm strength Faster gait Can use with walker	Partial weight bearing both feet Maximal support provided Requires constant shift of weight	Weight bearing both feet (or one foot) Requires arm strength Requires coordination/ balance Most advanced gait

FIGURE 22-2 Crutch-walking gaits.

It is estimated that 50% of ergonomic-related injuries are due to **repetitive movement injuries**, tissue damage, usually to the tendons or bursae, caused by frequent repetition of the same motion. Carpal tunnel is an example. These injuries are common in sports but also common and growing in the workplace and home related to computer and other electronic device practices. The design of the screen, the chair, and accessories may be evaluated for maximum fit to the individual employee. Table 22-1 is a posture guide and checklist for employers and employees.

TABLE 22-1 ▶ **Modified OSHA checklist for working postures at the computer**

The workstation should allow:	Y	N
1. **Head** and **neck** to be upright, or in line with the torso (not bent down/back)		
2. **Head**, **neck**, and **trunk** to face forward (not twisted)		
3. **Trunk** to be perpendicular to floor (may lean back into backrest but not forward)		
4. **Shoulders** and **upper arms** to be in line with the torso, generally about perpendicular to the floor and relaxed (not elevated or stretched forward)		
5. **Upper arms** and **elbows** to be close to the body (not extended outward)		
6. **Forearms**, **wrists**, and **hands** to be straight and in line (forearm at about 90 degrees to the upper arm)		
7. **Wrists** and **hands** to be straight (not bent up/down or sideways toward the little finger)		
8. **Thighs** to be parallel to the floor and the **lower legs** to be perpendicular to floor (thighs may be slightly elevated above knees)		
9. **Feet** rest flat on the floor or are supported by a stable footrest.		

www.osha.gov/SLTC/etools/computerworkstations/checklist

BODY MECHANICS

One aspect of ergonomics is **body mechanics** defined as the efficient use of the body to prevent injury to the health-care provider or patient. The general guidelines are:

- Keep the back straight
- Keep abdominal muscles tight
- Bend from knees, not back
- Maintain a broad base with one foot slightly forward
- Use the feet, not the body, to pivot
- Carry heavy objects close to your body
- Synchronize lifting, such as "on three—one, two, three"
- Know your limits

TERMS

PHYSICAL MODALITIES REVIEW

The following list reviews the terms discussed in this chapter and other important terms you may see on the exam.

activities of daily living (ADL) common acts performed during a person's normal day

body mechanics the efficient use of the body to prevent injury to the health-care provider or patient

cryotherapy (cold) causes blood vessels to constrict, preventing or minimizing swelling and reducing pain; used in the initial treatment of an injury

diathermy deep heat therapy using a mechanical energy source

ergonomics adaptation of the environment and use of techniques and equipment to prevent injury

gait person's way of walking

hydrotherapy hot- or cold-water regimens used for therapy

isometric exercise a type of exercise that contracts opposing muscles without the muscles shortening

passive exercise exercises performed on the patient by another person or a mechanical device

physical medicine (physiatry) deals with the diagnosis and treatment of disease and disability using physical means, such as diathermy

range of motion (ROM) passive or active; the patient or caregiver exercises joints by performing standard joint motions (e.g., flexion and rotation) to maintain or improve the movement

rehabilitative medicine deals with restoring or improving function impaired by disease or injury

repetitive movement injuries tissue damage, usually to the tendons or bursae, caused by frequent repetition of the same motion

resistance exercise exercises performed with counter pressure applied to increase the effectiveness and to determine improvement

thermotherapy (heat) reduces swelling and decreases pain by improving circulation; it is not used in acute phase of injury

ultrasound heat therapy using high-frequency sound waves; a special gel substance is placed on the head of the ultrasound attachment to improve conductivity

ultraviolet heat lamps to treat specific conditions (e.g., psoriasis, newborn jaundice)

whirlpool bath or other container in which water is continually circulated to provide massage and heat therapy

REVIEW QUESTIONS

All questions are relevant for all medical assisting and medical administrative certification exams.

1. Heat applied to a large part of the body will cause:
   A. vasoconstriction.
   B. vasodilation.
   C. decreased blood flow to the body part.
   D. increased blood pressure to the area.

   Answer: **B**
   Why: Cold application causes the blood vessels to constrict, or become smaller, thus increasing blood pressure in the area and decreasing blood flow to the body part or area. Heat application has the opposite effect on the area.
   Review: ◯ Yes   ◯ No

2. Infrared therapy uses heat produced by:
   A. electricity.
   B. water.
   C. chemicals.
   D. sound waves.
   E. wavelengths.

   Answer: **E**
   Why: Infrared therapy is treatment by exposure to various wavelengths of infrared radiation. Infrared treatment relieves pain and stimulates circulation of blood.
   Review: ◯ Yes   ◯ No

3. Cryotherapy is a form of treatment that uses:
   A. sound waves and microwaves.
   B. ice packs and cold packs.
   C. paraffin wax.
   D. hot compresses and hot water.

   Answer: **B**
   Why: The root *cryo* refers to the use of cold or freezing. Cryotherapy is a form of treatment that utilizes different forms of cold such as chemical ice bags, cold soaks, and ice packs.
   Review: ◯ Yes   ◯ No

4. Which of the following is necessary to do when measuring crutches so they fit properly?
   A. The patient should be fitted without shoes on, barefooted.
   B. With the patient standing normally, the crutch tips should be touching the sides of the shoes.
   C. There should be a gap of two- to three-finger widths between the underarm and the top of the crutch.
   D. When the hands are resting on the handgrips, the elbows should be straight, not flexed.
   E. The handgrips on the crutches should be at the same height as the patient's waist.

   Answer: **C**
   Why: There should be some space between the underarm and the top of the crutch to make sure the patient's underarms do not rest on the crutch. Two- to three-finger widths or approximately 2 inches is adequate. The patient should have shoes on, and the crutch tips should be placed at least 4 to 6 inches from the shoes. The elbows should be flexed slightly when the hands are on the handgrips. The handgrips are positioned slightly above the hip but not at the waist.
   Review: ◯ Yes   ◯ No

5. A device used to measure the extent of joint movement is a(n):
   A. diathermy machine.
   B. passive motion machine.
   C. electrical stimulation device.
   D. goniometer.

   Answer: **D**
   Why: A goniometer is used to perform goniometry, the measurement of degrees of joint movement. Diathermy is the use of shortwaves to heat the body tissues. A passive motion machine is a device that moves a body part without the patient assisting. Electrical stimulation is the use of intermittent electrical stimuli to cause muscles to contract.
   Review: ◯ Yes   ◯ No

6. The realignment of a dislocated finger is an example of which kind of therapy?
   A. Immobilization
   B. Manipulation
   C. Traction
   D. Resistance exercise
   E. Passive exercise

Answer: **B**
Why: Manipulation is the use of the hands in therapy to reduce a dislocation or move a body part into alignment. Immobilization of a body part does not allow movement. An example is placing a splint or cast on the body part. Traction is a method of applying force on a body part to pull or stretch the body part. Resistance exercise is the act of exercising while applying opposite force—for example, using weights while exercising. Passive exercise requires another person to perform the movement for the patient. The patient does not move the body part.
Review: Yes ○ No ○

7. When the tips of both crutches and one leg are advancing at the same time, it is referred to as a:
   A. three-point gait.
   B. two-point gait.
   C. swing-to gait.
   D. swing-through gait.

Answer: **A**
Why: A three-point gait refers to two crutch tips and one foot touching the ground at the same time.
Review: Yes ○ No ○

8. The type of exercise used when the patient is unable to move the affected body part without help is:
   A. range of motion.
   B. active exercise.
   C. isometric exercise.
   D. resistant exercise.
   E. passive exercise.

Answer: **E**
Why: In passive exercise, someone or something moves the body part without patient assistance. Passive exercise is frequently used after surgery to increase flexion and extension in joints.
Review: Yes ○ No ○

9. Kneading and tapping tissue with the hands is a form of:
   A. manipulation.
   B. traction.
   C. range of motion.
   D. massage.

Answer: **D**
Why: Massage is a type of passive treatment used to alleviate pain and improve function of body parts. Massage includes rubbing, stroking, kneading, and tapping tissue with the hands or with devices.
Review: Yes ○ No ○

10. When instructing a patient on the use of a cane, you should tell him or her to:
   A. use the cane only when using stairs.
   B. use the cane on his or her weaker side.
   C. go up steps with the stronger limb first.
   D. go down steps with the cane first.
   E. adjust the cane low enough so that the arm is straight when walking.

Answer: **C**
Why: Proper technique when using a cane includes using the cane on the stronger side. The cane will provide support on the strong side when moving the weak side. The patient then has a smoother gait and does not have the tendency to limp. When going up steps, the stronger side goes first; going down steps, the weaker limb goes first. When using the cane, the arm is slightly bent.
Review: Yes ○ No ○

11. Good body mechanics include the following guidelines except:
    A. when lifting, maintain a narrow base with feet together.
    B. carry heavy objects close to your body.
    C. bend from the knees, not the back.
    D. use feet to pivot, not the body.

Answer: **A**
Why: When lifting, the feet should be slightly apart with one foot forward. This provides a broad base to support the weight of the load.
Review: Yes ◯ No ◯

12. The area of medicine that deals with restoring or improving function impaired by disease is:
    A. preventive health.
    B. ergonomics.
    C. rehabilitative medicine.
    D. thermotherapy.
    E. disability management.

Answer: **C**
Why: Rehabilitative medicine deals with restoration of an individual or a part of the body to normal or near-normal function after a disabling disease or injury.
Review: ◯ Yes   ◯ No

13. Cold therapy is frequently applied to:
    A. increase blood flow to the affected part.
    B. promote healing by increasing circulation.
    C. increase nerve sensitivity.
    D. decrease swelling.

Answer: **D**
Why: Cold has the effect of decreasing pain by numbing the nerve pathways. Cold therapy decreases circulation (blood flow), thus decreasing swelling.
Review: ◯ Yes   ◯ No

14. The use of a whirlpool is an example of:
    A. diathermy.
    B. cryotherapy.
    C. hydrotherapy.
    D. thermotherapy.
    E. ultrasound therapy.

Answer: **C**
Why: The root word *hydro* means "water." A whirlpool is a tank in which warm water is circulated to provide massage and heat therapy.
Review: ◯ Yes   ◯ No

15. An example of a deep heating agent is:
    A. diathermy.
    B. hydrocollator pack.
    C. infrared lamp.
    D. paraffin bath.

Answer: **A**
Why: Deep heating agents produce heat through energy that will penetrate the tissues as deep as 30 to 50 mm. Superficial heating agents affect tissues approximately 10 mm beneath the skin's surface. Hydrocollator packs (hot packs), infrared lamps, and paraffin baths are all considered superficial heating agents.
Review: ◯ Yes   ◯ No

16. To evaluate the extent of movement of a patient's knee, the following exam would be performed:
    A. isometric exercise.
    B. range of motion.
    C. manipulation.
    D. gait evaluation.
    E. body mechanics.

Answer: **B**
Why: Range-of-motion testing is performed to determine the extent of movement of various joints. The patient is evaluated to see how many degrees of flexion and extension the joint will perform. Isometric exercises are exercises that contract opposing muscles without the muscles shortening. Manipulation involves maneuvers to realign affected areas such as joint dislocations or spinal injuries. Gait evaluation is the evaluation of the manner of walking. Body mechanics is defined as the efficient use of the body to prevent injury.
Review: ◯ Yes   ◯ No

17. The preferred method used in the initial treatment of an injury is:

A. hot compresses.
B. paraffin.
C. hydrotherapy.
D. ice pack.
E. ultrasound.

Answer: **D**

Why: Cold therapy is initially used after an injury to prevent swelling and reduce pain. There is decreased blood flow to the affected part, limiting the initial edema in the area.
Review: ○ Yes   ○ No

18. The type of gait in which the patient advances the left foot and right crutch and then the right foot and left crutch is a:

A. swing-through gait.
B. two-point gait.
C. three-point gait.
D. four-point gait.

Answer: **B**

Why: A two-point gait means there are two "points" on the ground at the same time. One crutch and the opposite foot are on the ground at the same time, followed by the other crutch and foot. This is used for a patient who is partially weight-bearing and can place some weight on both sides of his or her body.
Review: ○ Yes   ○ No

19. Exercises performed by the patient without assistance are:

A. active exercises.
B. passive exercises.
C. range-of-motion exercises.
D. water exercises.

Answer: **A**

Why: Active exercise refers to those movements the patient is able to perform without assistance. Passive exercise requires another person to move the body part. Range-of-motion and water exercises both can be performed passively.
Review: ○ Yes   ○ No

20. The common acts performed during a person's normal day are referred to as:

A. body mechanics.
B. activities of daily living.
C. ergonomics.
D. isometric exercises.
E. passive exercises.

Answer: **B**

Why: ADL, activities of daily living, are the common tasks that a person performs each day, such as brushing hair and opening doors. Body mechanics refers to the efficient use of the body while performing activities, and ergonomics is the adaptation of the environment and use of techniques and equipment to prevent injury—for example, equipment designed for better posture when sitting in a desk chair. Isometric and passive exercises are used in rehabilitative therapy.
Review: ○ Yes   ○ No

21. A therapeutic method used to treat jaundice in newborns is:

A. ultrasound.
B. infrared.
C. diathermy.
D. ultraviolet.

Answer: **D**

Why: Ultraviolet is light beyond the range of human vision. It occurs naturally in sunlight and burns or tans the skin. Ultraviolet lamps are also used to treat psoriasis and other skin conditions.
Review: ○ Yes   ○ No

22. Physiatry deals with:

A. prevention and treatment of sports injuries.
B. prevention of injury and impairment.
C. diagnosis and treatment of disease and disability using physical means.
D. restoring and improving function through rehabilitation.
E. diagnosis and treatment of mental disorders.

Answer: **C**

Why: Physiatry, or physical medicine, deals with the diagnosis and treatment of disease and disability using physical means, including such therapies as diathermy.
Review: ○ Yes   ○ No

23. Which of the following therapeutic methods uses melted wax?
    A. Chemical hot packs
    B. Paraffin bath
    C. Diathermy
    D. Cryotherapy

    Answer: **B**
    Why: Paraffin is a type of wax that is melted to create a liquid. The affected body part—usually a hand, a foot, or a joint—is submerged in the wax, or the wax is painted on the body part. The wax hardens, and the heat of the wax penetrates the skin and provides a soothing effect to the painful area. It is frequently used to treat arthritic joint pain and stiffness.
    Review: ○ Yes   ○ No

24. A method of physical therapy used to re-align fractured bones is:
    A. electrical stimulation.
    B. massage.
    C. passive exercise.
    D. infrared heat.
    E. traction.

    Answer: **E**
    Why: Traction is the application of a slow pulling force on a body part and is commonly used to re-align fractured bones.
    Review: ○ Yes   ○ No

25. The purpose of heat therapy includes the following *except*:
    A. relieve muscle spasm.
    B. decrease bleeding or hemorrhage.
    C. relieve pain.
    D. increase blood flow to the body part.

    Answer: **B**
    Why: Heat causes an increase in blood flow to an area of the body, causing muscles to relax, and relieves pain. Cold therapy is indicated for decreasing blood flow and controlling hemorrhage.
    Review: ○ Yes   ○ No

CRITICAL THINKING CASE REVIEW

Bobby is a 15-year-old patient of Dr. Clayton. He is involved in the sport of motor cross. In one of the competitions, he sustained a serious accident and fractured the two bones in his lower right leg.

1. The two bones of the lower leg are the:
   A. ulna and the tibia.
   B. tibia and the radius.
   C. femur and the fibula.
   D. femur and the ulna.
   E. tibia and the fibula.

   Answer: **E**
   Why: The ulna and the radius are the bones located in the forearm, and the femur is the large bone located in the thigh. The tibia and fibula are the bones in the lower leg (refer to Chapter 6).
   Review: ○ Yes   ○ No

2. Emergency Medical Services (EMS) were called to the scene of the accident, and after an assessment they:
   A. mobilized the fracture.
   B. immobilized the fracture.
   C. casted the fracture.
   D. gave Bobby crutches.

   Answer: **B**
   Why: A fracture should not be mobilized (moved about), since it is important to keep it as aligned as possible to avoid further damage and more pain. Casting and providing crutches are not the role of EMS (refer to Chapter 26). The correct procedure would be for EMS to immobilize or stabilize the fracture.
   Review: ○ Yes   ○ No

3. When Bobby was brought to the Emergency Department, _____ was used to attempt to prevent swelling.
   A. thermotherapy
   B. cryotherapy
   C. hydrotherapy
   D. physical therapy
   E. traction

Answer: **B**
Why: Thermotherapy is a form of heat used to reduce swelling after it is established; hydrotherapy uses hot and/or cold water to reduce swelling, but this is commonly done in physical therapy and not in the acute phase of an injury; physical therapy is also not done in the initial phase of an injury. Traction does not prevent swelling. Cryotherapy is correct because it is using cold to prevent or minimize swelling.
Review: ○ Yes   ○ No

4. After Bobby was treated, he was given crutches and taught the following gait:
   A. swing-to gait.
   B. four-point gait.
   C. three-point gait.
   D. two-point gait.

Answer: **C**
Why: A, B, and D gaits require weight bearing on the newly fractured leg which would not be appropriate in the early stages of healing. The three-point gait is the only choice that does not require some weight bearing on the injured leg.
Review: ○ Yes   ○ No

5. After several weeks and after the cast was removed, Bobby was sent for physical therapy which included:
   A. cryotherapy.
   B. hydrotherapy.
   C. traction.
   D. weight lifting.
   E. weight transfer.

Answer: **B**
Why: At this time in bobby's rehabilitation, it is appropriate to use a form of hydrotherapy to either massage the affected area with whirlpool or hot-to-cold plunges to contract and dilate vessels, improving circulation after several weeks of casting.
Review: ○ Yes   ○ No

CHAPTER

23

THAT'S NOT WHAT I MEANT BY A FOOD PYRAMID.

Nutrition

Review Tip:

Increasing emphasis is placed on nutrition in treating disease and maintaining wellness. The certification exams always include questions on therapeutic diets, as well as vitamins and minerals and their functions in the body.

Nutrition is the process of taking food into the body and using it.

STEPS OF NUTRITION

1. Ingestion—taking in of nutrients; eating and drinking
2. Digestion—physical and chemical changing of nutrients in the body to allow absorption
3. Absorption—transferring of digested nutrients from the gastrointestinal system to the blood circulation
4. Metabolism—synthesizing of nutrients from the bloodstream, producing energy

NUTRIENTS

Nutrients are components of food necessary for the body to perform physiologic functions.

ENERGY NUTRIENTS

Energy nutrients are those that produce calories, units of heat that convert into energy when metabolized. Table 23-1 lists calorie distribution for the three energy nutrients.

- Carbohydrates—sugars and starches, the body's primary energy source; they produce 4 calories per gram

- Proteins—nutrients with amino acids (building blocks); develop and heal body tissue; they produce 4 calories per gram
  - Complete—protein nutrient that contains all nine essential amino acids
  - Incomplete—protein nutrient that does not contain all nine essential amino acids

- Fats (lipids)—greasy material in nutrients; transport fat-soluble vitamins, insulate the body from the cold, and provide fatty acids; they produce 9 calories per gram
  - Saturated fats—primarily found in meat, butter, and egg yolks; usually solid at room temperature; increase blood cholesterol
  - Unsaturated fats—primarily found in vegetable and olive oils; usually liquid at room temperature; help decrease blood cholesterol
  - Trans fats (trans-fatty acids, hydrogenated fats)—manufactured fats created by hydrogenation of unsaturated fats; found in commercial baked goods, fried foods, and processed foods; usually solid at room temperature; increase blood cholesterol
  - Cholesterol—found in animal foods and manufactured by the body (Fig. 23-1); not a true fat or lipid but a lipoprotein; necessary for vitamin D and acid bile production
    - High-density lipoprotein, or HDL (good cholesterol)—works to stabilize LDL by transporting select amounts of it to the liver for elimination
    - Low-density lipoprotein, or LDL (bad cholesterol)—waxy material that clogs blood vessels, causing cardiovascular disease
  - Triglycerides—component molecule of fat found in fatty foods; a combination of fatty acids and glycerol; high levels clog blood vessels, causing cardiovascular disease

TABLE 23-1 ▶ Calorie distribution

Nutrient	Calories per Gram
Carbohydrate	4
Protein	4
Fat	9

Cholesterol is produced by your liver

Cholesterol comes from the food you eat (absorbed through the digestive tract)

FIGURE 23-1 Sources of cholesterol.

NONENERGY NUTRIENTS

- Water—a colorless, transparent, odorless, tasteless liquid that is the basis of living organisms and necessary for physiologic functions

- Fiber—nondigestible but edible portion of plants; necessary for the gastrointestinal elimination function

- Vitamins—organic substances found naturally in foods; needed in small amounts for metabolism and prevention of certain diseases (*Note:* The certification exams ask questions about which vitamins are water-soluble and which are fat-soluble.)

  - Vitamin B_1 (thiamin)—water-soluble vitamin primarily found in whole grains and beans necessary for carbohydrate metabolism
  - Vitamin B_2 (riboflavin)—water-soluble vitamin primarily found in animal products and broccoli; necessary for protein metabolism
  - Vitamin B_6—water-soluble vitamin primarily found in brewer's yeast, whole grains, and nuts; aids in regulation of central nervous system
  - Vitamin B_{12} (cyanocobalamin)—water-soluble vitamin primarily found in animal products and soybeans; promotes red blood cell (RBC) formation; a deficiency causes pernicious anemia
  - Vitamin C (ascorbic acid)—water-soluble vitamin primarily found in citrus fruits and tomatoes; promotes stress resistance, wound healing, and oral health
  - Vitamin A—fat-soluble vitamin primarily found in milk and yellow vegetables; promotes good eyesight and protects skin from infection; a deficiency causes night blindness
  - Vitamin D—fat-soluble vitamin primarily found in sunlight and dairy products; strengthens bone development; a deficiency causes rickets

- Vitamin E—fat-soluble vitamin primarily found in green leafy vegetables, nuts, and whole grains; protects RBCs; a deficiency causes anemia
- Vitamin K—fat-soluble vitamin primarily found in green leafy vegetables and tomatoes; promotes blood clotting

- Minerals—elements usually found in the earth's crust, the human body, and some foods; necessary to carry out bodily functions
  - Major minerals—essential elements needed by the body in larger amounts: calcium (Ca), chloride (Cl), magnesium (Mg), phosphorus (P), potassium (K), sodium (Na); Table 23-2 lists the major minerals, the recommended daily allowance (RDA) as established by the Food and Nutrition Board of the National Academy of Sciences, their sources, and their purposes
  - Trace minerals—essential elements needed by the body in very small amounts: copper, fluoride, iodine, iron, zinc; Table 23-3 lists the trace minerals, their sources, and their purposes

DIETARY GUIDELINES

The United States Department of Agriculture (USDA) developed guidelines to assist the general population in making healthy food choices. Prior to 2005, these guidelines were displayed in a food pyramid that divided foods into groups. The group with the most recommended servings per day was on the bottom, and the group with the fewest recommended servings per day was on the top, forming the pyramid shape. In 2011, the food pyramid

TABLE 23-2 ▸ Major minerals

Mineral	Major Food Source	Purpose
Calcium (Ca) *RDA 1,000–1,200 mg	Dairy products, salmon, sardines, dark leafy greens, fortified cereals	Bone and tooth development, nerve impulse transmission; disorders include osteoporosis and rickets
Chloride (Cl) *RDA 1,500 mg	Table salt, rye, tomatoes, lettuce, celery, olives	Acid–base balance; disorders include decreases in mental capacities
Magnesium (Mg) *RDA 320–420 mg	Green vegetables, whole grains, soy, avocado, most nuts	Enzyme activity, metabolism, heartbeat regulation; deficiencies include metabolic disorders
Phosphorus (P) *RDA 700 mg	Dairy products, meats, fish, nuts, protein-rich foods	Bone and tooth development, acid–base balance, protein and glucose metabolism; disorders include anemia, abnormal growth, bone loss
Potassium (K) *RDA 4,700 mg	Oranges, dried fruits, potatoes, green leafy vegetables, lentils, lima beans	Protein metabolism, acid–base balance correction, nerve impulse transmission, heartbeat regulation; disorders include hyperkalemia and hypokalemia
Sodium (Na) *RDA 1,500 mg	Tale salt, processed food, fast foods, sauces, soups	Fluid balance maintenance; disorders include hypertension

*RDA for normal, nonpregnant, nonlactating adult.

TABLE 23-3 ▸ Trace minerals

Mineral	Major Food Source	Purpose
Copper (Cu)	Organ meats, whole grains, nuts	Hemoglobin formation, iron absorption, enzyme function
Fluoride (Fl)	Fish, some water supplies	Tooth decay resistance; disorders from overuse include tooth mottling
Iodine (I)	Saltwater fish and crustaceans, iodized table salt	Metabolism regulation, element of thyroid hormone; disorders include goiter
Iron (Fe)	Organ meats, dark green leafy vegetables	Hemoglobin element, oxygen transport; disorders include anemia
Zinc (Zn)	Organ meats, other foods high in protein	Enzyme element, wound healing, growth; disorders include dwarfism

FIGURE 23-2 My Plate.

was replaced by My Plate (Fig. 23-2), but the food pyramid continues to be used by health-care educational facilities.

GENERAL USDA RECOMMENDATIONS

- Eat a variety of foods from each food group
- Combine healthy eating with physical activity
- Choose a diet low in saturated fat and cholesterol
- Eat plenty of grain products, fruit, and vegetables
- Note Na content in food products and use in moderation
- Use alcoholic beverages in moderation

FOOD GROUPS IN ORDER OF LARGEST TO SMALLEST

1. Grains
2. Vegetables
3. Milk
4. Fruits
5. Meats and beans
6. Oils

COMMON THERAPEUTIC (SPECIAL) DIETS

- Pregnancy/lactating diet
  - Calorie intake as recommended by health-care provider
  - Ca, iron, vitamin C, and folic acid intake should increase
  - Weight gain as recommended by health-care provider
- Clear liquid
  - Used in introducing foods back into diet (e.g., after illness or surgery and in preparation for specific procedures such as a colonoscopy)

- Rule of thumb—clear liquids are those you can see through, such as apple juice, tea, clear broth, or noncaffeinated sodas
- Soft
  - Normal foods in mashed or pureed form
  - Accommodation for patients with difficulty chewing
- Bland
  - Nonirritating foods (e.g., most dairy products, hot cereals, mashed potatoes, grits)
  - Used in gastrointestinal tract disorders, such as various ulcer forms, ulcerative colitis, or gastritis
- Diabetic
  - Goal is to prevent abnormal fluctuations in insulin and blood glucose levels
  - Simple sugars should be limited
  - Intake of complex carbohydrates, protein, and unsaturated fats should increase
  - Calorie intake is tailored per patient
- Low (restricted) Na
  - Used in hypertension, congestive heart failure, and other diseases that increase the body's normal fluid load
  - Educate patient to read Na contents in food ingredient labels
- Low cholesterol (low fat)
  - Used in patients with high cholesterol, increased triglycerides, and cardiovascular disease
  - Limitation of fat calories to less than 20% of total daily caloric intake
- Low purine
  - Used in patients who have gout or the inability to metabolize uric acid
  - Limitation of purine-rich foods such as organ meats, red meat, asparagus, salmon, and halibut
- Food sensitivity and intolerance
  - Gluten-free—avoid this protein found in processed wheat, oats, barley, and rye
  - Lactose-free—avoid or limit dairy products
- Food allergies
  - The most common food allergens—eggs, fish, milk, nuts from trees, peanuts, and shellfish
  - Elimination method—used to verify allergies by avoiding suspect foods then introducing them back into the diet one by one
  - Allergic reactions—vary in severity from mild intolerance symptoms to hives, facial swelling, difficulty breathing, and most severe are anaphylaxis and even death
  - Patient education, including avoidance of the food allergen; reading food labels for ingredients and

warnings and inquiring at restaurants, homes of others, and other eating establishments about food content

WEIGHT CONTROL

Generally, the condition of being overweight is a product of taking in more calories than the body burns or metabolizes. The clinical definition of **overweight** is an adult with a body mass index (BMI) of 25 or greater (Table 23-4). **Obesity** is an adult with a BMI of 30 or higher. The following are common guidelines for weight loss and control:

- Establish healthy eating habits
  - Eat regularly scheduled well-rounded meals based on the recommendations of the food pyramid
  - Eat smaller portions
  - Avoid processed foods and high-calorie foods (fatty, sugary)
  - Limit meals eaten outside the home, especially fast foods
  - Limit juices, sodas, sports drink, bottled teas, and other beverages with sugar
  - Drink plenty of water
- Engage in physical activity
  - Decrease time sitting in front of the television or computer or other electronic and sedentary activities
  - Increase physical activity (recommendations vary regarding time and frequency, general range is every day for 30–60 minutes to three times a week for 20–60 minutes)

CANCER AND DIET

Conversation and studies around diet and cancer prevention and treatment agree that while certain foods may be contributory, no definitive evidence proves that food causes cancer. It is thought that:

- Anti-cancer foods and foods recommended during treatment include plant-based foods—fruits and vegetables (especially those with bright colors), grains, nuts, legumes and fiber in general, unsaturated fats, and the omega-3 fatty acids

TABLE 23-4 Adult BMI	
BMI	**Weight Status**
Below 18.5	Underweight
18.5–24.9	Normal
25.0–29.9	Overweight
30.0 and Above	Obese

- Foods to avoid or keep to a minimum to help prevent cancer include saturated and trans fats found in animal products especially red meat and whole dairy products, sugars, white flour, foods with nitrites and nitrates (e.g., hot dogs), and alcohol

During cancer treatment such as chemotherapy or radiation, the immune system is weakened, causing an increased threat of infections. To help prevent foodborne infections,

- Wash hands before and after food preparation
- Wash foods well
- Maintain and prepare foods at the recommended temperatures
- Avoid raw foods, including salad bars and undercooked foods
- Clean utensils, counters, and food containers well

EATING DISORDERS

An abnormal eating habit that involves insufficient or excessive food ingestion to the detriment of one's health is considered an eating disorder. Women account for 85% to 90% of eating disorders. The two most serious were also addressed in Chapter 6.

- Anorexia nervosa—self-starvation for fear of becoming fat; often considers oneself fat no matter how thin or emaciated; hospitalization may be necessary to restore nutrition and treat resulting cardiac or other medical conditions; psychotherapy is needed
- Bulimia—large quantities of food are eaten in a short timeframe (binging) followed by self-induced vomiting, use of laxatives or diuretics (purging), and often excessive exercise in an effort to stay thin or of normal size; treatment is psychotherapy

ETHNIC CONSIDERATIONS

The demographics of the United States continue to change as diverse populations grow. Certain diseases prominent in specific races or cultures (e.g., hypertension in African Americans and diabetes in certain Native American tribes) are often controlled by diet. It is important for the patient educator to determine the dietary habits of the involved ethnic group. Every attempt should be made to maintain the foods of the specific culture with, perhaps, different methods of preparation—for example, baking instead of frying. The educator, who often is the medical assistant, must know the prescribed therapeutic diet and understand the fundamentals of nutrients. All healthcare workers are obligated to stay current as standards and guidelines change.

TERMS

NUTRITION REVIEW

The following list reviews the terms discussed in this chapter and other important terms you may see on the exam.

absorption the transfer of digested nutrients from the gastrointestinal system to the blood circulation

calorie unit of energy that produces heat

carbohydrates sugars and starches; the body's primary energy source

digestion physical and chemical changing of nutrients in the body to allow absorption

estimated energy requirement (EER) approximation of needed daily calories

fats (lipids) greasy material in nutrients; transport fat-soluble vitamins, insulate the body from the cold, and provide fatty acids

fiber nondigestible but edible portion of plants; necessary for the gastrointestinal elimination function

ingestion taking in of nutrients; eating and drinking

metabolism synthesizing of nutrients from the bloodstream, producing energy

nutrients components of food necessary for the body to perform physiologic functions

nutrition the process of taking food into the body and using it

obese an adult with a BMI of 30 or higher

proteins nutrients comprising amino acids (building blocks); produce and heal body tissue

recommended daily allowance (RDA) established by the Food and Nutrition Board of the National Academy of Sciences, quantities of nutrients needed daily for good health

trans fats (trans fatty acids, hydrogenated fats) manufactured fats created by hydrogenation of unsaturated fats; found in commercial baked goods, fried foods, and processed foods; usually solid at room temperature; increase blood cholesterol

triglycerides component molecule of fat found in fatty foods; a combination of fatty acids and glycerol; high levels clog blood vessels, causing cardiovascular disease

vitamins organic substances found naturally in foods and needed in small amounts for metabolism and prevention of certain diseases

REVIEW QUESTIONS

All questions are relevant for all medica assisting and medical administrative certification exams.

1. The process of taking nutrients into the body is called:
   A. digestion.
   B. ingestion.
   C. absorption.
   D. metabolism.

   Answer: **B**
   Why: Ingestion is the process of introducing food and drink into the stomach. Digestion, absorption, and metabolism are part of the digestive process after the food enters the body.
   Review: Yes ○ No ○

2. The cholesterol considered to be the "good" type is:
   A. triglycerides.
   B. high-density lipoprotein.
   C. low-density lipoprotein.
   D. saturated fat.
   E. unsaturated fat.

   Answer: **B**
   Why: High-density lipoproteins are considered the good cholesterol because they actually carry back to the liver cholesterol that has been deposited on arterial walls. Increased deposits on arterial walls can lead to blockage of arteries and result in a higher risk of heart disease or heart attack.
   Review: Yes ○ No ○

3. The nutrient that primarily builds and heals body tissue is:
   A. carbohydrate.
   B. fat.
   C. protein.
   D. triglyceride.

   Answer: **C**
   Why: Protein is a nutrient comprising amino acids, the building blocks of the body. The amino acids help build up tissue and promote healing of damaged tissue.
   Review: Yes ○ No ○

4. The vitamin that promotes red blood cell production is:
   A. vitamin A.
   B. vitamin C.
   C. vitamin D.
   D. vitamin K.
   E. vitamin B_{12}.

   Answer: **E**
   Why: Vitamin B_{12} is used to treat red blood cell deficiencies such as pernicious anemia. It promotes the production of red blood cells. Vitamin B_{12} is found in organ meats and dairy products.
   Review: Yes ○ No ○

5. The organization that developed guidelines to assist people in making healthy food choices is the:
   A. FDA.
   B. USDA.
   C. CDC.
   D. AMA.

   Answer: **B**
   Why: The United States Department of Agriculture (USDA) developed the food pyramid that emphasizes food from the major food groups: (1) grains, (2) vegetables, (3) fruits, (4) milk, (5) meat and beans, and (6) oils. The FDA is the Food and Drug Administration, the CDC is the Centers for Disease Control and Prevention, and the AMA is the American Medical Association.
   Review: Yes ○ No ○

6. A clear liquid diet includes the following EXCEPT:
   A. chicken broth.
   B. tea.
   C. milk.
   D. apple juice.
   E. water.

Answer: **C**
Why: Clear liquid means you can see through the liquid. Milk is not considered a clear liquid. A clear liquid diet is recommended for patients recovering from diarrhea or surgery.
Review: Yes ○ No ○

7. Metabolism is the process of:
   A. taking food into the body.
   B. physically changing nutrients to allow absorption.
   C. chemically changing nutrients in the body.
   D. using nutrients from the bloodstream to produce energy.

Answer: **D**
Why: Metabolism is the process by which nutrients are distributed into the blood and are used for growth and energy production.
Review: Yes ○ No ○

8. The fat-soluble vitamin that promotes blood clotting is:
   A. vitamin A.
   B. vitamin D.
   C. vitamin E.
   D. vitamin C.
   E. vitamin K.

Answer: **E**
Why: Vitamins A, D, E, and K are all fat-soluble vitamins, which means that they are stored in the body and can have a cumulative effect. Vitamin K has a chief function of production of prothrombin in the body. Prothrombin is one of the clotting factors.
Review: Yes ○ No ○

9. A person on a low-cholesterol diet should limit which of the following food groups?
   A. Fruits
   B. Meats
   C. Vegetables
   D. Grains

Answer: **B**
Why: Cholesterol is found in animal products. This includes chicken and fish, although these tend to be lower in cholesterol than red meat. The human liver also naturally produces cholesterol. An increase in cholesterol is associated with an increased risk for heart disease and atherosclerosis (cholesterol plaque in the blood vessels).
Review: Yes ○ No ○

10. The mineral responsible for proper bone and tooth development is:
   A. iron.
   B. sodium.
   C. calcium.
   D. potassium.
   E. zinc.

Answer: **C**
Why: Calcium is primarily found in milk and milk products. It is also found in dark green leafy vegetables and promotes the formation of teeth and bones.
Review: Yes ○ No ○

11. Which of the following nutrients has the highest amount of calories per gram?
   A. Carbohydrate
   B. Fat
   C. Protein
   D. Fiber

Answer: **B**
Why: Carbohydrates and proteins have 4 calories per gram of food. Fat contains 9 calories per gram. Fiber is a nondigestible nutrient but one necessary for gastrointestinal elimination.
Review: Yes ○ No ○

12. A patient diagnosed with hypertension will usually benefit from a diet low in:
    A. sodium.
    B. calcium.
    C. iodine.
    D. iron.
    E. protein.

Answer: **A**

Why: Sodium is found in table salt and processed food. Sodium is responsible for maintaining fluid balance, so a diet low in sodium may help lower blood pressure by decreasing the amount of fluid retained by the body.

Review: Yes ○ No ○

13. Which of the following diets is recommended for a patient diagnosed with gout?
    A. Low salt
    B. Low carbohydrate
    C. Low purine
    D. Low fiber

Answer: **C**

Why: Gout is a condition associated with the inability to metabolize uric acid. If there is an excess of uric acid in the body, it is converted to sodium urate crystals that deposit in the joints. A common joint affected by the pain of gout is the great toe. Purine-rich foods are primarily organ meats such as liver and kidney.

Review: Yes ○ No ○

14. The substance necessary for hemoglobin to transport oxygen in the blood is:
    A. zinc.
    B. iodine.
    C. potassium.
    D. iron.
    E. calcium.

Answer: **D**

Why: Iron is found in organ meats and dark green leafy vegetables and is responsible for increasing the ability of the red blood cells to transport oxygen by providing hemoglobin. Iron injections are administered to help treat disorders including iron-deficiency anemia.

Review: Yes ○ No ○

15. The process by which nutrients leave the gastrointestinal system and enter the bloodstream is:
    A. ingestion.
    B. digestion.
    C. absorption.
    D. metabolism.

Answer: **C**

Why: Ingestion is the process of taking nutrients into the body. Digestion is the process of breaking down the nutrients for absorption into the bloodstream. Metabolism is the synthesizing of nutrients from the bloodstream, producing energy.

Review: Yes ○ No ○

16. An example of a saturated fat is:
    A. butter.
    B. olive oil.
    C. egg whites.
    D. walnuts.
    E. salmon.

Answer: **A**

Why: Saturated fat is a type of fat that is found in a solid state when at room temperature and is responsible for increasing blood cholesterol. Unsaturated fats are usually liquid at room temperature and are helpful in decreasing blood cholesterol. Olive oil is an example of an unsaturated fat. Egg whites are not fats but rather are proteins. Walnuts and salmon are proteins that contain unsaturated fat.

Review: Yes ○ No ○

17. A patient diagnosed with hypokalemia should increase the intake of:
    A. copper.
    B. potassium.
    C. fluoride.
    D. calcium.

Answer: **B**

Why: Hypokalemia is a condition in which an inadequate amount of potassium is found in the bloodstream. The treatment includes increasing the intake of potassium through certain foods or medication. Foods rich in potassium include fruits, especially bananas and citrus fruits.

Review: Yes ○ No ○

18. The mineral iodine is an essential substance for the proper function of which one of the following organs?
   A. Kidneys
   B. Adrenal glands
   C. Thyroid gland
   D. Liver

Answer: **C**
Why: The thyroid gland requires adequate amounts of iodine to function properly. A decrease in the function of the thyroid gland may result in development of a goiter, an enlargement of the thyroid gland.
Review: Yes ◯ No ◯

19. Night blindness can be caused by a deficiency of:
   A. vitamin A.
   B. vitamin B.
   C. vitamin C.
   D. vitamin D.

Answer: **A**
Why: Vitamin A is a fat-soluble vitamin that promotes good eyesight and may cause night blindness when deficient in the body. Vitamin A is found in milk and yellow vegetables.
Review: Yes ◯ No ◯

20. The diet recommended for the treatment of ulcers is:
   A. low sodium.
   B. soft.
   C. clear liquid.
   D. bland.
   E. low cholesterol.

Answer: **D**
Why: A bland diet includes foods that are nonirritating, including dairy products, mashed potatoes, and hot cereals.
Review: Yes ◯ No ◯

21. A clear liquid diet is indicated for which of the following?
   A. A patient with an ulcer
   B. A patient with difficulty chewing
   C. A patient with diarrhea
   D. A patient who is limiting calories for weight loss

Answer: **C**
Why: A patient with diarrhea should initially limit intake to clear liquids and then gradually add foods back into the diet. A patient with an ulcer will usually benefit from a diet that is bland and nonirritating. A patient with difficulty chewing can usually eat soft foods but does not require only liquids. A patient who is limiting calories for weight loss should still eat balanced meals from all of the food groups; there is no indication for a clear liquid diet.
Review: Yes ◯ No ◯

22. A low-fat diet would be recommended to treat:
   A. hypertension.
   B. gallbladder disease.
   C. thyroid disease.
   D. gout.
   E. diabetes.

Answer: **B**
Why: The gallbladder is where bile is stored. Bile is necessary to break up fat particles that can be absorbed through the intestinal walls into the body. Patients with gallbladder disease will want to limit the intake of fat to decrease the need for bile. Most gallbladder disease is caused by obstruction of the bile ducts resulting from gallstones.
Review: Yes ◯ No ◯

23. Ascorbic acid is also known as vitamin:
   A. A.
   B. B.
   C. C.
   D. D.

Answer: **C**
Why: Ascorbic acid, also known as vitamin C, is a water-soluble vitamin present in citrus fruits, tomatoes, and green leafy vegetables. Vitamin C is essential for fighting bacterial infections and preventing scurvy. Scurvy is characterized by weakness, anemia, edema, soft bleeding gums with ulceration, and loosening of the teeth.
Review: Yes ◯ No ◯

24. Which of the following may be prevented with proper amounts of vitamin D in the diet?
    A. Diabetes
    B. Hemorrhage
    C. Blindness
    D. Heart disease
    E. Rickets

Answer: **E**
Why: Rickets is a condition characterized by weak bones. The disease usually is seen in infancy and childhood. The bones do not form properly because they are soft and pliable. Deformities may include bowlegs and knock-knees.
Review: Yes ◯ No ◯

25. Persons who need to limit their intake of iodine in the body will want to avoid:
    A. milk.
    B. seafood.
    C. bananas.
    D. eggs.

Answer: **B**
Why: Seafood, especially shellfish, is very high in iodine content. Some people are highly allergic to iodine and should avoid foods with iodine. Injected contrast media should also be avoided because of the high concentration of iodine.
Review: Yes ◯ No ◯

CRITICAL THINKING CASE REVIEW

Mr. White, a long-standing diabetic patient of Dr. Patel, was recently diagnosed with the comorbidity of hypertension. The medical assistant is providing patient education.

1. Dr. Patel wrote the order to review a _____ diet with the patient.
   A. low-sodium
   B. low-potassium
   C. low-carbohydrate
   D. low-fat
   E. low-protein

Answer: **C**
Why: Mr. White has been a diabetic, and he should have been on a low-carbohydrate diet. Since this is presumably the only prior condition and diet, it would be the only one to be reviewed or reexamined or checked. This is a question that requires careful reading.
Review: Yes ◯ No ◯

2. Dr. Patel also ordered the medical assistant to instruct the patient on a _____ diet for his hypertension.
   A. low-sodium
   B. low-potassium
   C. low-carbohydrate
   D. low-fat

Answer: **A**
Why: Excess sodium is contraindicated in hypertension because it often results in retention of fluid which increases the burden on the circulatory system and kidneys and, consequently, increases blood pressure or hypertension.
Review: Yes ◯ No ◯

3. A strategy used to assure that Mr. White understands what the medical assistant is teaching is to:
   A. listen carefully.
   B. use open language.
   C. observe boundaries.
   D. ask for feedback.
   E. exhibit a confident demeanor.

Answer: **D**
Why: While A, B, C, and E are important when communicating with patients, they are not strategies that will assure the patient understands what you are teaching. By asking for feedback (Chapters 7 and 8) such as paraphrasing, asking questions, you will be able to determine understanding.
Review: Yes ◯ No ◯

4. With the diagnoses of diabetes and hypertension, another type of diet appropriate for Mr. White is:

A. low cholesterol to control his HDL.

B. low cholesterol to control his LDL.

C. low cholesterol to control his trans-fatty acids.

D. low cholesterol to control sodium levels.

Answer: **B**

Why: The low-cholesterol diet is appropriate, since patients with diabetes and hypertension usually have resulting cardiac and circulatory problems due to clogged blood vessels. The "good" cholesterol is the HDL. The "bad" cholesterol is the LDL, which is the one that should be kept low and is the best answer. Low cholesterol does not control trans-fatty acids, which are hydrogenated fats that are ingested or sodium levels. This is another question that requires careful reading.

Review: Yes ○ No ○

5. Given the following lunch choices and assuming they were prepared using traditional methods and ingredients, which would be best for Mr. White?

A. Grilled cheese sandwich with a pickle and a bowl of berries

B. Grilled chicken with barbecue sauce, rice, salad, and a brownie

C. Grilled hamburger without a bun, salad, cottage cheese, and fruit

D. Caesar salad with a small dish of low-fat ice cream

E. Three egg white omelet with spinach, salsa, and a slice of watermelon

Answer: **E**

Why: A traditional grilled cheese sandwich is high in fat, and the pickle adds extra sodium. The B choice is loaded with carbohydrates contraindicated in diabetes and most likely high sodium content in the barbecue sauce. C would not be a bad choice, but it is not the best choice given the fat in the hamburger and cottage cheese. D is a poor choice because it contains very little protein which is important in a diabetic diet to control insulin level, and low-fat ice cream usually has added sugar. E is the correct answer because egg whites contain no cholesterol; nothing in this lunch, in ordinary amounts, is contraindicated for diabetes or hypertension.

Review: Yes ○ No ○

CHAPTER

24

Pharmacology and Medication Administration

Review Tip:

The national exams contain medication dosage calculation problems. Know how to multiply and divide fractions and decimals. Practice solving problems without a calculator, since you are not permitted to use one during the exam. The examiners usually provide scrap paper to work out the problem before listing the answer on the exam form. Practice problems follow the review terms in this chapter.

Pharmacology is the study of drugs. Two federal agencies regulate drugs and drug administration. The **Food and Drug Administration (FDA)** controls the drugs that are acceptable for use in the United States; the **Drug Enforcement Agency (DEA)** controls who may administer and use specific drugs. Both agencies hold enforcement powers, which may include imprisonment, fines, and revocation or suspension of professional licenses. Drugs are placed in five schedules for regulation and control, as described in Table 24-1. Visit RxList (www.rxlist.com) for a list of the 200 most current commonly used drugs. This list is recommended by the testing organizations and is subject to change. The recommendation is to review it close to your test date.

TABLE 24-1 ▸ Drug schedules		
Schedule	**Use**	**Example**
I	Illegal or restricted to research; dispensed with special permits; high potential for abuse	Heroin, marijuana in some states
II	Medical use with precautions and limitations; dispensed with written prescription; high potential for abuse	Cocaine, morphine, Demerol, oxycodone, Ritalin, marijuana in some states
III	Medical use with precautions and limitations; dispensed with written prescription; moderate potential for abuse	Barbiturates, small doses of codeine in combination with other drugs (e.g., Tylenol with codeine)
IV	Medical use with precautions and limitations; dispensed with written or oral prescription; low potential for abuse	Valium
V	Medical use with purchase over the counter; very low potential for abuse	Benadryl, Robitussin

ADMINISTRATION

MEDICAL DRUG USES

- Treatment—relieves symptoms of a disease or disorder (e.g., ibuprofen for fever and pain)
- Diagnosis—determine the presence of a specific disease by the body's reaction to specific drugs (e.g., Tensilon to aid in the diagnosis of myasthenia gravis)
- Restoration—remove the cause of the disease or disorder (e.g., an antibiotic)
- Replacement—substitute chemical agents normally found in the body (e.g., hormone replacement therapy [HRT])
- Prevention—block or weaken certain diseases (e.g., immunizations for vaccine-preventable diseases); see Box 6-7, "Types of Immunity," and Box 6-8, "Common Vaccine-Preventable Diseases," in Chapter 6

COMMON DRUG TYPES

Drugs are named and grouped for their uses—for example, *antiemetics* are used to combat emesis (vomiting). Table 24-2 lists common drug types and their trade names and uses.

COMMON DRUG ROUTES

- Buccal—placed between gum and cheek via tablet, gel, or spray (do not confuse with sublingual)
- Inhalation—inhaled into respiratory system via sprays, mists, masks (oxygen is considered a drug)
- Instillation—introduction of a solution, usually into a body cavity but sometimes used in relation to the eye and ear
- Intradermal (ID)—injected into dermal layer of skin at 15-degree angle via fine (25-G to 27-G) short needle, producing a small wheal; forearm site is most common, as with a tuberculin skin test
- Intramuscular (IM)—injected into muscle at 90-degree angle via an 18-G to 23-G long needle (1 to 3 inches); aspirate before injection to ensure that the needle is not in a blood vessel except with immunizations
  - Common IM sites; refer to Figure 24-1
    - Deltoids (upper arms)
    - Gluteus medius (the ventrogluteal area of this muscle is now recommended over the dorsogluteal area)
    - Vastus lateralis (thighs), usually for infants who are not walking
  - Z-track—used for specific IM medications that irritate subcutaneous tissue (e.g., Imferon and Kenalog); the skin at the injection site is pulled to one side before injection; the medication is administered and skin released; prevents medication from seeping into subcutaneous layers; refer to Figure 24-2, "Displacing the skin for Z-track injection"
- Intravenous (IV)—injected into vein via 18-G to 21-G needle (1 to 1½ inches)
- Nasal—usually a spray or ointment placed in the nostrils and absorbed through the mucous membranes; the head should be kept in neutral position, not tilted back
- Ophthalmic—placed into eye via ointment or drops
- Oral—placed in the mouth and swallowed via tablet, capsule, liquid, gel (most common medication route);

TABLE 24-2	Common drug types	
Drug Type	Common Use	Example
Analgesic	Lessens or relieves pain	Ibuprofen (Motrin) Acetaminophen (Tylenol)
Anesthetic (local)	"Deadens" an area to sensation, including pain	Lidocaine (Xylocaine)
Antacid	Neutralizes acid in gastrointestinal tract	Tums, Mylanta
Antibiotic	Eradicates or inhibits the growth of specific microbes	Penicillin, Augmentin
Anticoagulant	Prevents or decreases clotting	Heparin, Coumadin
Anticonvulsant	Prevents seizures	Dilantin, Tegretol
Antidepressant	Inhibits or decreases depression	Prozac, Cymbalta
Antidiarrheal	Inhibits or decreases diarrhea	Lomotil, Kaopectate
Antiemetic	Inhibits or decreases nausea	Compazine, Dramamine
Antihistamine	Inhibits or decreases symptoms of allergies	Benadryl, Claritin
Antihypertensive	Inhibits or controls high blood pressure	Aldomet, Lopressor
Anti-inflammatory ■ Steroidal ■ Nonsteroidal anti-inflammatory drug (NSAID)	Inhibits or decreases inflammation	Decadron Ibuprofen
Antipyretic	Decreases fever	Acetaminophen, ibuprofen
Antitussive	Inhibits or decreases cough	Codeine, Dimetapp
Bronchodilator	Dilates the bronchi	Albuterol
Decongestant	Decreases nasal congestion	Neo-Synephrine
Diuretic	Decreases body fluid by increasing urination	Lasix, Diuril
Immunization	Protects from specific communicable diseases	Hepatitis B, varicella, and polio vaccines

when pouring liquids hold the cup to eye level and measure from the **meniscus**, the crescent-shaped form at the top of the liquid

■ Otic—placed in ear via drops

■ Parenteral—nonoral, usually refers to injected medication: IM, IV, subcutaneous, ID

■ Rectal—placed in patient's rectum via suppository

■ Subcutaneous (Sub-Q or subQ; SC or SQ no longer used, per The Joint Commission)—injected in fatty tissue under the skin at a 45-degree angle via 23-G to 25-G needle (½ to 5/8 inches long); aspirate before injection to ensure that the needle is not in a blood vessel

• Used for allergic extracts administered with tuberculin needle and syringe to avoid entering muscle, and for insulin administration

• Common subcutaneous sites
○ Upper arms
○ Upper thighs
○ Upper medial back
○ Abdominal external obliques

■ Sublingual—placed under the tongue via tablets or gels

■ Topical—placed on skin or mucous membranes via ointments, creams, liquids, or sprays for direct treatment of skin or membranes

■ Transdermal—placed on skin via medicated patch for medication to absorb through skin and enter bloodstream

■ Urethral—placed into urethra and bladder via a urethral catheter

■ Vaginal—placed into vagina via applicator of cream or via douche

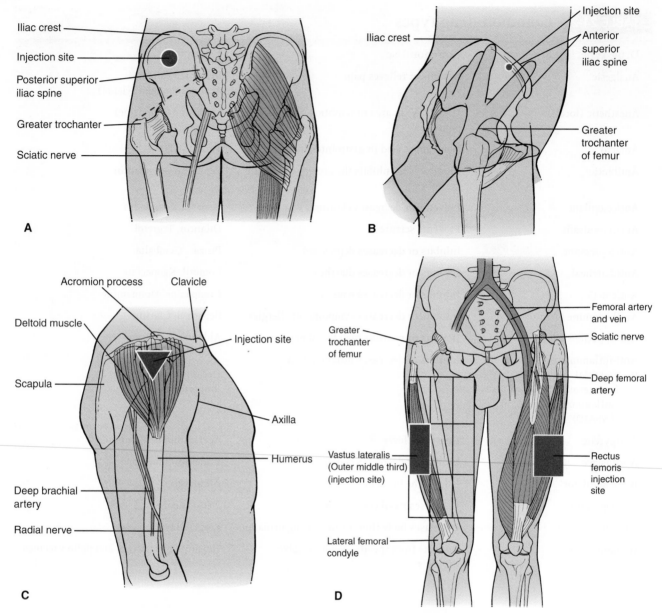

FIGURE 24-1 Intramuscular sites.

Note: Implantable medication devices and eye-curing lens devices are also available; national exam question probability is extremely low for these routes.

SYRINGES

Syringes are plastic or glass tube-like carriers used with an attached needle to administer substances into the body via injection.

- Insulin—small syringe with short, fine needle attached to administer insulin; measurements are in units (U is another abbreviation The Joint Commission recommends not to use); 100 units = 1 mL; syringes are supplied with 100-unit (most common), 80-unit, or 40-unit capacities

- Tuberculin—small syringe with short, fine needle attached to administer Mantoux tuberculin or other skin test intradermally; measurements are in tenths of a millimeter (0.1 mL) with a 1-mL capacity; usual amount is 0.1 mL of purified protein derivative (PPD); test results should be read in 48 to 72 hours

- Cartridges—individual-dose prefilled tubes with needles that screw onto or slide into a dispenser designed for that cartridge

OTHER MEDICATION PACKAGING

- Unit dose—a single dosage per container;

with the medication as with vaccines; do not interchange diluents

- Sterile technique is required for injectables, and the syringe used to reconstitute should not be used for administration if possible
- Refrigeration after reconstitution is often required

SEVEN PLUS "RIGHTS" OF DRUG ADMINISTRATION

These procedures must be carried out each time a drug is administered to avoid medication errors.

- Right patient—check the name on the physician's order and the medical record; ask the patient first and last name
- Right drug—check the drug label three times: when taking the drug container out (check drug expiration date at the same time), after placing the medication in the dispenser (e.g., syringe, medication cup), and before returning the drug container to storage
- Right route—check the route the physician ordered with the route you prepared (e.g., oral versus injectable)
- Right dose—check the dose on the physician's order with the dose prepared
- Right technique—ensure that the correct method is used throughout the procedure, including positioning the patient and aseptic technique
- Right time—check when the medication is to be given (e.g., now, with meals)
- Right documentation—record the procedure in the patient's medical record on completion, noting date, time, drug, dose, route, site (if injectable, topical, or transdermal), results/tolerance, patient education, medical assistant signature, and title

In addition to the seven generally accepted medication "rights," you may also see the following:

- Right reason—know why it is being given
- Right to know—does the patient know what is being given, the expected effect, and possible side effects
- Right to refuse—as with all treatments, the patient has the right to refuse which should be reported to the physician and documented

SAFETY

In addition to the medication "rights," when administering medication, general safety and Occupational Safety and Health Administration (OSHA) and The Joint Commission guidelines apply:

- Always check medication expiration date before administration
- Assure proper identification of the patient

FIGURE 24-2 Displacing the skin for Z-track injection.

- Multidose vials—a container of medication intended for parental use with more than one dosage; date and time bottles when first opened; should be discarded if
  - Sterility is compromised or questionable
  - It is not used within 28 days of opening or the manufacturer's recommendation
  - It is unopened but expired
  - Recommended storage has been breached such as refrigeration
- Ampules—glass or plastic unit dose vial of injectable solution:
  - Usually require breaking the top along a scored neck to open; recommend covering with a sterile gauze to execute
  - Solution should be drawn out with a filter needle to avoid small fragments of glass or plastic resulting from opening
- Powder for reconstitution; may be for oral, topical, or injectable medications
  - Use only the recommended diluent such as water, sterile normal saline, or the diluent that comes

- **Always** ask the patient if he or she is allergic to any medications
- Follow aseptic technique (Chapter 17)
- Prevent accidental needlesticks by using safety lock needles
- Discard needles and syringes immediately into biohazard containers
- Wear appropriate personal protective equipment (PPE)
- Have the patient wait 10 to 20 minutes after any injectable substance

DOSAGE CALCULATIONS

The majority of medical facilities maintain conversion charts to simplify medication dosage calculations when one unit (such as grams) must be changed to another unit (such as milligrams). In other instances, the amount of a medication ordered may be more or less than the medication on hand. The medical assistant is expected to determine the correct dosage. Table 24-3 contains the most common conversions used in dosage calculations.

METHODS

- Formula with like units—used when medication ordered is more than or less than the medication on hand but the units are the same (e.g., both in

TABLE 24-3 ▶ Common conversions

Component	Equivalent
1 gram (G, Gm, g, gm)	1,000 milligrams (mg) 5 grains (gr)
1 gr	60 mg
1 kilogram (kg)	2.2 pounds (lb) 1,000 g
1 milliliter (mL, ml)	15 drops (15 gtt) 1 cubic centimeter (the abbreviation of cc is no longer acceptable per The Joint Commission)
1 teaspoon (tsp)	5 mL 60 gtt

milligrams). Box 24-1 shows the steps involved in calculating a dosage for like units.

- Conversion ratio—used when the units of medication on hand are different from the units ordered (e.g., milligrams are ordered, but the medication on hand is in grams). The conversion is done first, then the formula for the dosage. Box 24-2 shows the steps involved in calculating a dosage for unlike units.
- Body weight—used in instances in which medication dosage is more closely calculated for the individual

---

BOX 24-1

Dosage calculation with like units

Problem 1: The physician ordered 800 mg ibuprofen po to be given now; the office stocks ibuprofen in 200 mg per tablet. How many tablets will you give?

$$\text{Formula}: \frac{\text{Dose ordered}}{\text{Dose on hand}} \times \frac{\text{Quantity}}{1} = \text{Amount desired}$$

(where "quantity" is the amount and form that contains the dose on hand)

Step 1: Set up formula.

$$\frac{800\,\text{mg}}{200\,\text{mg}} \times \frac{1\,\text{tablet}}{1} = \text{number of tablets desired}$$

Step 2: Multiply 800 × 1 and 200 × 1.

$$\frac{800}{200} = 4\,\text{tablets}$$

Answer: Four tablets of 200 mg each are to be given.

Problem 2: The physician ordered 250 mg amoxicillin po to be given now; the office stocks amoxicillin 500 mg per tsp. How many teaspoons will you give?

Use the same formula as above:

$$\frac{250\,\text{mg}}{500\,\text{mg}} \times \frac{1\,\text{tsp}}{1} = ½ \text{ or } 0.5\,\text{tsp to be given}$$

BOX 24-2

Dosage calculation with unlike units

Problem: The physician ordered 0.4 g of ibuprofen po now; the office stocks ibuprofen 200 mg per tablet. How many tablets will you give?

Step 1: Because the units of the available dosage (mg) differ from the units of the ordered dosage (g, they must be converted. Grams are converted to milligrams using the following ratio:

1,000 mg : 1 g

or

1,000 mg = 1 g

Step 2: Set up the proportion to find the dosage using the above ratio, x (the unknown, in milligrams), and 0.4 g, which is the dose ordered:

1,000 mg : 1 g = x mg : 0.4 g

or

1,000 mg : 1 g :: x mg : 0.4 g

(*Hint:* Use like units for the first and third numbers and the second and fourth numbers.)

Step 3: The product of the first and fourth numbers equals the product of the second and third numbers: 400 mg = x mg.

Step 4: Use the formula in Box 24-1:

$$\text{Formula}: \frac{\text{Dose ordered}}{\text{Dose on hand}} \times \frac{\text{Quantity}}{1} = \text{Amount desired}$$

$$\frac{400\,\text{mg}}{200\,\text{mg}} \times \frac{\text{tablet}}{1} = 2\,\text{tablets}$$

Answer: Two tablets of 200 mg each are to be given.

BOX 24-3

Dosage calculation with body weight

Problem: The physician ordered 15 mg Tylenol per kilogram (kg) of body weight. You weighed the child, who is 8 kg. How many milligrams of Tylenol will you give?

Formula:
Dose ordered × Weight in kg = Dose to be given

Set up formula.
15 mg × 8 kg = 120 mg

Answer: 120 mg Tylenol is to be given.

patient (e.g., pediatrics); pounds are converted to kilograms. Box 24-3 shows the steps involved in calculating a dosage based on body weight.

■ Body surface area—used to calculate pediatric medication doses; complicated formula rarely used in the medical office.

PRESCRIPTIONS

Prescriptions are written directions for therapeutic agents; the most common involve medications. Licensed physicians, licensed nurse practitioners with prescribing privileges, and properly credentialed physicians' assistants are the only persons authorized to write prescriptions. They provide a legal document, informing the pharmacist of the order to be filled. Many medical facilities use **e-prescribing**, electronically sending a prescription directly to the pharmacy through the EHR system.

The medical assistant with a physician's order may administer drugs but may *never* prescribe drugs. The medical assistant and administrative medical specialist may call a prescription into a pharmacy as written by one of the above legal entities. This is not considered prescribing.

Dispensing is defined as preparing and distributing medication. Only pharmacists, physicians, and properly credentialed nurse practitioners and physicians' assistants may dispense drugs. The medical assistant and administrative medical specialist may not dispense drugs but may give a patient prepackaged drugs (e.g., samples as ordered by the physician). This is not considered dispensing.

PRESCRIPTION INFORMATION

Box 24-4 lists common abbreviations used on prescriptions.

■ Physician name, address, phone number

■ Date of prescription

■ Patient name, address, and phone number

■ Drug, dose, and form

■ Number of doses to be dispensed

BOX 24-4

Common prescription abbreviations and instructions

Time

Once per day ("od" no longer used, per The Joint Commission) q: every	b.i.d.: twice per day	t.i.d.: three times per day	q.i.d.: four times per day
	Every day ("qd" no longer used, per The Joint Commission)	qh: every hour	q (2, 3, 4, etc.) h: every (2, 3, 4, etc.) hours

Select Administration Sites

Right ear ("AD" no longer used, per The Joint Commission)	Left ear ("AS" no longer used, per The Joint Commission)	Both ears ("AU" no longer used, per The Joint Commission)	Right eye ("OD" no longer used, per The Joint Commission)
Left eye ("OS" no longer used, per The Joint Commission)	Both eyes ("OU" no longer used, per The Joint Commission)	po: by mouth	top: topically

Amounts

<u>Always</u> use a zero before any stand alone decimal, for example 0.5mgs. NOT .5mgs.

Note: The Joint Commission eliminated a number of common abbreviations that resulted in medication errors.

- Patient instructions
- Number of refills
- Physician signature
- DEA number

MEDICAL ASSISTANT RESPONSIBILITY TO AVOID DRUG ABUSE

- Security of prescription pads
- Protection of signature stamps and physician's DEA number

IMMUNIZATIONS

Immunization is the process of making a person resistant to an infectious disease by the administration of a vaccine, a substance that stimulates the body's own immune system to create protection against a specific disease. The terms vaccines and immunizations are often used synonymously, although this is not technically correct. The vaccine is the substance that produces the immunity. The immunization occurs by administering the vaccine or putting the vaccine into the body system. Review to Chapter 6, "Anatomy and Physiology," Box 6-7, Types of Immunity, and Box 6-8, Common Vaccine-Preventable Diseases. Vaccines should be administered according to schedules published by the CDC, which change frequently based on ongoing research. The most current can be found on http://www.cdc.gov/vaccines/schedules/. The common schedules are:

- Childhood
- Adult

Refer to Table 24-4 for vaccine doses and routes.

TABLE 24-4 ▶ Administering vaccines

Vaccine	Dose	Route
Diphtheria, tetanus, pertussis (DTaP, DT, Tdap, Td)	0.5 mL	IM
Haemophilus influenzae **type b** (Hib)	0.5 mL	IM
Hepatitis A (HepA)	≤18 y; 0.5 mL ≥19 y; 1.0 mL	IM
Hepatitis B (HepB) *Persons 11–15 y may be given Recombivax HB (Merck) 1.0 mL adult formulation on a 2-dose schedule.*	<19 y; 0.5 mL ≥20 y;w 1.0 mL	IM
Human papillomavirus (HPV)	0.5 mL	IM
Influenza, live attenuated (LAIV)	0.2 mL	Intranasal spray
Influenza, trivalent inactivated (TIV)	6–35 mo: 0.25 mL ≥3 y: 0.5 mL	IM

TABLE 24-4 **Administering vaccines** (*Continued*)

Vaccine	Dose	Route
TIV: Fluzone intradermal (18–64 y)	0.1 mL	ID
Measles, mumps, rubella (MMR)	0.5 mL	Subcutaneous
Meningococcal—conjugate (MCV)	0.5 mL	IM
Meningococcal—polysaccharide (MPSV)	0.5 mL	Subcutaneous
Pneumococcal conjugate (PCV)	0.5 mL	IM
Pneumococcal polysaccharide (PPSV)	0.5 mL	IM or Subcutaneous
Polio, inactivated (IPV)	0.5 mL	IM or Subcutaneous
Rotavirus (RV)	Rotarix: 1.0 mL / Rotateq: 2.0 mL	Oral
Varicella (Var)	0.5 mL	Subcutaneous
Zoster (Zos)	0.65 mL	Subcutaneous
Combination Vaccines		
DTaP-HepB-IPV (Pediarix) DTaP-IPV/Hib (Pentacel) DTaP-IPV (Kinrix) Hib-HepB (Comvax)	0.5 mL	IM
MMRV (ProQuad)	≤12 y: 0.5 mL	Subcutaneous
HepA-HepB (Twinrix)	≥18 y: 1.0 mL	IM

Injections

Subcutaneous injection

Age	Injection Site
Infants (1–12 mo)	Fatty tissue over anterolateral thigh muscle
Children 12 mo or older, adolescents, and adults	Fatty tissue over anterolateral thigh muscle or fatty tissue over triceps

Intramuscular (IM) injection

Age	Injection Site
Newborns (first 28 d)	Anterolateral thigh muscle
Infants (1–12 mo)	Anterolateral thigh muscle
Toddlers (1–2 y)	Anterolateral thigh muscle or deltoid muscle of arm
Children & teens (3–18 y)	Deltoid muscle of arm or anterolateral thigh muscle
Adults 19 y or older	
Male or female less than 130 lb	Deltoid muscle of arm
Female 130–200 lb Male 130–260 lb	Deltoid muscle of arm
Female 200 + lb Male 260 + lb	Deltoid muscle of arm

(Continued)

TABLE 24-4 ▸ Administering vaccines (*continued*)

Intramuscular (IM) injection

Intradermal (ID) administration of Fluzone ID vaccine

Subcutaneous injection

Intranasal (IN) administration

Excerpted from Immunization Action Coalition, 1573 Selby Ave, St. Paul, MN 55104; Phone: (651) 647-9009 (http://www.immunize.org, www.vaccineinformation.org)

VACCINE INFORMATION STATEMENT

Vaccine information statements (VISs), sometimes called vaccine information *sheets*, explain the benefits and risks of a vaccine. Federal law requires a VIS for the appropriate vaccine(s) to be given to the responsible party such as a parent or the adult receiving the vaccine prior to administration. VISs are published by the CDC and translated into approximately 40 languages.

VACCINE ADVERSE EVENT REPORTING SYSTEM

Vaccine Adverse Event Reporting System (VAERS) provides a nationwide mechanism by which adverse events following immunization may be reported, analyzed, and made available to the public. VAERS also provides a vehicle for disseminating vaccine safety-related information

to parents and guardians, health care providers, vaccine manufacturers, state vaccine programs, and other constituencies.

The primary objectives of VAERS are to:

- Detect new, unusual, or rare vaccine adverse events (VAEs)
- Monitor increases in known adverse events
- Identify potential patient risk factors for particular types of adverse events
- Identify vaccine lots with increased numbers or types of reported adverse events
- Assess the safety of newly licensed vaccines

VACCINE STORAGE

Vaccine storage is usually the responsibility of a specified medical assistant or medical administrative assistant called a vaccine coordinator. Everyone who administers vaccine or has reason to go into the refrigerator storing the vaccine has a responsibility to be aware of the correct temperature or any potential risk to the integrity of the vaccine. Storage and handling errors result in the following:

■ Reduced effectiveness of vaccine and exposure to the disease

■ Wasted vaccine and additional cost

■ Necessity of revaccination

■ Loss of patient confidence in you and your organization

■ Potential malpractice litigation

Review Figure 24-3 for vaccine storage guidelines.

Cold Chain
(A temperature-controlled supply chain)
Vaccines must be stored properly from the time they are manufactured until they are administered to patients

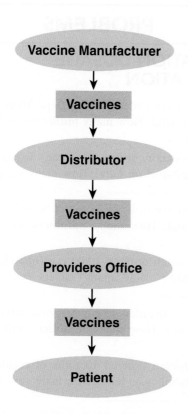

Recommended Temperatures	
Freezer	Between −58°F and +5°F (−50°C to −15°C)
Refrigerator	Between 35°F and 46°F (2°C to 8°C)
Average	40°F (5°C)

Vaccine Storage Temperatures
• Live vaccines
  - Most tolerate freezing
  - Deteriorate rapidly after removal from cold storage
• Inactivated vaccines
  - Damaged by exposure to temperature extremes (extreme heat or freezing temperatures)
  - Potency negatively affected by extended or multiple temperature excursions

Vaccine Storage and Handling Plans
• Develop and maintain written routine plan for:
  - Ordering and accepting vaccine deliveries
  - Storing and handling vaccines
  - Managing inventory
  - Managing potentially compromised vaccines
• Develop and maintain written emergency vaccine retrieval and storage plan
  - Backup storage location with appropriate storage units, temperature monitoring capability, and backup generator
  - Adequate coolers or refrigerated trucks

Vaccine Coordinator Responsibilities
• Ordering vaccines
• Overseeing proper receipt and storage of shipments
• Organizing vaccines within storage unit(s)
• Temperature monitoring of storage unit(s) at least twice daily
• Recording temperature readings on log
• Daily physical inspection of storage unit(s)
• Rotating stock so that vaccine closest to its expiration date will be used first
• Monitoring expiration dates and removing expired vaccines
• Responding to potential temperature fluctuations
• Overseeing proper vaccine transport
• Maintaining storage equipment and records
• Maintaining VFC program documentation in participating clinics
• Ensuring adequate staff training

FIGURE 24-3 Vaccine storage. (Adapted from http://www.cdc.gov/vaccines/recs/storage/.)

TERMS

PHARMACOLOGY AND MEDICATION ADMINISTRATION REVIEW

The following list reviews the terms discussed in this chapter as well as other important terms that you may see on the exam.

dispensing preparing and distributing medication

Drug Enforcement Agency (DEA) federal agency that controls who may administer and use specific drugs

e-prescribing electronically sending a prescription directly to the pharmacy through the EHR

Food and Drug Administration (FDA) federal agency that controls the drugs that are acceptable for use in the United States

immunization the process of making a person resistant to an infectious disease by the administration of a vaccine; often used synonymously with vaccine which is not correct

instillation introduction of a solution, usually into a body cavity

intramuscular (IM) injected into muscle at 90-degree angle via 18-G to 23-G long needle

meniscus in medication administration, the crescent-shaped form at the top of the liquid

parenteral substances administered by intramuscular, intradermal, intravenous, or subcutaneous routes

patient-controlled analgesia (PCA) an electronic infusion device that allows the patient to self-administer IV pain medication through an open IV line

pharmacology the study of drugs

prescriptions written directions for therapeutic agents; the most common involve medications

Rx most commonly found on prescription forms, meaning treatment or recipe

subcutaneous injected in fatty tissue under the skin at a 45-degree angle

syringes plastic or glass tube-like carriers used with an attached needle to administer substances into the body via injection

topical placed on skin or mucous membranes via ointments, creams, liquids, or sprays for direct treatment to skin or membranes

transdermal drug route in which medication is placed on skin via a patch for medication to absorb through skin and enter bloodstream

vaccine a substance that stimulates the body's own immune system to create protection against a specific disease

Vaccine Adverse Event Reporting System (VAERS) a mechanism by which adverse events following immunization may be reported, analyzed, and made available to the public

Vaccine Information Statement (VIS) sometimes called vaccine information sheet; explain the benefits and risks of a vaccine and are required by federal law

Z-track a method of intramuscular (IM) medication administration used for specific IM medications that irritate subcutaneous tissue (e.g., Imferon, Kenalog); the skin is pulled to one side of the injection site before the injection; the medication is administered, and the skin is released; prevents medication from seeping into subcutaneous layers

PROBLEMS

MEDICATION DOSAGE CALCULATION

1. The physician orders 40 mg Depo-Medrol; 80 mg/mL is on hand. How many milliliters will you give?

   _____

2. The physician orders 750 mg Tagamet liquid; 1,500 mg/tsp is on hand. How many teaspoons will you give? _____

3. The physician ordered 75 mg of Seconal; 50 mg/mL is on hand. How many milliliters will you give?

   _____

4. The physician ordered 1,500 mg Duricef; 1 g/tablet is on hand. How many tablets will you give?

   _____

5. The physician orders 15 mg morphine sulfate; 1 gr/mL is on hand. How many milliliters will you give?

   _____

6. The physician ordered 10 units of regular insulin; 100 units/mL is on hand. How many millimeters will you give? _____

7. The physician ordered 5 mg Coumadin; 5 mg/tablet is on hand. How many tablets will you give?

   _____

8. The physician ordered 20 mg Tylenol/kg of body weight; on hand is 80 mg/tablet. The child weighs 12 kg. How many tablets will you give? _____

9. The physician ordered 20 mg Tylenol/kg of body weight; on hand is 80 mg/tablet. The child weighs 44 lb. How many tablets will you give? _____

10. The physician ordered 3,000 units of heparin; 5,000 units/mL is on hand. How many milliliters will you give? _____

Answers: (1) 0.5 mL, (2) 0.5 tsp, (3) 1.5 mL, (4) 1.5 tab, (5) 0.25 mL, (6) 0.1 mL, (7) 1 tab, (8) 3 tab, (9) 5 tab, (10) 0.6 mL

REVIEW QUESTIONS

All questions are relevant for all medical assisting certification exams. Questions 1 through 15 are relevant for all medical administrative specialist certification exams.

1. The agency that controls who may administer and use specific drugs is the:
   A. FDA.
   B. CDC.
   C. DEA.
   D. PDR.

   Answer: **C**
   Why: The Drug Enforcement Agency (DEA) is a federal branch of the Justice Department. Their responsibilities include overseeing the prescribing, refilling, and storing of controlled substances in the medical office. The FDA is the Food and Drug Administration, the CDC is the Centers for Disease Control and Prevention, and the PDR is the *Physician's Desk Reference.*
   Review: ○ Yes   ○ No

2. Which of the following is not included in the "rights" of drug administration?
   A. Right drug
   B. Right physician
   C. Right patient
   D. Right route
   E. Right time

   Answer: **B**
   Why: The "rights" of drug administration are the procedures to be carried out each time a drug is administered to a patient to avoid medication errors. The "rights" include the right patient, drug, route, dose, technique, time, and documentation.
   Review: ○ Yes   ○ No

3. Drugs that can be purchased over the counter are classified as schedule:
   A. I.
   B. II.
   C. IV.
   D. V.

   Answer: **D**
   Why: Drugs are placed in five schedules for regulation and control. Schedule I drugs are illegal or restricted to research. Schedule II and III drugs must be used with precautions and limitations and are dispensed with a written prescription. Schedule II drugs have a high potential for abuse, and Schedule III drugs have a moderate potential for abuse. Schedule IV drugs are dispensed with written or oral prescription and have a low potential for abuse.
   Review: ○ Yes   ○ No

4. Parenteral administration of medication generally means that the medication is:
   A. administered through a suppository.
   B. injected.
   C. in liquid form to swallow.
   D. dissolved in and absorbed through the mouth.
   E. placed under the tongue.

   Answer: **B**
   Why: **Parenteral** is a term used to describe the administration of medication by injection so the medication does not pass through the gastrointestinal tract. This method includes intramuscular, subcutaneous, and intravenous routes.
   Review: ○ Yes   ○ No

5. To convert grams to milligrams:
   A. divide by 100.
   B. divide by 1,000.
   C. multiply by 100.
   D. multiply by 1,000.

   Answer: **D**
   Why: Grams is a single unit of measure; *milli* is the prefix used for 1,000; 1,000 mg = 1 g.
   Review: ○ Yes   ○ No

6. Information found on a prescription includes the following EXCEPT:
   A. patient instructions.
   B. number of doses to be dispensed.
   C. patient's date of birth.
   D. patient's name and address.
   E. number of refills.

Answer: **C**
Why: The patient's birth date is usually not included on a prescription. Most prescription forms are preprinted with the physician's name, address, phone number, and DEA number. The physician completes the prescription with the prescription date, drug requested, dose, drug form, and number of refills. There is also a space for the patient's name and address.
Review: ◯ Yes ◯ No

7. Which of the following is an appropriate task for a medical assistant or administrative medical specialist?
   A. Call a drug renewal to a pharmacy.
   B. Prescribe drugs.
   C. Authorize reorder of drugs.
   D. Dispense drugs.

Answer: **A**
Why: A medical assistant or administrative medical specialist may call in a prescription for a drug that a physician has ordered for a patient. Only a physician can prescribe and authorize the reorder or refill of drugs. Dispensing drugs is only permitted by licensed pharmacists, physicians, or other credentialed medical personnel.
Review: ◯ Yes ◯ No

8. The prescription directions "ii gtt q4h" mean:
   A. one drop every hour.
   B. one drop every 4 hours.
   C. two drops every hour.
   D. two drops every 4 hours.
   E. four drops every 4 hours.

Answer: **D**
Why: The abbreviation gtt means "drops." The Roman numeral ii means "two." "Every 4 hours" is abbreviated q4h.
Review: ◯ Yes ◯ No

9. Which of the following classifications of medication is used to control high blood pressure?
   A. Antipyretic
   B. Antiemetic
   C. Antihypertensive
   D. Antihistamine

Answer: **C**
Why: The prefix *anti* means "to work against." Hypertension is the medical term for elevated or high blood pressure. Antipyretics are used to decrease fever, antiemetics to decrease nausea, and antihistamines to decrease symptoms of allergies.
Review: ◯ Yes ◯ No

10. Of the following drugs, which one can be dispensed only with a written prescription?
   A. Valium
   B. Robitussin
   C. Tylenol
   D. Morphine
   E. Benadryl

Answer: **D**
Why: Morphine is classified as a Schedule II drug. Drugs in this category cannot be called in and require a written prescription with precautions and limitations ordered. They have a high potential for abuse.
Review: ◯ Yes ◯ No

11. The method of administration of medication under the tongue is:
   A. topical.
   B. sublingual.
   C. parenteral.
   D. subcutaneous.

Answer: **B**
Why: Sublingual means "beneath the tongue." Nitroglycerin, used to treat angina, is an example of a medication administered sublingually. It is dissolved beneath the tongue and absorbed through the mucous membranes.
Review: ◯ Yes ◯ No

12. The physician orders 300 mg of medication t.i.d. × 10 days. The medication is available in 150-mg capsules. How many capsules will the patient need to complete the course of therapy?
    A. 60
    B. 45
    C. 30
    D. 20
    E. 10

Answer: **A**
Why: The patient will need to take two capsules three times a day for 10 days. The total is 60 capsules for the entire course of therapy. The abbreviation t.i.d. means three times per day. To receive 300 mg of the medication with each dose, the patient will have to take two 150-mg capsules for each dose.
Review: ○ Yes   ○ No

13. The agency that controls the drugs that are acceptable for safe use and sale in the United States is the:
    A. DEA.
    B. AMA.
    C. FDA.
    D. CDC.

Answer: **C**
Why: The Food and Drug Administration (FDA) reviews drug applications and petitions for food additives and removes unsafe drugs from the sales market. The FDA also oversees the proper labeling of food, drugs, and cosmetics.
Review: ○ Yes   ○ No

14. The equivalent of 5 cubic centimeters^3 is:
    A. 5 mg.
    B. 5 mL.
    C. 5 cm.
    D. 5 drops.
    E. 5 g.

Answer: **B**
Why: The measurement of 1 cubic centimeter^3 is the same as 1 mL. One cubic centimeter is a square cube 1 centimeter long by 1 cm wide by 1 cm high. One milliliter of fluid will equally fill 1 cm^3 of space; therefore, 5 cm^3 equals 5 mL.
Review: ○ Yes   ○ No

15. The physician orders 2.5 mg of Compazine, IM. Available is Compazine 5 mg/mL provided in a 10-mL multidose vial. How many milliliters will you give the patient?
    A. 0.1 mL
    B. 0.25 mL
    C. 0.5 mL
    D. 1.0 mL

Answer: **C**
Why: That the medication is provided in a 10-mL multidose vial is not important when performing the calculation. This information states the total number of milliliters in the container. If there are 5 mg of Compazine in 1 mL, then to give 2.5 mg, which is one-half of 5 mg, give one-half milliliter, or 0.5 mL.
Review: ○ Yes   ○ No

16. The classification of drugs that prevent or decrease clotting is:
    A. antiemetic.
    B. antipyretic.
    C. antineoplastic.
    D. antitussive.
    E. anticoagulant.

Answer: **E**
Why: Anticoagulants are used to prevent the formation of blood clots. Antiemetics are used to inhibit nausea. Antipyretics are used to decrease fever. Antineoplastics are indicated to slow the rate of tumor growth and delay metastasis (cancer). Antitussives are used to control coughing.
Review: ○ Yes   ○ No

17. The proper angle of the needle to the skin when administering an intramuscular injection is:
    A. 30 degree.
    B. 45 degree.
    C. 60 degree.
    D. 90 degree.

Answer: **D**
Why: The needle should be at a 90 degree angle to ensure that the beveled tip of the needle is placed within the muscle. If a lesser angle is used, the medication may be deposited within the subcutaneous or fatty layer of tissue.
Review: ○ Yes   ○ No

18. The muscle used for injection in the thigh is the:
   A. gluteus maximus.
   B. gluteus medius.
   C. vastus lateralis.
   D. rectus abdominis.
   E. rectus femoris.

Answer: **C**

Why: The vastus lateralis is the large (*vastus*) muscle on the side (*lateralis*, lateral) of the thigh. This is the preferred site for injections for infants.

Review: ○ Yes   ○ No

----

19. Which of the following is proper technique when administering a tuberculin skin test?
   A. Massage the injection site to lessen the pain of the procedure.
   B. Place a bandage over the injection site.
   C. After inserting the needle beneath the skin, aspirate to ensure the needle is not in a blood vessel.
   D. Leave the injection site uncovered.

Answer: **D**

Why: Massaging or covering the site may cause the medication to be pressed into the tissues or out of the wheal, and the results, if any, will be unreliable. Aspiration is not required for an intradermal injection.

Review: ○ Yes   ○ No

----

20. The physician orders ampicillin 0.5 g. Available is ampicillin 250 mg/mL. How many milliliters will you give the patient?
   A. 0.25 mL
   B. 0.5 mL
   C. 1 mL
   D. 1.5 mL
   E. 2 mL

Answer: **E**

Why: The first step to calculate the dose is to convert grams to milligrams. 0.5 g (grams) is equal to 500 mg (1 g equals 1,000 mg). The dose ordered is 500 mg, and available is 250 mg in each milliliter. Two milliliters of this medication contains 500 mg.

Review: ○ Yes   ○ No

----

21. A subcutaneous injection is injected into:
   A. muscle tissue.
   B. dermal tissue.
   C. fatty tissue.
   D. epidermal tissue.

Answer: **C**

Why: The subcutaneous tissue lies beneath the skin or dermis. It is the fatty layer. Medications injected in this tissue are absorbed slower than those given by the intramuscular method.

Review: ○ Yes   ○ No

----

22. A solution administered through the ID method is:
   A. Keflex.
   B. penicillin.
   C. hepatitis B vaccine.
   D. tuberculin solution.
   E. Imferon.

Answer: **D**

Why: ID is the abbreviation for intradermal. This is the injection method of placing a minute amount of solution just beneath the surface of the skin, within the dermis. Tuberculin solution is used to perform tuberculosis skin testing.

Review: ○ Yes   ○ No

----

23. Imferon, an iron preparation, is administered by which method?
   A. Subcutaneous
   B. Z-track
   C. Intravenous
   D. Sublingual

Answer: **B**

Why: Z-track is an intramuscular method of injection. Iron is a medication that will cause irritation and discoloration if deposited in the subcutaneous tissue. The Z-track method requires that the skin be pulled to one side before injection. After the injection is given, the skin is released, and there is no trailing or seeping of medication into the tissues.

Review: ○ Yes   ○ No

24. A subcutaneous injection is given using which technique?
    A. 90-degree angle, 21-G needle
    B. 15-degree angle, 25-G needle
    C. 60-degree angle, 21-G needle
    D. 45-degree angle, 25-G needle
    E. 30-degree angle, 23-G needle

Answer: **D**
Why: The subcutaneous injection is administered into the fatty tissue. To avoid entering the muscle, a 45-degree angle is required. Solutions used for subcutaneous method are aqueous (watery), so they can be injected into the fatty tissue and absorbed slowly.
Review: ○ Yes   ○ No

25. The reason for aspirating before injecting a medication is to ensure that the:
    A. patient receives all the medication.
    B. injection will be deposited in the muscular tissue.
    C. needle is not in a blood vessel.
    D. injection will be less painful.

Answer: **C**
Why: Aspiration is the process of pulling back on the syringe plunger to ensure the needle is not positioned in a blood vessel. If blood appears in the syringe, the injection is discontinued and a new syringe is prepared. If the medication is injected into a blood vessel, the patient could have a serious adverse reaction to the medication. The exception is vaccine, since injection into the blood system is not harmful and may speed up immunity.
Review: ○ Yes   ○ No

26. Which medication amount is correctly stated?
    A. .5mgs.
    B. 0.5mgs.
    C. 00.5mgs.
    D. .50mgs.
    E. 1/2 mgs.

Answer: **B**
Why: To avoid medication errors, The Joint Commission requires all stand alone decimals to have a zero before the decimal mark; fractions are not commonly used when working with milligrams
Review: ○ Yes   ○ No

CRITICAL THINKING CASE REVIEW

The medical assistant in Dr. Jones office gave Ms. Anick the medication that was ordered for Mr. Ortiz. Fortunately, no harm came to the patient.

1. In addition to the medical assistant not following one of the important seven medication rights of "the right patient," she most likely did not properly identify the patient which is a safety guideline of:
    A. FDA.
    B. CDC.
    C. TJC.
    D. AMA.
    E. PDR.

Answer: **C**
Why: FDA or Food and Drug Administration has the job of assuring that the drug is safe and does not deal with the individual patient; the CDC or Centers for Disease Control and Prevention has the job of disease surveillance; the American Medical Association does not issue guidelines for drug administration for medical assistants. TJC or The Joint Commission issues patient safety guidelines, one of which is to always properly identify the patient.
Review: ○ Yes   ○ No

2. When an event that compromises safety occurs in the medical office:
   A. an incident report should be completed.
   B. the practice's attorney should be notified.
   C. the event should be reported to the local medical board.
   D. no further action is required since no harm came to the patient.

Answer: **A**

Why: An incident report should **always** be completed when issues of safety are involved (Chapter 4). These are used for trending and remediating problems either with processes or personnel and for documentation that is not appropriate in the medical record. In certain circumstances, the practice's attorney and the medical board may also be notified, but the best answer is A.
Review: ◯ Yes   ◯ No

3. If the patient decided to bring suit against the practice, it is unlikely that it would be successful since there was no:
   A. duty.
   B. dereliction of duty.
   C. direct cause.
   D. damage.
   E. diagnosis.

Answer: **D**

Why: There was a duty since Ms. Anick was a patient of the practice, and there was dereliction of the duty since the medication should not have been administered to that patient. IF Ms. Ancik had a reaction or bad outcome, it would have been a direct cause of the injection. The key is that there were no damages, and therefore, the four "Ds" (Chapter 4) could not be satisfied. "E," diagnosis, is a detractor and not one of the four "Ds."
Review: ◯ Yes   ◯ No

4. In addition to properly identifying the patient and the seven commonly accepted rights, the medical assistant learned that the error probably would have been avoided if the use of which additional right had been carried out?
   A. Right to refuse
   B. Right to know—does the patient know what is being given
   C. Right reason—know why it is being given
   D. Right to an attorney

Answer: **B**

Why: Although following "A" and "C" could have avoided the error, the most likely or best answer is "B." If the medical assistant had asked the patient if she knew why the medication was being given, the patient could not respond, which should have alerted the assistant.
Review: ◯ Yes   ◯ No

5. After the error was discovered, the first person the medical assistant should have told was the:
   A. patient.
   B. supervisor.
   C. biller to avoid a charge to the patient.
   D. coworker in case help was needed.
   E. provider.

Answer: **E**

Why: The provider should be notified first to determine if the medication may be harmful and if there is another medication that should be given to counteract it. Also, the provider should be the person to explain the error to the patient and answer any questions for potential side effects and other risks. This is compliance in disclosing errors in patient care as discussed in Chapter 16.
Review: ◯ Yes   ◯ No

CHAPTER 25

Emergency Preparedness

Review Tip:

After you complete the chapter, check your cardiopulmonary resuscitation (CPR) certification card and ensure it is current. If not, sign up for a course and bring a friend or relative. CPR is a separate certification, and the national exams contain only general questions.

The focus of this chapter is not to teach general first aid but to discuss emergency preparedness and provide an overview of recognizing and dealing with emergencies that may occur within the medical office or the community. Please note that the AAMA often refers to "emergency preparedness" as "protective practices."

Emergency preparedness or protective practices may be divided into three categories:

- The individual (patient, staff member, visitor)
- The medical office (emergency within the office such as fire or chemical exposure)
- The community (natural disaster, act of terrorism, horrific event such as a school fire)

THE INDIVIDUAL

Before proceeding, review the section on the Good Samaritan Act in Chapter 4, which discusses an individual's liability in emergency situations. No matter the location or the emergency, always ask the victim's permission before touching him or her, even though it is in the context of providing first aid. A **medical emergency** is the occurrence of a sudden injury or illness that requires immediate medical intervention. **First aid** is the immediate care rendered in an emergency until definitive or advanced care is available if needed. Being prepared is a major component in effectively dealing with emergencies that arise in the medical office. The medical office generally has guidelines, policies, and procedures for office emergencies and documentation. These should be reviewed and revised on a regular basis and followed when needed. Many of the elements of preparedness come under the roles of the medical assistant and medical administrative specialist.

ACTIVATION OF EMERGENCY MEDICAL SYSTEM

- Dial 911 (in most areas)
- Know the correct number if there is no 911 system in the area (e.g., the emergency number for some rural areas may be the police or fire department)
- Know if an alternative to 911, such as 311, is available for less urgent situations
- Have readily available the numbers for poison control center, suicide hotlines, abuse shelters, emergency food banks, and other services that may be used in an emergency
- Know the capacity of the office telephone system (e.g., can you keep a patient on the line *and* activate emergency medical system (EMS)?)
- Know when your physicians and other medical staff are on site

MEDICAL ASSISTANT AND MEDICAL ADMINISTRATIVE SPECIALIST ROLES IN EMERGENCIES

- Recognizing emergencies and responding
- Monitoring emergency supplies, equipment, and drug readiness (includes expiration dates on drugs and sterile packs; functioning of battery-operated equipment)
- Knowing the location of emergency supplies
- Restocking equipment after each use
- Maintaining up-to-date emergency phone numbers
- Keeping CPR and other first aid skills current
- Providing personal protection for self, patient, and other involved individuals
- Documenting the event and the first aid rendered
- Observing the environment for possible risks, such as frayed wiring or loose carpeting (risk management)

COMMON EMERGENCY EQUIPMENT AND SUPPLIES IN THE MEDICAL OFFICE

- Oxygen with nasal cannulas and various sizes of oxygen masks
- Various sizes of blood pressure cuffs
- Code cart containing cardiac monitor and defibrillator, emergency drugs, intravenous (IV) solutions with tubing and IV cannulas, tourniquets and tapes, bandage scissors, pen light, Ambu bag, airways, and intubation equipment per physician's preferences and training
- Automatic external defibrillator (AED)
- Personal protective equipment (PPE) (refer to Chapter 17)
- Materials for wound care: antiseptic solution, sterile dressings
- Cold packs
- Emergency childbirth delivery pack (for offices that practice obstetrics) with gloves, blankets, two Kelly clamps, cord clamp, scissors, nasal suction bulb, and plastic bag or container for placenta

RECOGNIZING EMERGENCIES

A four-pronged approach is used in recognizing medical emergencies and determining their seriousness. The first is the ability to determine an emergency exists; the second is to be sure the health-care responder or others are not in danger. Health-care personnel will then perform primary and secondary assessments.

SIGNS OF EMERGENCIES

- Respiratory distress
- Unconsciousness
- Hemorrhage
- Chest pain
- Wounds or penetrating objects
- Bone protrusions or deformities
- Skin burns
- High or low body temperatures
- Severe pain
- Abnormal skin color
- Abnormal behavior

SCENE MANAGEMENT

The guidelines here apply to the medical office in addition to other sites.

- Ensure dangers do not exist for responder (e.g., wet floor, "hot" wire)
- Remove hazard if this does not pose a danger to the responder
- Remove others in the vicinity of danger if appropriate
- Assign tasks; for example, have someone activate EMS while you are rendering first aid

PRIMARY ASSESSMENT AND TREATMENT PRIORITIES (ABCs)

- A—airway: check open airway using head-tilt/chin-lift method or jaw thrust (for suspected neck injuries) if needed
- B—breathing: ensure patient is breathing by looking for chest movement
- C—circulation: ensure patient has a pulse

SECONDARY ASSESSMENT, IF INDICATED

- Vital signs (pulse, respirations, blood pressure, temperature)
- Skin (color, temperature, degree of moisture)
- Head-to-toe observation and palpation for pain, abnormalities, and bleeding (usually done by physician, midlevel provider, or EMS personnel)
- Level of consciousness

COMMON EMERGENCIES

Common emergencies are listed, along with the first aid treatment generally administered by the medical assistant.

BURNS

Burns are tissue damage caused by exposure to heat, chemicals, or electricity. The extent of burns is estimated using the **rule of nines**, in which each body part is considered 9% of the body: the affected parts are added to determine the percentage of body burned (Fig. 25-1).

- First degree (superficial)—involves epidermis; red appearance with minimal or no edema (such as sunburn)
  - Immerse in cool water or provide cool water compresses
  - Avoid ointments or other greasy substances (e.g., butter, which is a home remedy for some cultures)·
- Second degree (partial thickness)—involves epidermis and part of dermis; blistered red appearance with edema
  - Immerse in cool (not cold) water or provide cool (not cold) compresses

FIGURE 25-1 Rule of nines. (Reprinted with permission from Hosley JB, Jones SA, Molle-Matthews EA. *Lippincott's Textbook for Medical Assistants.* Philadelphia PA: Lippincott-Raven Publishers, 1997.)

- Avoid ointments or other greasy substances
- May apply dry, sterile dressing
- Third degree (full thickness)—involves epidermis, entire dermis, and often underlying tissues; pale white or charred appearance with broken skin and edema
  - Activate EMS
  - Check ABCs
  - Use sterile gloves and other PPE if indicated
  - Cover affected areas with sterile dressings soaked in sterile saline
  - Observe for shock

SHOCK

Shock is a life-threatening condition related to inadequate oxygen supply. It is often characterized by heavy blood loss; lowered blood pressure; weak, increased pulse; cool, clammy skin; increased respiratory rate; anxiety; and agitation. The most common types of shock are as follows:

- Hypovolemic—shock resulting from hemorrhage (excessive bleeding)
  - Use PPE
  - Cover wound with sterile dressing (if possible) and apply direct pressure
  - Elevate bleeding area
  - Keep head lower than body (except in cases of head wounds)

- Apply pressure to nearest pressure point (Refer to Fig. 18-1) between bleeding and heart if bleeding does not stop
- Keep patient warm

■ Anaphylactic (anaphylaxis)—shock caused by a severe allergic reaction that results in respiratory distress and, in some instances, cardiac arrest
  - Activate EMS
  - Check ABCs
  - Remove allergen if possible
  - Keep patient warm
  - Prepare to administer medication such as epinephrine per physician or mid-level provider order

■ Septic—shock caused by an overwhelming infection affecting major body systems
  - Activate EMS
  - Check ABCs

■ Cardiogenic—shock caused by impaired cardiac function; first aid is the same as for septic shock

■ Neurogenic—shock caused by trauma or other insult (e.g., toxin) to the nervous system
  - Activate EMS
  - Check ABCs
  - Immobilize head for spinal injury
  - Keep patient warm
  - Prepare to assist with administration of antitoxin if known and available

■ Insulin (see "Diabetic Emergencies")

DIABETIC EMERGENCIES

Box 25-1 contains a mnemonic to help differentiate between insulin shock and diabetic coma.

■ Insulin shock or ketoacidosis—severe hypoglycemia in diabetic patients, characterized by rapid heart rate; cold, clammy skin; and confusion
  - Administer sugar (e.g., Insta-Glucose, a glucose gel rapidly absorbed through oral mucosa)
  - Keep patient quiet and at rest

■ Diabetic coma—severe hyperglycemia in diabetic patients, characterized by rapid respirations; warm, dry skin; thirst; "fruity" breath (sometimes mistaken for alcohol); and confusion
  - Activate EMS

BOX 25-1

Mnemonic to help differentiate between diabetic coma and insulin shock

Hot and dry; blood glucose high (diabetic coma)
Cold and clammy; needs some candy (insulin shock)

- Prepare to bring the insulin and appropriate needle and syringe or administer insulin with the physician's order if within the scope of practice in your state

CARDIAC EMERGENCIES

Myocardial infarction (MI, heart attack) is the most common and is necrosis of the cardiac muscle caused by blockage in the coronary artery. It is characterized by chest, left arm, or jaw pain; sweating; rapid respirations; and often nausea and vomiting.

■ Activate EMS
■ Check ABCs if needed
■ Position code cart and AED
■ Initiate cardiac monitor
■ Take vital signs
■ Keep patient calm
■ Prepare to assist with administration of oxygen and other drugs with physician's order

CEREBROVASCULAR ACCIDENT

A **cerebrovascular accident** (CVA, stroke) is the occlusion of a blood vessel or vessels in the brain or hemorrhage in the brain characterized by one or more of the following symptoms: weakness, paralysis of one or more areas, dysphasia or aphasia, and confusion.

■ Activate EMS
■ Check ABCs, if needed
■ Take vital signs
■ Keep patient calm
■ Prepare to assist with administration of oxygen with physician's order

RESPIRATORY EMERGENCIES

Respiratory emergencies involve the impairment or absence of breathing.

■ Respiratory arrest—total absence of breathing
  - Activate EMS
  - Check ABCs
  - Head-tilt/chin-lift maneuver (Fig. 25-2)
  - Support breathing by health-care provider "breathing" for victim (CPR guidelines) or using an Ambu bag
  - Prepare for cardiac arrest (have code cart, AED, emergency drugs, and cardiac monitor ready; begin chest compressions if pulse/heartbeat stops); refer to algorithm in Figure 25-3

■ Asthma—inflammatory lung disease characterized by difficulty breathing caused by airway obstruction
  - Check ABCs
  - Maintain sitting position if conscious

FIGURE 25-2 Lateral view for head-tilt/chin-lift maneuver for airway management and CPR.

- Keep patient calm
- Assist patient with his or her inhaler if available
- Prepare to initiate small-volume nebulizer with physician order
- Monitor oxygen saturation by using a pulse oximeter

■ Hyperventilation—increased ventilation leading to decreased carbon dioxide, dizziness, and possible unconsciousness; usually stress-induced

- Keep patient calm
- Seal paper bag over patient's mouth and nose
- Assist patient with taking slow, deep breaths into paper bag

■ Choking—laryngospasms, usually caused by obstruction of the airway with a foreign object, such as food

- Allow patient to cough
- Use Heimlich maneuver if coughing, speaking, or breathing ceases (Fig. 25-4)
  - Standing—get behind victim; rescuer's arms come around to below victim's xiphoid process;

FIGURE 25-3 Resuscitation algorithm.

FIGURE 25-4 Heimlich maneuver.

rescuer makes fist with dominant hand and administers inward and upward thrusts until foreign object is expelled

- Lying—if patient loses consciousness, lower him or her to floor, check mouth for foreign objects and, if seen, sweep objects out with fingers; rescuer kneels beside patient, places closed dominant hand below xiphoid process, and administers inward and upward abdominal thrusts until foreign object is expelled

SEIZURES

A **seizure**, or **convulsion**, is an abnormal generalized series of involuntary muscle contraction and relaxation. There are many causes, including brain injury or high fever.

- Activate EMS
- Lower patient to floor
- Protect from injury by furniture or other obstacles
- Loosen tight clothing
- Log roll patient if he or she is vomiting
- Avoid restricting patient or putting *anything* in patient's mouth
- Assist with breathing if necessary when seizure is over

SYNCOPE

Syncope, also called *fainting* or *swooning*, is transient unconsciousness, usually caused by a sudden decrease in blood pressure or oxygen. **Do not confuse syncope and vertigo which is a specific kind of dizziness and is a symptom not a condition.**

- Assist the patient in lying down or sitting with head to knees
- Loosen tight clothing
- Use ammonia capsule at least 6 inches from nose and avoiding eyes (office policy permitting)
- Place cool cloth on forehead

COMMON INJURIES

- Wounds (always use PPE with open wounds)
  - Contusion (bruise)—a closed wound usually caused by blunt trauma
    - Apply ice pack or cold compress
    - Observe for increased swelling
  - Abrasion—an open wound resulting from scraping off of skin layer(s) by trauma; may or may not produce bleeding
    - Cleanse with soap and water or antiseptic
    - Apply sterile dressing if needed
    - Determine patient's tetanus immunization status
  - Avulsion—an open wound caused by forceful tearing away of skin from bony structure by trauma, sometimes leaving a skin flap and causing excessive bleeding
    - Replace skin flap if present
    - Treat the same as an abrasion
  - Laceration—a jagged cut into the body tissue
    - Treat the same as an abrasion
    - May require sutures or Steri-Strips
  - Puncture—an open wound caused by an object piercing the skin (first aid for bites and stings is the same as punctures and abrasions)
    - Treat the same as an abrasion
  - Puncture with fixed penetrating object
    - Activate EMS
    - Leave object imbedded
    - Stabilize object to prevent movement
  - Traumatic amputation—the removal of a body part by traumatic event
    - Treat the same as an avulsion
    - Wrap amputated part in sterile moist dressing and transport with patient (do not place on ice)
- Fracture—broken bones; see Figure 6-10, "Types of fractures," in Chapter 6

- Open fracture—broken bone that protrudes through skin
  - Immobilize with a splint
  - Cover wound with sterile dressing
  - Arrange transport to hospital
- Closed fracture—broken bone without an open wound
  - Immobilize with a splint
  - Apply ice pack or cold compress
  - Elevate; sling may be used to elevate and support hand and lower arm; tie knot off to the side of the neck, avoiding spine
- Joint dislocation—the ends of two or more bones that normally meet are forced from their normal positions, usually by a trauma
  - Do not move the affected bones
  - Seek medical care
  - Splint in place if care is not available within a reasonable time
  - Place ice wrapped in cloth to prevent swelling
- Sprain—stretching or tearing of a ligament caused by a wrench or twist; most common at the ankle
- Strain—stretching or tearing of a tendon; most common in back or hamstring
  - First aid is the same for sprain and strain **RICE**.
    - Rest
    - Ice
    - Compress (ace bandage)
    - Elevate
- Concussion or mild head injury (MHI) or mild traumatic brain injury (MTBI) usually caused by some sort of blow to the head with temporary symptoms such as headache, difficulty concentrating, sometimes unconsciousness, temporary memory loss, drowsiness
  - Call EMS if unconscious or very drowsy, seizure, vomiting, unequal pupils, confusion or agitation, one-sided body weakness, slurred speech, neck pain
  - If symptoms to activate EMS are absent, have person stop activity and remain at rest
  - Apply ice wrapped in cloth to injured area
  - If possible have someone stay with person and monitor level of consciousness for 24 hours

POISONINGS AND BITES

- **Poisoning** the injection, respiration, or ingestion of a toxic substance (may be natural or chemical).
  - Remove substance or victim from the area where the substance is while protecting rescuer (PPE)

- Check ABCs
- Call poison control center for specific instructions
- Do not induce vomiting or administer ipecac unless instructed to do so by poison control center or provider
- **Animal bites**
  - Activate EMS if the victim is seriously wounded or severe or steady bleeding
  - Notify the local health department or animal control immediately if rabies vaccine status of the animal (domestic or wild) is not up to date or unknown
  - Clean with soap and warm water; rinse for several minutes
  - Apply antibiotic cream and cover with sterile dressing
  - Assure the victim's tetanus vaccine is up to date
  - Follow up with health-care provider
- **Insect bite (severe)**
  - Activate EMS for the following:
    - Nausea
    - Facial swelling
    - Difficulty breathing
    - Nausea, vomiting, cramps
    - Decrease in blood pressure and circulation (shock)
    - Rapid heart rate
    - Hives
    - Dizziness, faintness
  - Monitor ABCs and initiate CPR if necessary
  - Check patient for allergy bracelet and epinephrine injector (EpiPen) and administer per directions
- **Insect bite (mild)**
  - Remove the stinker if appropriate
  - Apply ice wrapped in cloth
  - Apply a topical cream to ease pain or itch
  - Call poison control with concerns such as for scorpion bite

EXTREME TEMPERATURE EMERGENCIES

- Hyperthermia—abnormally high body temperature (e.g., heat exhaustion and heat stroke [most serious])
  - Remove from heat source
  - Check ABCs and activate EMS for heat stroke
  - Cool body with wet cloths
  - Slowly administer cool liquids if patient is alert
- Hypothermia—abnormally low body temperature
  - Check ABCs
  - Activate EMS

- Remove any wet clothing
- Warm with blankets
- Slowly administer warm liquids if patient is alert (no alcoholic beverages)

■ Frostbite—freezing of body parts; usually affects fingers, toes, ears, and nose
- Gently wrap affected part in warm material, such as a blanket
- Do not submerge in water or other liquid or rub
- Transport to hospital

THE MEDICAL OFFICE

Risk management in Chapter 4 is also a part of medical office safety such as observing for frayed electrical cords. In addition to common hazards, the medical office is at risk for emergencies and safety hazards encompassing more than a single person such as fire or chemical or infectious disease exposures (refer to Chapter 17). The H1N1 influenza in 2009 was an example. Common Occupational Safety and Health Administration (OSHA), The Joint Commission and state-specific emergency preparedness guidelines recommend that facilities have the following:

■ An **exposure-control plan** that describes personnel protective equipment (PPE) and other safety engineering devices and processes; it provides instructions of what an employee should do if an exposure occurs. The plan should be reviewed annually and contain the following:
- Definitions such as biohazardous waste
- Responsibilities
- Availability of recommended immunizations
- Availability and disposal mechanisms of PPE and safety engineering devices
- Procedures to follow for prevention and exposures
- Training guidelines
- Record-keeping and reporting

■ Adequate PPE and safety engineering devices
■ Contract for disposal of biohazardous material
■ Safety Data Sheets (SDS), formerly called Material Data Sheets (MSDS)
■ Common safety features
- Fire extinguishers; serviced annually; standard acronym for use PASS
  ○ **P**—pull the pin
  ○ **A**—aim the nozzle at the base of the fire
  ○ **S**—squeeze the trigger while keeping the extinguisher upright
  ○ **S**—sweep the area using the nozzle and covering the fire with the extinguisher material
- Proper labeling for safety equipment such as biohazardous waste material and eyewash stations (Fig. 25-5)
- Evacuation plan
  ○ Establish and post evacuation routes
  ○ Keep hallways and stairways unobstructed at all times
  ○ Move those closest to danger first
  ○ Initiate alarm
  ○ Move those requiring the most assistance last unless in immediate danger
  ○ Establish area to store mobility-assistive devices such as wheelchairs
  ○ Establish the chain of command; specifically who is in charge
  ○ Avoid delaying to "grab" valuables
  ○ Designate responsibility for moving or shutting down flammable substances such as oxygen unless it places the person in danger
  ○ Designate a preestablished assembly place
  ○ Designate who leaves last and assures the facility is empty
  ○ Establish a means of accounting for all staff, patients, and visitors

Automatic Electronic Defibrilator

Emergency Eye Wash

Emergency Shower

Fire Extinguisher

Biohazard Material

FIGURE 25-5 Examples of standard safety signs and symbols.

○ Do not return until instructed by the appropriate emergency services personnel

○ Conduct evacuation drills (frequency of drills may be required by local authorities; for example, some cities require evacuation in high-rise buildings quarterly)

- Clearly marked and lighted exits

THE COMMUNITY

Health-care providers often feel a responsibility to the community in times of disaster; the "community" may be local, national, or global. Many accrediting bodies such as The Joint Commission require emergency preparedness. This section addresses considerations for response to a local disaster. The medical assistant and medical administrative assistant may be involved in community emergency preparedness on two fronts: within the medical facility and directly within the community emergency preparedness system as a volunteer.

THE MEDICAL FACILITY RESPONSE

The medical facility may agree to take incoming "**walking wounded**" persons who have been triaged at a disaster command center, have minor injuries, and are capable of walking. It requires previous coordination and agreements with the local emergency preparedness authorities and the hospital or other facilities that provide a higher level of care. These agreements are updated at specified intervals. Generally, a medical office emergency preparedness committee is appointed. The committee develops and implements an emergency preparedness plan that, at a minimum, includes the following:

- Designation of roles such as triage officer, area coordinators, recorders, and runners

- Designation of medical office areas such as triage, holding, and treatment

- Readiness of emergency supplies such as PPE, dressings, splints, cots, and blankets; these should be stored and used only for disasters, not for general operation, and checked on a regular basis

- Preassembled "to-go box" with pens, pads, tape, clips, vests or large name tags identifying staff roles, and emergency charts with specially designed emergency forms (to date, these forms are hard copy, not electronic, and move with the patient)

- Staff training and drills (usually semi-annually and coordinated by the local emergency preparedness agency or hospital)

- Response call list for staff if a disaster occurs after hours

- Ancillary services and needs such as rapidly accessing more doses of tetanus toxoid, nearby child care for victims and staff, transport to a facility for higher level of care if needed

- Plan evaluation mechanism

INDIVIDUAL COMMITMENT

Health-care providers, including medical assistants and medical administrative specialists, may volunteer, as individuals, with the local emergency preparedness authority or affiliates such as the local department of health to respond to a disaster or emergency. An example is pandemic flu requiring rapid mass immunization. For the individual volunteer, this usually involves the following:

- Completion of an application

- Verification of credentials and requirements (may include specific immunizations and fingerprinting or other clearance for working with vulnerable populations)

- Training (may be conducted online)

This community involvement is not covered by the Good Samaritan Act. The volunteer should check with the sponsoring agency to assure inclusion in their liability coverage.

TERMS

EMERGENCY PREPAREDNESS REVIEW

The following list reviews the terms discussed in this chapter and other important terms that you may see on the exam.

ABCs (airway, breathing, circulation) primary assessment in emergencies to determine whether the patient's airway is open, breathing is occurring, and blood is appropriately circulating

abrasion open wound resulting in scraping off of skin layer(s) by trauma; may or may not produce bleeding

anaphylaxis shock caused by a severe allergic reaction that results in respiratory distress and, in some instances, cardiac arrest

avulsion open wound caused by forceful tearing away of skin from bony structure by trauma, sometimes leaving a skin flap and causing excessive bleeding

burns tissue damage from exposure to heat, chemicals, or electricity

cardiopulmonary resuscitation (CPR) a standardized approach to providing first aid in a situation in which the victim is not breathing and the heart may have stopped beating

contusion (bruise) closed wound usually caused by blunt trauma

epistaxis nosebleed

exposure-control plan plan that describes personnel protective equipment (PPE) and other safety engineering devices and processes; it provides instructions of what an employee should do if an exposure occurs

first aid the immediate care rendered in a medical emergency until definitive or advanced care is available

hemorrhage excessive bleeding that may result in hypovolemic shock

hyperglycemia abnormally high blood glucose level

hyperthermia abnormally high body temperature (e.g., heat exhaustion and heat stroke [most serious])

hypoglycemia abnormally low blood glucose level

hypothermia abnormally low body temperature

laceration straight or jagged cut into the body tissue

medical emergency the occurrence of a sudden injury or illness that requires immediate medical intervention

PASS pull, aim, squeeze, sweep; acronym for using a fire extinguisher

poisoning the injection, respiration, or ingestion of a toxic substance (may be natural or chemical)

rule of nines formula used to determine extent of the body burned; each body part is considered 9% of the body; the affected parts are added to determine the percentage of body burned

seizure convulsion generalized series of involuntary muscle contractions

shock life-threatening condition related to inadequate oxygen supply and often characterized by heavy blood loss; lowered blood pressure; weak, increased pulse; cool, clammy skin; increased respiratory rate; anxiety; and agitation

sprain stretching or tearing of a ligament caused by a wrench or twist

strain stretching or tearing of a tendon or muscle

syncope transient unconsciousness, usually caused by a sudden decrease in blood pressure or oxygen; also called *fainting* or *swooning*

vertigo a specific kind of dizziness and a symptom, not a condition

walking wounded persons in a disaster who have been triaged at a command center of the community disaster, have minor injuries, and are capable of walking.

REVIEW QUESTIONS

All questions are relevant for all medical assisting and medical administrative specialist certification exams.

1. The type of shock caused by severe allergic reaction is:
   A. traumatic.
   B. septic.
   C. cardiogenic.
   D. anaphylactic.

   Answer: **D**
   Why: Anaphylactic shock is an immediate type of allergic reaction resulting from hypersensitivity to an antigen. Substances may include drugs, vaccines, certain foods, serum and allergen extracts, insect venom, or chemical products such as latex.
   Review: ○ Yes   ○ No

2. The type of soft tissue injury that is a closed wound occurring from blunt trauma to the body is a(n):
   A. abrasion.
   B. avulsion.
   C. contusion.
   D. laceration.
   E. puncture.

   Answer: **C**
   Why: Abrasions, avulsions, lacerations, and punctures are all types of open wounds. A contusion is a closed wound that appears as a bruise on the skin. Blood collects under the skin and causes the discoloration.
   Review: ○ Yes   ○ No

3. The type of fracture that is common in children and is a partial or incomplete break in the bone is:
   A. comminuted.
   B. greenstick.
   C. open.
   D. spiral.

   Answer: **B**
   Why: A greenstick fracture is named because the bone breaks like a green branch, only bending and causing a few of the fibers to separate. It is not an open or compound fracture. A spiral fracture is caused by the twisting of a bone.
   Review: ○ Yes   ○ No

4. To control bleeding or hemorrhage, you should initially:
   A. place ice over the wound.
   B. apply direct pressure.
   C. apply a tourniquet above the injury.
   D. immobilize the body part.
   E. place the bleeding body part lower than the victim's heart.

   Answer: **B**
   Why: Application of direct pressure over the wound will stop hemorrhage in most cases. Use a tourniquet as a last resort if direct pressure does not stop the bleeding or if the wound is too large to apply direct pressure. If possible, the body part that is bleeding should be elevated higher than the victim's heart.
   Review: ○ Yes   ○ No

5. The ABCs of CPR include management of:
   A. airway, breathing, circulation.
   B. assessment, breathing, compressions.
   C. alertness, bleeding, circulation.
   D. airway, bleeding, circulation.

   Answer: **A**
   Why: The ABCs of CPR include an assessment of the major systems of the body that can result in life-threatening situations. First, check the airway to make sure it is open and unobstructed. Second, if the airway is open, ensure that the victim is breathing. Third, determine that the victim's heart is pumping and proper circulation is taking place in the body. This is important to deliver oxygen to the vital body organs.
   Review: ○ Yes   ○ No

6. The medical term used to describe a victim who has fainted is:
   A. epistaxis.
   B. shock.
   C. anaphylaxis.
   D. febrile.
   E. syncope.

Answer: **E**
Why: Syncope is usually caused by a sudden fall in blood pressure or loss of oxygen to the brain resulting in loss of consciousness.
Review: ○ Yes ○ No

7. A stroke is also known as:
   A. CVD.
   B. CVA.
   C. CHF.
   D. COPD.

Answer: **B**
Why: The abbreviation CVA means cerebrovascular accident; this occurs when there is damage in the blood vessels in the brain, blocking circulation to that part of the brain. Blockage can be caused by a thrombus (blood clot) or embolus (any other abnormal particle). CVD means cardiovascular disease, CHF means congestive heart failure, and COPD means chronic obstructive pulmonary disease.
Review: ○ Yes ○ No

8. Another term for a heart attack is:
   A. cardiovascular disease.
   B. coronary artery disease.
   C. myocardial infarction.
   D. congestive heart failure.
   E. cardiogenic shock.

Answer: **C**
Why: Myocardial infarction means the myocardium, or heart muscle, has experienced damage because of blocked arteries. The blockage is usually the result of plaque buildup in the vessels.
Review: ○ Yes ○ No

9. The treatment of third-degree burns includes:
   A. immersing body part in cold water.
   B. applying an ice pack to the affected part.
   C. removing any blisters that form.
   D. covering the victim and notifying EMS.

Answer: **D**
Why: Third-degree burns are the most invasive type of burn, involving the epidermis, the entire dermis, and sometimes subcutaneous tissue, muscle, and bone. Treatment includes covering the victim with a blanket to conserve warmth and transporting for further treatment, including management of shock.
Review: ○ Yes ○ No

10. Treatment of a victim experiencing convulsions includes the following EXCEPT:
    A. placing the victim on the floor.
    B. providing privacy to the victim.
    C. clearing nearby objects.
    D. not restraining the victim.
    E. placing an airway in the mouth.

Answer: **E**
Why: Nothing should be placed in the victim's mouth during seizure activity. The object may break teeth or obstruct the airway.
Review: ○ Yes ○ No

11. In some cases of poisoning, it is necessary to induce vomiting. The agent used is:
    A. iodine.
    B. ipecac.
    C. adrenalin.
    D. epinephrine.

Answer: **B**
Why: Syrup of ipecac is used to induce vomiting when the victim has ingested a poison that is noncorrosive. It is used because of the emetic (vomit-inducing) effect it has.
Review: ○ Yes ○ No

12. The type of shock caused from bacterial infection is:
A. anaphylactic.
B. cardiogenic.
C. psychogenic.
D. septic.
E. hypovolemic.

Answer: **D**
Why: Sepsis is a condition of something being dirty or unclean. Septic shock is caused from bacteria invading the body and causing a systemic infection, which leads to septicemia, or blood poisoning. The patient will ultimately go into shock.
Review: ◯ Yes   ◯ No

13. A victim experiencing a body temperature below 95°F is:
A. hypothermic.
B. hyperthermic.
C. febrile.
D. hypovolemic.

Answer: **A**
Why: Hypothermia is an abnormally low body temperature. The external environment can lead to hypothermia. Treatment of hypothermia is internal warming of the body.
Review: ◯ Yes   ◯ No

14. Which of the following is a sign or symptom of shock?
A. Warm skin
B. Slow pulse
C. High blood pressure
D. Pale skin
E. Slow respiration

Answer: **D**
Why: Signs of shock include cool, clammy skin, low blood pressure, increased respiratory rate, and rapid pulse. The skin is pale and may appear cyanotic (a blue or purplish coloration) because of decreased oxygen of the blood.
Review: ◯ Yes   ◯ No

15. Characteristics of a first-degree burn include:
A. blistered skin.
B. charred skin.
C. reddened skin.
D. edema of the skin.

Answer: **C**
Why: First-degree burns are the least serious type of burn. Sunburn is an example of a first-degree burn. The skin is only reddened, with no blisters or broken skin.
Review: ◯ Yes   ◯ No

16. The type of soft tissue injury that causes a jagged wound that bleeds is a(n):
A. abrasion.
B. contusion.
C. puncture.
D. hematoma.
E. laceration.

Answer: **E**
Why: A laceration results from tearing of tissues partly or completely. Lacerations are frequently caused by broken glass or metal objects.
Review: ◯ Yes   ◯ No

17. Diabetic coma is caused by:
A. overproduction of insulin.
B. low blood glucose level.
C. lack of insulin.
D. normal glucose with high insulin level.

Answer: **C**
Why: Diabetic coma results from a lack of insulin causing high blood glucose levels, which results in severe acidosis. A patient with low blood glucose could be in insulin shock, which is the opposite of diabetic coma.
Review: ◯ Yes   ◯ No

18. To control bleeding from a laceration of the palm of the hand, direct pressure should be placed over the:
A. subclavian artery.
B. brachial artery.
C. medial artery.
D. radial artery.
E. cephalic artery.

Answer: **D**
Why: To control bleeding, direct pressure should be placed over the artery closest to the injury and between the injury and the heart.
Review: ○ Yes   ○ No

19. To transport a victim with a compound fracture, it is important to:
A. apply a splint to the limb without repositioning the limb.
B. straighten the limb and apply a splint.
C. wrap the extremity with an elastic bandage.
D. place the fractured bone in alignment and apply an elastic bandage.

Answer: **A**
Why: A compound fracture is a break in the bone with the bone protruding through broken skin. This type of fracture is to be managed without realigning, repositioning, or moving the fractured bone. Apply a splint to the limb in the position of the fracture and seek medical care.
Review: ○ Yes   ○ No

20. When applying a triangular sling to support an injured arm, it is important to do all the following EXCEPT:
A. tie the sling at the neck off to the side of the spine to avoid nerve injury.
B. elevate the hand slightly to promote better circulation in the hand.
C. instruct the patient how to reapply the sling if removed.
D. secure the sling at the elbow to better support the injured limb.
E. position the hand lower than the level of the heart to avoid accumulation of fluid in the extremity.

Answer: **E**
Why: A triangular sling is used in first aid to immobilize an injured limb. If used to support an injured arm, the sling must be applied so the hand is slightly elevated to encourage good circulation and avoid accumulation of fluid in the extremity. If the hand is lower than the heart, edema can develop in the limb and cause further injury or pain.
Review: ○ Yes   ○ No

21. First aid treatment for a puncture wound with a fixed penetrating object includes the following EXCEPT:
A. removing the object if it is still imbedded in the body.
B. activating EMS.
C. applying a sterile dressing around the puncture site.
D. keeping the victim calm.

Answer: **A**
Why: It is important not to remove the imbedded object but to leave it, stabilize it, and transport the victim to an emergency medical facility for treatment. If the object is removed, further damage may occur to surrounding tissue. Hemorrhage may also be initiated if the object is removed and a blood vessel is opened.
Review: ○ Yes   ○ No

22. The type of wound that results from scraping off layer(s) of skin is a(n):
A. bruise.
B. laceration.
C. avulsion.
D. abrasion.
E. contusion.

Answer: **D**
Why: An abrasion is described as a rubbing away of a surface. An example is a skinned knee.
Review: ○ Yes   ○ No

23. The emergency treatment for a conscious patient with hypoglycemia is to:
  A. monitor the patient and eventually he or she will recover after the body has produced more insulin.
  B. give the patient some form of sugar by mouth after you have notified and received instructions from the physician or EMS.
  C. give an insulin injection immediately.
  D. immediately transport the victim to his or her own physician's office for treatment.

Answer: **B**
Why: If the patient is conscious, you can give sugar by mouth, but you should always contact the physician or EMS for instructions for treatment. If a victim is unconscious, you will never give anything by mouth. If insulin is injected into a patient with a low blood glucose level (hypoglycemia), the blood glucose level will drop even lower. If it is necessary to transport the patient, use the closest emergency medical facility available, because the victim's medical provider may be too far away.
Review: ◯ Yes ◯ No

24. Which of the following is a fracture of the radius bone at the wrist?
  A. Compound
  B. Closed
  C. Colles
  D. Greenstick
  E. Spiral

Answer: **C**
Why: A compound fracture occurs when the bone is broken and punctures through the skin. A closed fracture is a fracture of the bone without puncture of the skin. A greenstick is a partial or incomplete fracture of a bone, and a spiral fracture is caused from twisting of a bone. All of these fractures are not specific to a certain bone of the body, but a Colles fracture always involves the radial bone at the wrist.
Review: ◯ Yes ◯ No

25. It is necessary to perform the Heimlich maneuver if:
  A. the victim is coughing.
  B. the victim says he or she is choking.
  C. the victim is conscious but cannot speak or cough.
  D. the victim becomes unconscious.

Answer: **C**
Why: The Heimlich maneuver is performed to dislodge an object that is obstructing the airway. It is performed when a person is conscious but cannot speak or cough. If he or she can speak or cough, there is an airway or at least a partial airway open and the object may dislodge by itself with enough coughing. The universal sign for choking is a person who is unable to talk or cough and is clutching his or her throat.
Review: ◯ Yes ◯ No

26. The acronym PASS for using a fire extinguisher means:
  A. point, assess, squeeze, and squirt.
  B. pin, aim, squirt, and sweep.
  C. pull, aim, squeeze, and sweep.
  D. point, assess, squeeze, and sweep.
  E. pull, assert, squirt, and stop.

Answer: **C**
Why: Pull the pin, aim the extinguisher, squeeze the trigger, and sweep the fire is the process for using a fire extinguisher that is correct and has become a standard through common usage.
Review: ◯ Yes ◯ No

27. Fire extinguishers should be serviced:
  A. monthly.
  B. quarterly.
  C. semi-annually.
  D. annually.

Answer: **D**
Why: Annually is the recommendation from the National Fire Protection Association unless in a "severe environment" such as a chemistry laboratory.
Review: ◯ Yes ◯ No

28. Exposure-control plan guidelines are recommended by:
   A. SDS.
   B. OSHA.
   C. EEOC.
   D. ADA.
   E. HIPAA.

Answer: **B**
Why: OSHA is the Occupational Safety and Health Administration under which safety in the workplace falls. SDS are safety data sheets and provide information related to chemicals; EEOC is the Equal Employment Opportunity Commission and addresses discrimination in the workplace; the Americans with Disabilities Act (ADA) addresses equal accommodations for people with special needs, and the Healthcare Insurance Portability and Accountability Act (HIPAA) involves confidentiality in health care.
Review: ◯ Yes   ◯ No

29. An element of evacuation of a facility is to:
   A. evacuate those closest to danger first.
   B. take valuables with you.
   C. avoid using wheelchairs or other mobility devices.
   D. return as often as possible to assist.

Answer: **A**
Why: To prevent the most harm, you would evacuate those closest to the danger first. You should not take anything with you, and you would want to use mobility devices to assist with the evacuation of persons with mobility limitations. You should not return to a facility that is in the process of evacuation. You place yourself and emergency responders in danger.
Review: ◯ Yes   ◯ No

30. An exposure-control plan would include:
   A. fire extinguisher servicing.
   B. the evacuation route.
   C. first aid for closed fractures.
   D. storage of mobility devices.
   E. recommended immunizations.

Answer: **E**
Why: The exposure control plan describes personnel protective equipment (PPE) and other safety engineering devices and processes. Recommended immunizations will protect an employee from specific blood-borne diseases and are included in the OSHA guidelines. Fire extinguisher servicing, mobility device storage, and an evacuation route are safety issues that do not fall under exposure control. First aid is not part of an exposure plan with the exception of how employees should protect themselves and others from the spread of pathogens.
Review: ◯ Yes   ◯ No

CRITICAL THINKING CASE REVIEW

The All Care Community Health Center is building a larger facility very close to the current one. During the construction, scaffolding collapses with several workers on it. The sound can be heard in the community health center, the medical administrative specialist notifies the Emergency Medical System and other staff members rush out to help. Fortunately, EMS responds within ten minutes.

1. When the staff from All Care arrived on the scene, the first thing was to:
   A. Check the injured for the ABCs;
   B. Assure that they and others were save from any additional harm;
   C. Put on PPE;
   D. Apply direct pressure to any injuries with severe bleeding.

Answer: **B**
Why: In any type of emergency the first response is to survey the scene to assure there are no hazards for rescuers or others on the scene. In this case, it may be the danger of more scaffolding or other material falling on rescuers or victims.
Review: ◯ Yes   ◯ No

2. One of the victims has a bone protruding from above the knee and the wound is bleeding profusely. One of the medical assistants always keeps gloves in her pocket and the physician instructs her to put them on and place pressure at the pressure point located at which pulse pressure point?
   A. Radial
   B. Brachial
   C. Femoral
   D. Patellar
   E. Popliteal

Answer: **C**
Why: The radial and brachial pulses are located in the arms; the patellar and popliteal are below the break and pressure would not stop bleeding above the break. The femoral is above the break and is the correct answer (Chapter 18).
Review: ○ Yes   ○ No

3. If the bleeding continued the victim would most likely experience:
   A. Hypovolemia
   B. Hypothermia
   C. Hyperthermia
   D. Hypertension

Answer: **A**
Why: Hypovolemia is a type of shock caused by extensive blood loss. Hypothermia is a condition caused by cold; hyperthermia is a condition caused by heat and hypertension is a condition caused by high blood pressure. With severe bleeding the blood pressure decreases not increases and results in hyovolemia.
Review: ○ Yes   ○ No

4. One of the victims is not breathing and his heart stopped. The physician begins CPR and instructs the medical assistant to go back to the community health center for the:
   A. IV solution and cardiac medications
   B. Cardiac monitor and AED
   C. Phone number of the cardiologist
   D. Stretcher
   E. Ambu-bag and AED

Answer: **E**
Why: ABCs are the priority for life support; the ambu-bag helps to deliver fuller and more efficient breaths than a rescuer and is less exhausting for the rescuer. The AED also acts as a cardiac monitor and will deliver life-saving defibrillation if indicated.
Review: ○ Yes   ○ No

5. This type of emergency situation is:
   A. Considered a medical office emergency since the building was a medical office;
   B. Covered under the Good Samaritan Act;
   C. Not covered under the Good Samaritan Act;
   D. An example of an evacuation plan.

Answer: **B**
Why: It was not part of the jobs of the All Care Community Health Center staff to respond to this accident and they were not required to provide aid. It would have been the same as if they were passing by when the accident occurred and they stopped to render aid. Therefore, the staff was covered by the Good Samaritan Act (Chapter 4)
Review: ○ Yes   ○ No

Exam Preparation

CHAPTER

26

Certification Exam Day Advice

Here are a few simple strategies to help relieve the stress of exam day and increase your preparedness. Read them before taking the practice exam.

- Do not cram or study the night before.
- Do what works for you to get a good night's rest.
- Know the exact location of the exam site, including the room (do not guess; consider a trip to the site before exam day).
- Know the parking situation at the testing center.
- Know the intensity of the traffic for the route and for the time of day of the exam and allow plenty of time to get there.
- Place your exam acceptance letter or permit, photo identification, and other instructions where you will not forget them.
- Wear layered clothes; exam rooms may be cold or hot regardless of the outside temperature.
- Eat a meal or snack that contains protein 30 to 60 minutes before the exam.

ADVICE FOR TAKING THE EXAM

- *Read* the exam instructions carefully; if you are taking the computerized version, know how to get back to answer questions you have not completed. DO NOT forget to *submit* the exam at the end.

- *Guess* if you do not know an answer. The national exams do not penalize for guessing.

- *Review* the strategies for solving multiple-choice questions found in Chapter 1.

Best wishes and remember the words of Sara Henderson, a writer and outpost manager in the Australian outback: *All the strength you need to achieve anything is within you!*

Practice Exam

This timed exam is your opportunity to take a practice exam within a specific period. This will help determine your readiness to sit for the actual exam. Follow these instructions carefully and then proceed with the exam.

1. There are 100 questions and you have 1 hour to complete the practice exam. Set a timer or have someone time the exam for you. Be honest and stop the exam when the hour is completed. Unanswered questions are counted as wrong answers.

2. Use the answer sheet provided. You may photocopy the sheet so you can retake the exam.

3. Do not look at the answer key until you have completed the exam; then compare your answers with the answer key.

4. Choose a quiet, comfortable place to take the exam. Make sure others are aware that you are taking the practice exam so they will not interrupt you.

PRACTICE EXAM—CMA (AAMA)

1. Pathogens that thrive in the absence of oxygen are called:
   A. antitoxins.
   B. anaerobes.
   C. spores.
   D. aerobes.
   E. deoxygenators.

2. A communicable disease that does not have to be reported to the county health department is:
   A. tuberculosis.
   B. streptococcus.
   C. rubella.
   D. syphilis.
   E. rabies.

3. The term **esophagogastritis** means inflammation of the:
   A. larynx and pharynx.
   B. stomach and small intestine.
   C. small intestine and stomach.
   D. esophagus and stomach.
   E. esophagus and small intestine.

4. The structure in the body that lays over the larynx like a lid and prevents food from entering the trachea is the:
   A. pharynx.
   B. uvula.
   C. epiglottis.
   D. glottis.
   E. esophagus.

5. Proper interaction with pediatric patients includes the following EXCEPT:
   A. allowing them to handle safe medical equipment to see that it will not harm them.
   B. using words the child will understand to describe the procedure.
   C. telling a child that a procedure will not hurt at all.
   D. talking in the same tone and volume as you would use with an adult.
   E. positioning yourself at the same level when speaking to the child.

6. A urine test that compares the weight of urine to that of distilled water is:
   A. specific gravity.
   B. clarity.
   C. sedimentation rate.
   D. pH.
   E. ketone analysis.

7. A patient is noncompliant if he or she:
   A. follows the instructions exactly as they were provided.
   B. does not progress as quickly as expected to the treatment plan.
   C. refuses to follow prescribed orders.
   D. has a reaction to prescribed medication.
   E. asks his or her family to participate in the plan.

8. A telephone call that the medical assistant can handle is:
   A. authorizing a prescription refill in the absence of the physician.
   B. advising a patient who is complaining of chest pain after taking new medication.
   C. taking results from a referring physician about a patient's abnormal electrocardiogram results.
   D. a hospital admitting clerk with the room number for a newly admitted patient.
   E. ordering examinations for a hospitalized patient.

9. If a certain number of patients are scheduled to come in for an appointment at the beginning of the same clock hour, this is:
   A. modified wave scheduling.
   B. wave scheduling.
   C. block scheduling.
   D. group scheduling.
   E. tidal wave scheduling.

10. When alphabetically filing, which of the following is last?
    A. John A. Hall
    B. John A. Hale
    C. John A. Haley
    D. John A. Halee
    E. John A. Halley

11. The salutation of a letter is placed:
    A. two lines below the inside address.
    B. two lines below the signature line.
    C. before the inside address.
    D. after the complimentary closing.
    E. before the date of the letter.

12. Medical expenses resulting from a back injury while at work are submitted to:
    A. Medicare.
    B. HMO.
    C. workers' compensation.
    D. employee's health insurance.
    E. Blue Cross/Blue Shield.

13. A ledger is also used as the patient's:
    A. receipt.
    B. charge slip.
    C. statement.
    D. posting.
    E. claim.

14. The book containing procedure and service codes performed by doctors and medical personnel is the:
    A. International Classification of Diseases.
    B. Current Procedural Terminology.
    C. Physician's Desk Reference.
    D. Insurance Payment Manual.
    E. AMA Journal.

15. Ringworm is an example of a disease caused by:
    A. bacteria.
    B. fungus.
    C. virus.
    D. parasite.
    E. yeast.

16. The faint tapping sounds heard as the blood pressure cuff initially deflates are recorded as the:
    A. pulse pressure.
    B. diastolic pressure.
    C. rhythm pressure.
    D. systolic pressure.
    E. apical pressure.

17. A forceps is an instrument used to:
    A. grasp tissue.
    B. retract tissue.
    C. cut tissue.
    D. suture tissue.
    E. clamp a blood vessel.

18. The ECG lead that measures the difference in electrical potential between the right arm and left arm is:
    A. lead II.
    B. lead I.
    C. aVR.
    D. aVF.
    E. V6.

19. Medicare Part B does not cover:
    A. doctor's office visits.
    B. diagnostic laboratory services.
    C. hospital charges.
    D. X-rays in an outpatient facility.
    E. durable medical equipment.

20. The vacuum tube used to collect blood so the blood will clot in the tube is:
    A. red.
    B. lavender.
    C. gray.
    D. green.
    E. blue.

21. An intravenous pyelogram is used to examine the:
    A. liver and gallbladder.
    B. stomach and large intestine.
    C. kidneys and bladder.
    D. colon and ileum.
    E. kidneys and pelvis.

22. Passive exercise means that the patient:
    A. does not move the body part without assistance.
    B. can move the joints freely.
    C. has full range of motion.
    D. cannot move the joints freely.
    E. uses weights when exercising.

23. When nutrients are initially taken into the body, it is called:
    A. digestion.
    B. ingestion.
    C. absorption.
    D. metabolism.
    E. salivation.

24. The muscle used for an injection located in the thigh is the:
    A. gluteus medius.
    B. gluteus maximus.
    C. rectus femoris.
    D. vastus lateralis.
    E. gastrocnemius.

25. Emergency treatment for third-degree burns is:
    A. immersing the body part in cold water.
    B. applying an ice pack to the affected part.
    C. removing any blisters that form.
    D. covering the victim and notifying EMS.
    E. applying an antibiotic ointment.

26. A patient's implied consent usually covers:
    A. organ donation.
    B. biopsy.
    C. blood transfusion.
    D. appendectomy.
    E. electrocardiogram.

27. The medical term that means "within a vessel" is:
    A. intercellular.
    B. interarterial.
    C. intravascular.
    D. intravalvular.
    E. intervascular.

28. An organ located in the left upper quadrant is the:
    A. thymus.
    B. spleen.
    C. appendix.
    D. liver.
    E. gallbladder.

29. Which of the following is an example of nonverbal communication?
    A. Clarification
    B. Feedback
    C. Body language
    D. Messages
    E. E-mail

30. A patient who is sight impaired would benefit from patient educational training materials that are produced as:
    A. Braille materials.
    B. videotapes.
    C. posters.
    D. pamphlets.
    E. brochures.

31. When the medical assistant is dealing with a difficult caller on the phone, he or she should first:
    A. ask the physician to handle the call.
    B. forward the call to the office manager.
    C. tell the caller you will hang up if he or she continues to be difficult.
    D. determine the problem and the appropriate staff who can help.
    E. alert another staff member to witness the call.

32. The abbreviation used in an appointment book to indicate a patient is coming in to see the physician about a medical problem already treated is:
    A. F/U.
    B. CPX.
    C. NP.
    D. BE.
    E. NS.

33. An outguide used in filing is a:
    A. file that is no longer in use.
    B. file of a patient who is not a patient in the office any longer.
    C. guide to alphabetizing file.
    D. folder inserted in the file to hold the place of a file in use.
    E. tickler to remind the staff of something missing from that file.

34. The inside address of a professional letter includes the:
    A. address of the sending physician.
    B. recipient's address written with abbreviation to save space.
    C. physician's residence address printed at the left margin.
    D. recipient's address written without abbreviations.
    E. recipient's insurance company address.

35. The person covered by a benefits plan is the:
    A. administrator.
    B. carrier.
    C. employee.
    D. insured.
    E. payer.

36. The listing of charges for a medical practice is the:
    A. coding chart.
    B. customary charges.
    C. value scale.
    D. value unit.
    E. fee schedule.

37. The withholding from an employee's paycheck for Social Security and Medicare is required under which law?
    A. FICA
    B. FCC
    C. HCFA
    D. IRA
    E. FUTA

38. A yeast infection that causes vaginitis is:
    A. *Candida*.
    B. staphylococci.
    C. *Trichomonas*.
    D. tinea.
    E. scabies.

39. A respiration rate that falls within the average adult range is:
    A. 10 per minute.
    B. 20 per minute.
    C. 25 per minute.
    D. 30 per minute.
    E. below 10 per minute.

40. Proper technique to ensure package sterility includes using:
    A. a sterile package with only a small tear.
    B. sterile packages up to 30 days after the expiration date.
    C. a dry, undamaged sterile package.
    D. sterile gloves to transport sterile packages.
    E. a sterile pack still damp from the autoclave.

41. AC interference in an ECG tracing means:
    A. the patient is having a muscle tremor.
    B. there is a loose electrode connection.
    C. there is electrical interference in the room.
    D. the electrodes are too tight on the patient.
    E. the power to the machine is off.

42. The clear liquid portion of whole blood is:
    A. serum.
    B. thrombin.
    C. hemoglobin.
    D. fibrinogen.
    E. plasma.

43. To convert milligrams to grams:
    A. divide by 100.
    B. divide by 1,000.
    C. multiply by 100.
    D. multiply by 1,000.
    E. subtract the numerator from the denominator.

44. Diabetic coma is due to:
    A. overproduction of insulin.
    B. low blood glucose level.
    C. lack of insulin.
    D. normal glucose with high insulin level.
    E. increased metabolism of glucose.

45. An arthrogram is the radiographic visualization of:
    A. a joint.
    B. a blood vessel.
    C. the gallbladder.
    D. the spinal column.
    E. an artery.

46. Diathermy is an example of an agent that incorporates the use of:
    A. paraffin wax.
    B. cold water.
    C. ultraviolet light.
    D. deep heat.
    E. hot water.

47. Which of the following conditions would benefit from a low-purine diet?
    A. Gout
    B. Obesity
    C. High blood pressure
    D. Constipation
    E. Coronary artery disease

48. Antihypertensive medications are associated with the treatment of:
    A. fever.
    B. vomiting.
    C. high blood pressure.
    D. allergies.
    E. gout.

49. A laceration appears as a:
    A. scrape on the skin.
    B. bruise.
    C. jagged cut.
    D. swelling on the skin.
    E. hematoma.

50. *Res ipsa loquitur* is a Latin term that means which of the following?
    A. Let the buyer beware.
    B. The thing speaks for itself.
    C. The employer is responsible for the employee.
    D. The patient is always first.
    E. The physician is responsible.

51. The medical term meaning "inflammation of the bone" is:
    A. arthritis.
    B. bursitis.
    C. chondritis.
    D. osteitis.
    E. tendonitis.

52. The superior vena cava is the:
    A. vein that carries blood from the lower extremities to the aorta.
    B. artery that carries blood between the heart and lungs.
    C. vein that carries blood between the heart and lungs.
    D. artery that carries blood from the aorta to the kidneys.
    E. vein that carries blood from the upper body back to the heart.

53. Basic communication requires a message and:
    A. sender and receiver.
    B. feedback and body language.
    C. clarification and feedback.
    D. receiver and body language.
    E. a decoder.

54. The term **facsimile** refers to:
    A. fax.
    B. photocopy.
    C. e-mail.
    D. voice mail.
    E. Internet.

55. A matrix is a(n):
    A. form of billing.
    B. appointment book schedule with blocked out periods of time.
    C. form used for insurance filing.
    D. timed laboratory test.
    E. document used for patient billing.

56. The most common method used to chart the patient's medical record is:
    A. CPT.
    B. SOMR.
    C. SOAP.
    D. HCFA.
    E. ICD.

57. The salutation of a letter is the:
    A. closing.
    B. reference line.
    C. enclosure.
    D. greeting.
    E. purpose for writing.

58. Coordination of benefits means:
    A. the amount of money paid by the patient for medical services before the insurance pays.
    B. one insurance plan will work with other insurance plans to determine how much each plan pays.
    C. there is a flat fee paid for each service.
    D. there is a deductible required by the patient before payment from the insurance is made.
    E. each insurance company will pay an equal amount of the patient's bill.

59. ICD-9 codes that identify medical problems for reasons other than illness or injury are known as:
    A. E codes.
    B. M codes.
    C. CPT codes.
    D. V codes.
    E. neoplasms.

60. When a bank uses the term NSF, it means that:
    A. the check is voided and not to be used.
    B. the account is a newly opened account.
    C. there is not enough money to cover the amount of the check.
    D. the bank will issue a cashier's check in the amount of the check.
    E. the bank must wait 1 week before depositing the check.

61. The proper time and temperature for sterilizing instruments is:
    A. 30 minutes at 150°F.
    B. 45 minutes at 250°F.
    C. 60 minutes at 150°F.
    D. 30 minutes at 250°F.
    E. 20 minutes at 150°F.

62. The Fowler's position is used for:
    A. female pelvic examination.
    B. examination of the abdomen.
    C. patient with difficulty breathing.
    D. sigmoidoscopy.
    E. examination of the spine.

63. The abbreviation OU is no longer in use. Instead of using OU, which of the following should be written?
    A. Both eyes
    B. Right ear
    C. Both ears
    D. Left eye
    E. Optical unit

64. Which of the following is the finer or smaller suture?
    A. 2-0
    B. 4-0
    C. 0-0
    D. 10-0
    E. 1-0

65. The V1 ECG lead is located:
    A. between the fourth and fifth intercostal space.
    B. over the left nipple.
    C. between the second and third intercostal space.
    D. at the fourth intercostal space to the right of the sternum.
    E. at the fourth intercostal space to the left of the sternum.

66. Which of the following is a proper site for a capillary puncture?
    A. Tip of ring finger
    B. Heel of an adult
    C. Tip of index finger
    D. Tip of little finger
    E. Earlobe of an infant

67. The abbreviation used to indicate that a patient should be fasting for an examination is:
    A. NPO.
    B. AC.
    C. PC.
    D. NOS.
    E. CBC.

68. KUB is an X-ray examination of the:
    A. heart and lungs.
    B. spinal column.
    C. liver and gallbladder.
    D. abdomen.
    E. urinary system.

69. Cold applied to part of the body causes the effect of:
    A. vasoconstriction.
    B. vasodilation.
    C. increased blood flow to the body part.
    D. increased blood pressure to the area.
    E. muscle rigor.

70. A patient with arteriosclerosis would benefit from which of the following diets?
    A. Low salt
    B. Low carbohydrate
    C. Low protein
    D. Low cholesterol
    E. High protein

71. The first action to control bleeding or hemorrhage is to:
    A. place ice over the wound.
    B. apply direct pressure.
    C. apply a tourniquet above the injury.
    D. immobilize the body part.
    E. elevate the head.

72. The term **enteritis** means inflammation of the:
    A. colon.
    B. small intestine.
    C. stomach.
    D. esophagus.
    E. gallbladder.

73. An example of active immunity is:
    A. maternal antibodies passed through the uterus to the baby.
    B. immunization with antibodies.
    C. maternal antibodies acquired by the baby from breast milk.
    D. producing antibodies as a result of having a disease.
    E. avoiding an infected person.

74. When a person refuses to acknowledge the loss of a loved one, the type of behavior is:
    A. sympathy.
    B. mourning.
    C. denial.
    D. depression.
    E. withdrawal.

75. The computer device that displays the written data is the:
    A. disk drive.
    B. monitor.
    C. hard drive.
    D. floppy disk.
    E. software.

76. When the doctor is late and not yet at the office, the medical assistant should:
    A. offer waiting patients an opportunity to reschedule.
    B. cancel all remaining appointments for the day.
    C. reschedule all the patients for another day.
    D. offer to refer the patients to another physician's practice.
    E. close the office and notify the answering service.

77. The "O" in the SOAP method of charting includes the:
    A. blood pressure reading.
    B. opinion of a family member.
    C. symptoms the patient states.
    D. prior complaints from the patient.
    E. patient's demographics.

78. To retain insurance coverage, the individual must pay the cost of the insurance, which is the:
    A. premium.
    B. copayment.
    C. coinsurance.
    D. deductible.
    E. reimbursement.

79. CPT is an abbreviation of the reference manual used for:
    A. ordering laboratory tests.
    B. billing insurance companies for procedures.
    C. reporting diseases to the CDC.
    D. selecting the fees for each examination.
    E. providing the diagnosis on a claim.

80. The best way to ensure that patients pay for services is to:
    A. ask patients where they would like the bill mailed.
    B. give a copy of the bill to patients when they leave the office.
    C. confirm the name of the patient's insurance company.
    D. accept checks only, not credit cards.
    E. ask for payment of services at the time of the office visit.

81. Acquired immunodeficiency syndrome is caused by:
    A. yeast.
    B. fungi.
    C. bacteria.
    D. a virus.
    E. a parasite.

82. The pulse point located on the top of the foot is the:
    A. femoral.
    B. dorsalis pedis.
    C. temporal.
    D. popliteal.
    E. ulnar.

83. An instrument required on a suture tray is a:
    A. dilator.
    B. scalpel.
    C. retractor.
    D. needle holder.
    E. stapler remover.

84. The ECG grounding lead is attached to the:
    A. RA.
    B. LA.
    C. RL.
    D. LL.
    E. AV.

85. A urine specimen that is collected after eating is called:
    A. clean catch.
    B. random.
    C. voided.
    D. postprandial.
    E. timed.

86. A myelogram is an X-ray examination of the:
    A. spinal cord.
    B. brain.
    C. muscles.
    D. heart.
    E. abdomen.

87. A physician orders amoxicillin 1 g to be divided into four equal doses. Available is amoxicillin 250 mg/5 mL. How many milliliters will the patient receive for each dose?
    A. 0.5 mL
    B. 1 mL
    C. 5 mL
    D. 10 mL
    E. 2 mL

88. Anaphylaxis refers to a:
    A. nose bleed.
    B. type of shock.
    C. hemorrhage disorder.
    D. congenital disorder.
    E. heart attack.

89. Dyspepsia refers to:
    A. difficulty speaking.
    B. difficult digestion.
    C. difficulty breathing.
    D. abnormal pain.
    E. difficulty swallowing.

90. The perineum is the:
    A. lining of the abdomen.
    B. covering of the spinal cord.
    C. floor of the pelvis.
    D. outside lining of the lungs.
    E. lining of the heart.

91. *Respondeat superior* refers to:
    A. a subpoena.
    B. a physician's responsibility for the actions of his staff.
    C. something for something, a favor for a favor.
    D. responding to your superiors.
    E. the thing speaks for itself.

92. The proper angle of the needle to the skin when administering a subcutaneous injection is:
    A. 10 degrees.
    B. 15 degrees.
    C. 45 degrees.
    D. 75 degrees.
    E. 90 degrees.

93. Which of the following is not considered for use on the skin for cleansing?
    A. Acetone
    B. Povidone–iodine
    C. Betadine
    D. Alcohol
    E. Hibiclens

94. Which of the following instruments is used to evaluate lung capacity?
    A. Audiometer
    B. Goniometer
    C. Sphygmomanometer
    D. Spirometer
    E. Doppler

95. The process by which nutrients transfer from the gastrointestinal system into the blood is referred to as:
    A. ingestion.
    B. digestion.
    C. absorption.
    D. metabolism.
    E. mastication.

96. The classification of drugs used to relieve pain is:
    A. antidepressant.
    B. analgesic.
    C. antibiotic.
    D. antidote.
    E. antihypertensive.

97. The device used to check vision is a(n):
    A. otoscope.
    B. ophthalmoscope.
    C. Snellen chart.
    D. tuning fork.
    E. flashlight.

98. A wound that results from scraping the skin is a(n):
    A. laceration.
    B. avulsion.
    C. contusion.
    D. evisceration.
    E. abrasion.

99. When several tubes of blood are to be drawn, which is drawn first?
    A. Anticoagulant tubes
    B. Blood culture tubes
    C. Tubes with no additive
    D. Heparinized tubes
    E. EDTA tubes

100. The parenteral method of administration of medication means that the drug is:
    A. rubbed on the skin.
    B. inserted rectally.
    C. swallowed.
    D. dissolved in the mouth.
    E. injected.

Answers to Practice Exam—CMA (AAMA)

1. B	26. E	51. D	76. A
2. B	27. C	52. E	77. A
3. D	28. B	53. A	78. A
4. C	29. C	54. A	79. B
5. C	30. A	55. B	80. E
6. A	31. D	56. C	81. D
7. C	32. A	57. D	82. B
8. D	33. D	58. B	83. D
9. B	34. D	59. D	84. C
10. E	35. D	60. C	85. D
11. A	36. E	61. D	86. A
12. C	37. A	62. C	87. C
13. C	38. A	63. A	88. B
14. B	39. B	64. D	89. B
15. B	40. C	65. D	90. C
16. D	41. C	66. A	91. B
17. A	42. E	67. A	92. C
18. B	43. B	68. E	93. A
19. C	44. C	69. A	94. D
20. A	45. A	70. D	95. C
21. C	46. D	71. B	96. B
22. A	47. A	72. B	97. C
23. B	48. C	73. D	98. E
24. D	49. C	74. C	99. B
25. D	50. B	75. B	100. E

PRACTICE EXAM—RMA (AMT)

1. Pathogens that thrive in the absence of oxygen are called:
   A. antitoxins.
   B. anaerobes.
   C. spores.
   D. aerobes.

2. A communicable disease that does not have to be reported to the county health department is:
   A. tuberculosis.
   B. streptococcus.
   C. rubella.
   D. syphilis.

3. The term **esophagogastritis** means inflammation of the:
   A. larynx and pharynx.
   B. stomach and small intestine.
   C. small intestine and stomach.
   D. esophagus and stomach.

4. The structure in the body that lays over the larynx like a lid and prevents food from entering the trachea is the:
   A. pharynx.
   B. uvula.
   C. epiglottis.
   D. glottis.

5. Proper interaction with pediatric patients includes the following EXCEPT:
   A. allowing them to handle safe medical equipment to see that it will not harm them.
   B. using words the child will understand to describe the procedure.
   C. telling a child that a procedure will not hurt at all.
   D. talking in the same tone and volume as you would use with an adult.

6. A urine test that compares the weight of urine to that of distilled water is:
   A. specific gravity.
   B. clarity.
   C. sedimentation rate.
   D. pH.

7. A patient is noncompliant if he or she:
   A. follows the instructions exactly as they were provided.
   B. does not progress as quickly as expected to the treatment plan.
   C. refuses to follow prescribed orders.
   D. has a reaction to prescribed medication.

8. A telephone call that the medical assistant can handle is:
   A. authorizing a prescription refill in the absence of the physician.
   B. advising a patient who is complaining of chest pain after taking new medication.
   C. taking results from a referring physician about a patient's abnormal electrocardiogram results.
   D. a hospital admitting clerk with the room number for a newly admitted patient.

9. If a certain number of patients are scheduled to come in for an appointment at the beginning of the same clock hour, this is:
   A. modified wave scheduling.
   B. wave scheduling.
   C. block scheduling.
   D. group scheduling.

10. When alphabetically filing, which of the following is last?
    A. John A. Hall
    B. John A. Hale
    C. John A. Halley
    D. John A. Halee

11. The salutation of a letter is placed:
    A. two lines below the inside address.
    B. two lines below the signature line.
    C. before the inside address.
    D. after the complimentary closing.

12. Medical expenses resulting from a back injury while at work are submitted to:
    A. Medicare.
    B. HMO.
    C. workers' compensation.
    D. employee's health insurance.

13. A ledger is also used as the patient's:
    A. receipt.
    B. charge slip.
    C. statement.
    D. posting.

14. The book containing procedure and service codes performed by doctors and medical personnel is the:
    A. International Classification of Diseases.
    B. Current Procedural Terminology.
    C. Physician's Desk Reference.
    D. Insurance Payment Manual.

15. Ringworm is an example of a disease caused by:
    A. bacteria.
    B. fungus.
    C. virus.
    D. parasite.

16. The faint tapping sounds heard as the blood pressure cuff initially deflates are recorded as the:
    A. pulse pressure.
    B. diastolic pressure.
    C. rhythm pressure.
    D. systolic pressure.

17. A forceps is an instrument used to:
    A. grasp tissue.
    B. retract tissue.
    C. cut tissue.
    D. suture tissue.

18. The ECG lead that measures the difference in electrical potential between the right arm and left arm is:
    A. lead II.
    B. lead I.
    C. aVR.
    D. aVF.

19. Medicare Part B does not cover:
    A. doctor's office visits.
    B. diagnostic laboratory services.
    C. hospital charges.
    D. X-rays in an outpatient facility.

20. The vacuum tube used to collect blood so the blood will clot in the tube is:
    A. red.
    B. lavender.
    C. gray.
    D. green.

21. An intravenous pyelogram is used to examine the:
    A. liver and gallbladder.
    B. stomach and large intestine.
    C. kidneys and bladder.
    D. colon and ileum.

22. Passive exercise means that the patient:
    A. does not move the body part without assistance.
    B. can move the joints freely.
    C. has full range of motion.
    D. cannot move the joints freely.

23. When nutrients are initially taken into the body, it is called:
    A. digestion.
    B. ingestion.
    C. absorption.
    D. metabolism.

24. The muscle used for an injection located in the thigh is the:
    A. gluteus medius.
    B. gluteus maximus.
    C. rectus femoris.
    D. vastus lateralis.

25. Emergency treatment for third-degree burns is:
    A. immersing the body part in cold water.
    B. applying an ice pack to the affected part.
    C. removing any blisters that form.
    D. covering the victim and notifying EMS.

26. A patient's implied consent usually covers:
    A. organ donation.
    B. electrocardiogram.
    C. blood transfusion.
    D. appendectomy.

27. The medical term that means "within a vessel" is:
    A. intercellular.
    B. interarterial.
    C. intravascular.
    D. intravalvular.

28. An organ located in the left upper quadrant is the:
    A. thymus.
    B. spleen.
    C. appendix.
    D. liver.

29. Which of the following is an example of nonverbal communication?
    A. Clarification
    B. Feedback
    C. Body language
    D. Messages

30. A patient who is sight impaired would benefit from patient educational training materials that are produced as:
    A. Braille materials.
    B. videotapes.
    C. posters.
    D. pamphlets.

31. When the medical assistant is dealing with a difficult caller on the phone, he or she should first:
    A. ask the physician to handle the call.
    B. forward the call to the office manager.
    C. tell the caller you will hang up if he or she continues to be difficult.
    D. determine the problem and the appropriate staff that can help.

32. The abbreviation used in an appointment book to indicate a patient is coming in to see the physician about a medical problem already treated is:
    A. F/U.
    B. CPX.
    C. NP.
    D. BE.

33. An outguide used in filing is a:
    A. file that is no longer in use.
    B. file of a patient that is not a patient in the office any longer.
    C. guide to alphabetizing file.
    D. folder inserted in the file to hold the place of a file in use.

34. The inside address of a professional letter includes the:
    A. address of the sending physician.
    B. recipient's address written with abbreviation to save space.
    C. physician's residence address printed at the left margin.
    D. recipient's address written without abbreviations.

35. The person covered by a benefits plan is the:
    A. administrator.
    B. carrier.
    C. employee.
    D. insured.

36. The listing of charges for a medical practice is the:
    A. fee schedule.
    B. customary charges.
    C. value scale.
    D. value unit.

37. The withholding from an employee's paycheck for Social Security and Medicare is required under which law?
    A. FICA
    B. FCC
    C. HCFA
    D. IRA

38. A yeast infection that causes vaginitis is:
    A. *Candida*.
    B. staphylococci.
    C. *Trichomonas*.
    D. tinea.

39. A respiration rate that falls within the average adult range is:
    A. 10 per minute.
    B. 20 per minute.
    C. 25 per minute.
    D. 30 per minute.

40. Proper technique to ensure package sterility includes using:
    A. a sterile package with only a small tear.
    B. sterile packages up to 30 days after the expiration date.
    C. a dry, undamaged sterile package.
    D. sterile gloves to transport sterile packages.

41. AC interference in an ECG tracing means:
    A. the patient is having a muscle tremor.
    B. there is a loose electrode connection.
    C. there is electrical interference in the room.
    D. the electrodes are too tight on the patient.

42. The clear liquid portion of whole blood is:
    A. serum.
    B. thrombin.
    C. hemoglobin.
    D. plasma.

43. To convert milligrams to grams:
    A. divide by 100.
    B. divide by 1,000.
    C. multiply by 100.
    D. multiply by 1,000.

44. Diabetic coma is due to:
    A. overproduction of insulin.
    B. low blood glucose level.
    C. lack of insulin.
    D. normal glucose with high insulin level.

45. An arthrogram is the radiographic visualization of:
    A. a joint.
    B. a blood vessel.
    C. the gallbladder.
    D. the spinal column.

46. Diathermy is an example of an agent that incorporates the use of:
    A. paraffin wax.
    B. cold water.
    C. ultraviolet light.
    D. deep heat.

47. Which of the following conditions would benefit from a low-purine diet?
    A. Gout
    B. Obesity
    C. High blood pressure
    D. Constipation

48. Antihypertensive medications are associated with the treatment of:
    A. fever.
    B. vomiting.
    C. high blood pressure.
    D. allergies.

49. A laceration appears as a:
    A. scrape on the skin.
    B. bruise.
    C. jagged cut.
    D. swelling on the skin.

50. *Res ipsa loquitur* is a Latin term that means which of the following?
    A. Let the buyer beware.
    B. The thing speaks for itself.
    C. The employer is responsible for the employee.
    D. The patient is always first.

51. The medical term meaning "inflammation of the bone" is:
    A. arthritis.
    B. bursitis.
    C. chondritis.
    D. osteitis.

52. The superior vena cava is the:
    A. vein that carries blood from the lower extremities to the aorta.
    B. artery that carries blood between the heart and lungs.
    C. vein that carries blood from the upper body back to the heart.
    D. vein that carries blood between the heart and lungs.

53. Basic communication requires a message and:
    A. sender and receiver.
    B. feedback and body language.
    C. clarification and feedback.
    D. receiver and body language.

54. The term **facsimile** refers to:
    A. fax.
    B. photocopy.
    C. e-mail.
    D. voice mail.

55. A matrix is a(n):
    A. form of billing.
    B. appointment book schedule with blocked out periods of time.
    C. form used for insurance filing.
    D. timed laboratory test.

56. The most common method used to chart the patient's medical record is:
    A. CPT.
    B. SOMR.
    C. SOAP.
    D. HCFA.

57. The salutation of a letter is the:
    A. closing.
    B. reference line.
    C. enclosure.
    D. greeting.

58. Coordination of benefits means:
    A. the amount of money paid by the patient for medical services before the insurance pays.
    B. one insurance plan will work with other insurance plans to determine how much each plan pays.
    C. each insurance company will pay an equal amount of the patient's bill.
    D. there is a deductible required by the patient before payment from the insurance is made.

59. ICD-9 codes that identify medical problems for reasons other than illness or injury are known as:
    A. E codes.
    B. M codes.
    C. CPT codes.
    D. V codes.

60. When a bank uses the term NSF, it means that:
    A. the check is voided and not to be used.
    B. the account is a newly opened account.
    C. there is not enough money to cover the amount of the check.
    D. the bank will issue a cashier's check in the amount of the check.

61. The proper time and temperature for sterilizing instruments is:
    A. 30 minutes at 150°F.
    B. 45 minutes at 250°F.
    C. 60 minutes at 150°F.
    D. 30 minutes at 250°F.

62. The Fowler's position is used for:
    A. female pelvic examination.
    B. examination of the abdomen.
    C. patient with difficulty breathing.
    D. sigmoidoscopy.

63. The abbreviation OU is no longer in use. Instead of using OU, which of the following should be written?
    A. Both eyes
    B. Right ear
    C. Both ears
    D. Left eye

64. Which of the following is the finer or smaller suture?
    A. 2-0
    B. 4-0
    C. 0-0
    D. 10-0

65. The V1 ECG lead is located:
    A. between the fourth and fifth intercostal space.
    B. at the fourth intercostal space to the left of the sternum.
    C. between the second and third intercostal space.
    D. at the fourth intercostal space to the right of the sternum.

66. Which of the following is a proper site for a capillary puncture?
    A. Tip of ring finger
    B. Heel of an adult
    C. Tip of index finger
    D. Tip of little finger

67. The abbreviation used to indicate that a patient should be fasting for an examination is:
    A. NPO.
    B. AC.
    C. PC.
    D. NOS.

68. KUB is an X-ray examination of the:
    A. urinary system.
    B. spinal column.
    C. liver and gallbladder.
    D. abdomen.

69. Cold applied to part of the body causes the effect of:
    A. vasoconstriction.
    B. vasodilation.
    C. increased blood flow to the body part.
    D. increased blood pressure to the area.

70. A patient with arteriosclerosis would benefit from which of the following diets?
    A. Low salt
    B. Low carbohydrate
    C. Low protein
    D. Low cholesterol

71. The first action to control bleeding or hemorrhage is to:
    A. place ice over the wound.
    B. apply direct pressure.
    C. apply a tourniquet above the injury.
    D. immobilize the body part.

72. The term **enteritis** means inflammation of the:
    A. colon.
    B. small intestine.
    C. stomach.
    D. esophagus.

73. An example of active immunity is:
    A. maternal antibodies passed through the uterus to the baby.
    B. immunization with antibodies.
    C. maternal antibodies acquired by the baby from breast milk.
    D. producing antibodies as a result of having a disease.

74. When a person refuses to acknowledge the loss of a loved one, this type of behavior is:
    A. sympathy.
    B. mourning.
    C. denial.
    D. depression.

75. The computer device that displays the written data is the:
    A. disk drive.
    B. monitor.
    C. hard drive.
    D. floppy disk.

76. When the doctor is late and not yet at the office, the medical assistant should:
    A. offer waiting patients an opportunity to reschedule.
    B. cancel all remaining appointments for the day.
    C. reschedule all the patients for another day.
    D. offer to refer the patients to another physician's practice.

77. The "O" in the SOAP method of charting includes the:
    A. blood pressure reading.
    B. opinion of a family member.
    C. symptoms the patient states.
    D. prior complaints from the patient.

78. To retain insurance coverage, the individual must pay the cost of the insurance, which is the:
    A. premium.
    B. copayment.
    C. coinsurance.
    D. deductible.

79. CPT is an abbreviation of the reference manual used for:
    A. ordering laboratory tests.
    B. billing insurance companies for procedures.
    C. reporting diseases to the CDC.
    D. selecting the fees for each examination.

80. The best way to ensure that patients pay for services is to:
    A. ask patients where they would like the bill mailed.
    B. ask for payment of services at the time of the office visit.
    C. confirm the name of the patient's insurance company.
    D. accept checks only, not credit cards.

81. Acquired immunodeficiency syndrome is caused by:
    A. yeast.
    B. fungi.
    C. bacteria.
    D. a virus.

82. The pulse point located on the top of the foot is the:
    A. femoral.
    B. dorsalis pedis.
    C. temporal.
    D. popliteal.

83. An instrument required on a suture tray is a:
    A. dilator.
    B. scalpel.
    C. retractor.
    D. needle holder.

84. The ECG grounding lead is attached to the:
    A. RA.
    B. LA.
    C. RL.
    D. LL.

85. A urine specimen that is collected after eating is called:
    A. clean catch.
    B. random.
    C. voided.
    D. postprandial.

86. A myelogram is an X-ray examination of the:
    A. spinal cord.
    B. brain.
    C. muscles.
    D. heart.

87. A physician orders amoxicillin 1 g to be divided into four equal doses. Available is amoxicillin 250 mg/5 mL. How many milliliters will the patient receive for each dose?
    A. 0.5 mL
    B. 1 mL
    C. 5 mL
    D. 10 mL

88. Anaphylaxis refers to a:
    A. nose bleed.
    B. type of shock.
    C. hemorrhage disorder.
    D. congenital disorder.

89. Dyspepsia refers to:
    A. difficulty speaking.
    B. difficult digestion.
    C. difficulty breathing.
    D. abnormal pain.

90. The perineum is the:
    A. lining of the abdomen.
    B. covering of the spinal cord.
    C. floor of the pelvis.
    D. outside lining of the lungs.

91. *Respondeat superior* refers to:
    A. a subpoena.
    B. a physician's responsibility for the actions of his staff.
    C. something for something, a favor for a favor.
    D. responding to your superiors.

92. The proper angle of the needle to the skin when administering a subcutaneous injection is:
    A. 10 degrees.
    B. 15 degrees.
    C. 45 degrees.
    D. 75 degrees.

93. Which of the following is not considered for use on the skin for cleansing?
    A. Acetone
    B. Povidone-iodine
    C. Betadine
    D. Alcohol

94. Which of the following instruments is used to evaluate lung capacity?
    A. Audiometer
    B. Goniometer
    C. Sphygmomanometer
    D. Spirometer

95. The process by which nutrients transfer from the gastrointestinal system into the blood is referred to as:
    A. ingestion.
    B. digestion.
    C. absorption.
    D. metabolism.

96. The classification of drugs used to relieve pain is:
    A. antidepressant.
    B. analgesic.
    C. antibiotic.
    D. antidote.

97. The device used to check vision is a(n):
    A. otoscope.
    B. ophthalmoscope.
    C. Snellen chart.
    D. tuning fork.

98. A wound that results from scraping the skin is a(n):
    A. laceration.
    B. avulsion.
    C. contusion.
    D. abrasion.

99. When several tubes of blood are to be drawn, which is drawn first?
    A. Anticoagulant tubes
    B. Blood culture tubes
    C. Tubes with no additive
    D. Heparinized tubes

100. The parenteral method of administration of medication means that the drug is:
    A. rubbed on the skin.
    B. inserted rectally.
    C. swallowed.
    D. injected.

Answers to Practice Exam—RMA (AMT)

1. B	26. B	51. D	76. A
2. B	27. C	52. C	77. A
3. D	28. B	53. A	78. A
4. C	29. C	54. A	79. B
5. C	30. A	55. B	80. B
6. A	31. D	56. C	81. D
7. C	32. A	57. D	82. B
8. D	33. D	58. B	83. D
9. B	34. D	59. D	84. C
10. C	35. D	60. C	85. A
11. A	36. A	61. D	86. A
12. C	37. A	62. C	87. C
13. C	38. A	63. A	88. B
14. B	39. B	64. D	89. B
15. B	40. C	65. D	90. C
16. D	41. C	66. A	91. B
17. A	42. D	67. A	92. C
18. B	43. B	68. A	93. A
19. C	44. C	69. A	94. D
20. A	45. A	70. D	95. C
21. C	46. D	71. B	96. B
22. A	47. A	72. B	97. C
23. C	48. C	73. D	98. D
24. D	49. C	74. C	99. B
25. D	50. B	75. B	100. D

PRACTICE EXAM—CMAS (AMT)

1. Pathogens that thrive in the absence of oxygen are called:
   A. antitoxins.
   B. anaerobes.
   C. spores.
   D. aerobes.

2. A communicable disease that does not have to be reported to the county health department is:
   A. tuberculosis.
   B. streptococcus.
   C. rubella.
   D. syphilis.

3. The term **esophagogastritis** means inflammation of the:
   A. larynx and pharynx.
   B. stomach and small intestine.
   C. small intestine and stomach.
   D. esophagus and stomach.

4. The structure in the body that lays over the larynx like a lid and prevents food from entering the trachea is the:
   A. pharynx.
   B. uvula.
   C. epiglottis.
   D. glottis.

5. Proper interaction with pediatric patients includes the following EXCEPT:
   A. allowing them to handle safe medical equipment to see that it will not harm them.
   B. using words the child will understand to describe the procedure.
   C. telling a child that a procedure will not hurt at all.
   D. talking in the same tone and volume as you would use with an adult.

6. A urine test that compares the weight of urine to that of distilled water is:
   A. specific gravity.
   B. clarity.
   C. sedimentation rate.
   D. pH.

7. A patient is noncompliant if he or she:
   A. follows the instructions exactly as they were provided.
   B. does not progress as quickly as expected to the treatment plan.
   C. refuses to follow prescribed orders.
   D. has a reaction to prescribed medication.

8. A telephone call that the medical assistant can handle is:
   A. authorizing a prescription refill in the absence of the physician.
   B. advising a patient who is complaining of chest pain after taking new medication.
   C. taking results from a referring physician about a patient's abnormal electrocardiogram results.
   D. a hospital admitting clerk with the room number for a newly admitted patient.

9. If a certain number of patients are scheduled to come in for an appointment at the beginning of the same clock hour, this is:
   A. modified wave scheduling.
   B. wave scheduling.
   C. block scheduling.
   D. group scheduling.

10. When alphabetically filing, which of the following is last?
    A. John A. Hall
    B. John A. Hale
    C. John A. Halley
    D. John A. Halee

11. The salutation of a letter is placed:
    A. two lines below the inside address.
    B. two lines below the signature line.
    C. before the inside address.
    D. after the complimentary closing.

12. Medical expenses resulting from a back injury while at work are submitted to:
    A. Medicare.
    B. HMO.
    C workers' compensation.
    D. employee's health insurance.

13. A ledger is also used as the patient's:
    A. receipt.
    B. charge slip.
    C. statement.
    D. posting.

14. The book containing procedure and service codes performed by doctors and medical personnel is the:
    A. International Classification of Diseases.
    B. Current Procedural Terminology.
    C. Physician's Desk Reference.
    D. Insurance Payment Manual.

15. Ringworm is an example of a disease caused by:
    A. bacteria.
    B. fungus.
    C. virus.
    D. parasite.

16. The faint tapping sounds heard as the blood pressure cuff initially deflates are recorded as the:
    A. pulse pressure.
    B. diastolic pressure.
    C. rhythm pressure.
    D. systolic pressure.

17. A forceps is an instrument used to:
    A. grasp tissue.
    B. retract tissue.
    C. cut tissue.
    D. suture tissue.

18. An evacuation plan requires:
    A. keeping hallways unobstructed at all times.
    B. maintaining SDS.
    C. using a fire extinguisher.
    D. returning to the building to help others.

19. Medicare Part B does not cover:
    A. doctor's office visits.
    B. diagnostic laboratory services.
    C. hospital charges.
    D. X-rays in an outpatient facility.

20. PASS is an acronym for:
    A. using a fire extinguisher.
    B. keeping hallways unobstructed at all times.
    C. maintaining MSDS.
    D. returning to the building during an evacuation to help others.

21. An intravenous pyelogram is used to examine the:
    A. liver and gallbladder.
    B. stomach and large intestine.
    C. kidneys and bladder.
    D. colon and ileum.

22. Passive exercise means that the patient:
    A. does not move the body part without assistance.
    B. can move the joints freely.
    C. has full range of motion.
    D. cannot move the joints freely.

23. When nutrients are initially taken into the body, it is called:
    A. digestion.
    B. ingestion.
    C. absorption.
    D. metabolism.

24. The term that demonstrates how each rank is accountable to those directly superior is called:
    A. the agenda.
    B. autocratic management style.
    C. participatory management.
    D. the chain of command.

25. Emergency treatment for third-degree burns is:
    A. immersing the body part in cold water.
    B. applying an ice pack to the affected part.
    C. removing any blisters that form.
    D. covering the victim and notifying EMS.

26. A patient's implied consent usually covers:
    A. organ donation.
    B. electrocardiogram.
    C. blood transfusion.
    D. appendectomy.

27. The medical term that means "within a vessel" is:
    A. intercellular.
    B. interarterial.
    C. intravascular.
    D. intravalvular.

28. An organ located in the left upper quadrant is the:
    A. thymus.
    B. spleen.
    C. appendix.
    D. liver.

29. Which of the following is an example of nonverbal communication?
    A. Clarification
    B. Feedback
    C. Body language
    D. Messages

30. A patient who is sight impaired would benefit from patient educational training materials that are produced as:
    A. Braille materials.
    B. videotapes.
    C. posters.
    D. pamphlets.

31. When the medical assistant is dealing with a difficult caller on the phone, he or she should first:
    A. ask the physician to handle the call.
    B. forward the call to the office manager.
    C. tell the caller you will hang up if he or she continues to be difficult.
    D. determine the problem and the appropriate staff that can help.

32. The abbreviation used in an appointment book to indicate a patient is coming in to see the physician about a medical problem already treated is:
    A. F/U.
    B. CPX.
    C. NP.
    D. BE.

33. An outguide used in filing is a:
    A. file that is no longer in use.
    B. file of a patient that is not a patient in the office any longer.
    C. guide to alphabetizing file.
    D. folder inserted in the file to hold the place of a file in use.

34. The inside address of a professional letter includes the:
    A. address of the sending physician.
    B. recipient's address written with abbreviation to save space.
    C. physician's residence address printed at the left margin.
    D. recipient's address written without abbreviations.

35. The person covered by a benefits plan is the:
    A. administrator.
    B. carrier.
    C. employee.
    D. insured.

36. The listing of charges for a medical practice is the:
    A. fee schedule.
    B. customary charges.
    C. value scale.
    D. value unit.

37. The withholding from an employee's paycheck for Social Security and Medicare is required under which law?
    A. FICA
    B. FCC
    C. HCFA
    D. IRA

38. A yeast infection that causes vaginitis is:
    A. *Candida*.
    B. staphylococci.
    C. *Trichomonas*.
    D. tinea.

39. A respiration rate that falls within the average adult range is:
    A. 10 per minute.
    B. 20 per minute.
    C. 25 per minute.
    D. 30 per minute.

40. A plan that describes personnel protective equipment (PPE) and other safety engineering devices and processes and provides instructions of what an employee should do if a related incident occurs is called:
    A. risk management.
    B. quality assurance.
    C. exposure control.
    D. aseptic technique.

41. Medicare Part B provides coverage for:
    A. home health services.
    B. hospital services.
    C. outpatient services.
    D. pharmaceutical supplies.

42. The first aid for frostbite is to:
    A. vigorously rub the affected body part.
    B. immerse the affected body part in water.
    C. gently wrap the affected body part in warm material.
    D. instruct the person to move around to increase circulation.

43. Facilities management includes all the following EXCEPT:
    A. hiring and firing disposable waste contractors.
    B. negotiating contracts with insurance companies.
    C. maintaining carpeting, elevators, and other structures.
    D. complying with the Americans with Disabilities Act.

44. Diabetic coma is due to:
    A. overproduction of insulin.
    B. low blood glucose level.
    C. lack of insulin.
    D. normal glucose with high insulin level.

45. An arthrogram is the radiographic visualization of:
    A. a joint.
    B. a blood vessel.
    C. the gallbladder.
    D. the spinal column.

46. Diathermy is an example of an agent that incorporates the use of:
    A. paraffin wax.
    B. cold water.
    C. ultraviolet light.
    D. deep heat.

47. Which of the following conditions would benefit from a low-purine diet?
    A. Gout
    B. Obesity
    C. High blood pressure
    D. Constipation

48. Antihypertensive medications are associated with the treatment of:
    A. fever.
    B. vomiting.
    C. high blood pressure.
    D. allergies.

49. A laceration appears as a:
    A. scrape on the skin.
    B. bruise.
    C. jagged cut.
    D. swelling on the skin.

50. *Res ipsa loquitur* is a Latin term that means which of the following?
    A. Let the buyer beware.
    B. The thing speaks for itself.
    C. The employer is responsible for the employee.
    D. The patient is always first.

51. The medical term meaning "inflammation of the bone" is:
    A. arthritis.
    B. bursitis.
    C. chondritis.
    D. osteitis.

52. The superior vena cava is the:
    A. vein that carries blood from the lower extremities to the aorta.
    B. artery that carries blood between the heart and lungs.
    C. vein that carries blood from the upper body back to the heart.
    D. vein that carries blood between the heart and lungs.

53. Basic communication requires a message and:
    A. sender and receiver.
    B. feedback and body language.
    C. clarification and feedback.
    D. receiver and body language.

54. The term **facsimile** refers to:
    A. fax.
    B. photocopy.
    C. e-mail.
    D. voice mail.

55. A matrix is a(n):
    A. form of billing.
    B. appointment book schedule with blocked out periods of time.
    C. form used for insurance filing.
    D. timed laboratory test.

56. The most common method used to chart the patient's medical record is:
    A. CPT.
    B. SOMR.
    C. SOAP.
    D. HCFA.

57. The salutation of a letter is the:
    A. closing.
    B. reference line.
    C. enclosure.
    D. greeting.

58. Coordination of benefits means:
    A. the amount of money paid by the patient for medical services before the insurance pays.
    B. one insurance plan will work with other insurance plans to determine how much each plan pays.
    C. each insurance company will pay an equal amount of the patient's bill.
    D. there is a deductible required by the patient before payment from the insurance is made.

59. ICD-9 codes that identify medical problems for reasons other than illness or injury are known as:
    A. E codes.
    B. M codes.
    C. CPT codes.
    D. V codes.

60. When a bank uses the term NSF, it means that:
    A. the check is voided and not to be used.
    B. the account is a newly opened account.
    C. there is not enough money to cover the amount of the check.
    D. the bank will issue a cashier's check in the amount of the check.

61. Supplies that are stored and maintained for emergencies in the medical office are:
    A. available for daily use.
    B. used and replaced on a routine basis.
    C. often kept off site to better utilize space.
    D. unintended for routine use.

62. The Fowler's position is used for:
    A. female pelvic examination.
    B. examination of the abdomen.
    C. patient with difficulty breathing.
    D. sigmoidoscopy.

63. The abbreviation OU is no longer in use. Instead of using OU, which of the following should be written?
    A. Both eyes
    B. Right ear
    C. Both ears
    D. Left eye

64. A fire extinguisher should be serviced at least:
    A. daily.
    B. monthly.
    C. every 6 months.
    D. annually.

65. The role of the practice manager generally includes all the following EXCEPT:
    A. negotiating insurance contracts.
    B. evaluating personnel.
    C. reviewing policies and procedures.
    D. developing treatment protocols.

66. An exposure control plan should be reviewed at least:
    A. annually.
    B. monthly.
    C. every 6 months.
    D. quarterly.

67. The abbreviation used to indicate that a patient should be fasting for an examination is:
    A. NPO.
    B. AC.
    C. PC.
    D. NOS.

68. KUB is an X-ray examination of the:
    A. urinary system.
    B. spinal column.
    C. liver and gallbladder.
    D. abdomen.

69. A medical office would not send a memorandum to the:
    A. patient.
    B. physician.
    C. practice manager.
    D. human resources department.

70. A patient with arteriosclerosis would benefit from which of the following diets?
    A. Low salt
    B. Low carbohydrate
    C. Low protein
    D. Low cholesterol

71. The first action to control bleeding or hemorrhage is to:
    A. place ice over the wound.
    B. apply direct pressure.
    C. apply a tourniquet above the injury.
    D. immobilize the body part.

72. The term **enteritis** means inflammation of the:
    A. colon.
    B. small intestine.
    C. stomach.
    D. esophagus.

73. An example of active immunity is:
    A. maternal antibodies passed through the uterus to the baby.
    B. immunization with antibodies.
    C. maternal antibodies acquired by the baby from breast milk.
    D. producing antibodies as a result of having a disease.

74. When the person refuses to acknowledge the loss of a loved one, the type of behavior is:
    A. sympathy.
    B. mourning.
    C. denial.
    D. depression.

75. The computer device that displays the written data is the:
    A. disk drive.
    B. monitor.
    C. hard drive.
    D. floppy disk.

76. When the doctor is late and not yet at the office, the medical assistant should:
    A. offer waiting patients an opportunity to reschedule.
    B. cancel all remaining appointments for the day.
    C. reschedule all the patients for another day.
    D. offer to refer the patients to another physician's practice.

77. The "O" in the SOAP method of charting includes the:
    A. blood pressure reading.
    B. opinion of a family member.
    C. symptoms the patient states.
    D. prior complaints from the patient.

78. To retain insurance coverage, the individual must pay the cost of the insurance, which is the:
    A. premium.
    B. copayment.
    C. coinsurance.
    D. deductible.

79. CPT is an abbreviation of the reference manual used for:
    A. ordering laboratory tests.
    B. billing insurance companies for procedures.
    C. reporting diseases to the CDC.
    D. selecting the fees for each examination.

80. The best way to ensure that patients pay for services is to:
    A. ask patients where they would like the bill mailed.
    B. ask for payment of services at the time of the office visit.
    C. confirm the name of the patient's insurance company.
    D. accept checks only, not credit cards.

81. Acquired immunodeficiency syndrome is caused by:
    A. yeast.
    B. fungi.
    C. bacteria.
    D. a virus.

82. The pulse point located on the top of the foot is the:
    A. femoral.
    B. dorsalis pedis.
    C. temporal.
    D. popliteal.

83. Ensuring a system is in place to review and report results of all diagnostic tests is an example of:
    A. exposure control.
    B. incident reporting.
    C. facility management.
    D. risk management.

84. Another term for an occurrence report is a(n):
    A. subpoena.
    B. civil suit.
    C. torte.
    D. incident report.

85. When the physician improperly terminates his or her contract with the patient, this is called:
    A. patient abandonment.
    B. breach of confidentiality.
    C. noncompliance.
    D. reciprocity.

86. A myelogram is an X-ray examination of the:
    A. spinal cord.
    B. brain.
    C. muscles.
    D. heart.

87. The term used when an outside entity examines the practice's medical records to ensure accuracy, completeness, and sequence of the documents is:
    A. medical records management.
    B. accreditation.
    C. audit.
    D. aging analysis.

88. Anaphylaxis refers to a:
    A. nose bleed.
    B. type of shock.
    C. hemorrhage disorder.
    D. congenital disorder.

89. Dyspepsia refers to:
    A. difficulty speaking.
    B. difficult digestion.
    C. difficulty breathing.
    D. abnormal pain.

90. The perineum is the:
    A. lining of the abdomen.
    B. covering of the spinal cord.
    C. floor of the pelvis.
    D. outside lining of the lungs.

91. *Respondeat superior* refers to:
    A. a subpoena.
    B. a physician's responsibility for the actions of his staff.
    C. something for something, a favor for a favor.
    D. responding to your superiors.

92. Management of the electronic health record does not require:
    A. archiving.
    B. retrieving.
    C. conditioning.
    D. security.

93. The medical record provides all the following EXCEPT a:
    A. resource for public education.
    B. legal document.
    C. tool for quality monitoring.
    D. method for continuity of care.

94. The telecommunications device for the deaf is what type of communication?
    A. Closed
    B. Body language
    C. Verbal
    D. Nonverbal

95. The process by which nutrients transfer from the gastrointestinal system into the blood is referred to as:
    A. ingestion.
    B. digestion.
    C. absorption.
    D. metabolism.

96. The classification of drugs used to relieve pain is:
    A. antidepressant.
    B. analgesic.
    C. antibiotic.
    D. antidote.

97. The device used to check vision is a(n):
    A. otoscope.
    B. ophthalmoscope.
    C. Snellen chart.
    D. tuning fork.

98. A wound that results from scraping the skin is a(n):
    A. laceration.
    B. avulsion.
    C. contusion.
    D. abrasion.

99. In the medical office, the electronic medical record will decrease the need for:
    A. security.
    B. transcription.
    C. a release of information form.
    D. staff.

100. Retention of medical records for minors is generally:
    A. 7 to 10 years.
    B. 7 to 10 years after reaching 18 years old.
    C. 7 to 10 years after becoming an emancipated minor.
    D. 7 to 10 years after the age of majority.

Answers to Practice Exam—CMAS (AMT)

1. B	26. B	51. D	76. A
2. B	27. C	52. C	77. A
3. D	28. B	53. A	78. A
4. C	29. C	54. A	79. B
5. C	30. A	55. B	80. B
6. A	31. D	56. C	81. D
7. C	32. A	57. D	82. B
8. D	33. D	58. B	83. D
9. B	34. D	59. D	84. D
10. C	35. D	60. C	85. A
11. A	36. A	61. D	86. A
12. C	37. A	62. C	87. C
13. C	38. A	63. A	88. B
14. B	39. B	64. D	89. B
15. B	40. C	65. D	90. C
16. D	41. C	66. A	91. B
17. A	42. C	67. A	92. C
18. A	43. B	68. A	93. A
19. C	44. C	69. A	94. D
20. A	45. A	70. D	95. C
21. C	46. D	71. B	96. B
22. A	47. A	72. B	97. C
23. C	48. C	73. D	98. D
24. D	49. C	74. C	99. B
25. D	50. B	75. B	100. D

Answer Sheet

1. (A) (B) (C) (D) (E)
2. (A) (B) (C) (D) (E)
3. (A) (B) (C) (D) (E)
4. (A) (B) (C) (D) (E)
5. (A) (B) (C) (D) (E)
6. (A) (B) (C) (D) (E)
7. (A) (B) (C) (D) (E)
8. (A) (B) (C) (D) (E)
9. (A) (B) (C) (D) (E)
10. (A) (B) (C) (D) (E)
11. (A) (B) (C) (D) (E)
12. (A) (B) (C) (D) (E)
13. (A) (B) (C) (D) (E)
14. (A) (B) (C) (D) (E)
15. (A) (B) (C) (D) (E)
16. (A) (B) (C) (D) (E)
17. (A) (B) (C) (D) (E)
18. (A) (B) (C) (D) (E)
19. (A) (B) (C) (D) (E)
20. (A) (B) (C) (D) (E)
21. (A) (B) (C) (D) (E)
22. (A) (B) (C) (D) (E)
23. (A) (B) (C) (D) (E)
24. (A) (B) (C) (D) (E)
25. (A) (B) (C) (D) (E)

26. (A) (B) (C) (D) (E)
27. (A) (B) (C) (D) (E)
28. (A) (B) (C) (D) (E)
29. (A) (B) (C) (D) (E)
30. (A) (B) (C) (D) (E)
31. (A) (B) (C) (D) (E)
32. (A) (B) (C) (D) (E)
33. (A) (B) (C) (D) (E)
34. (A) (B) (C) (D) (E)
35. (A) (B) (C) (D) (E)
36. (A) (B) (C) (D) (E)
37. (A) (B) (C) (D) (E)
38. (A) (B) (C) (D) (E)
39. (A) (B) (C) (D) (E)
40. (A) (B) (C) (D) (E)
41. (A) (B) (C) (D) (E)
42. (A) (B) (C) (D) (E)
43. (A) (B) (C) (D) (E)
44. (A) (B) (C) (D) (E)
45. (A) (B) (C) (D) (E)
46. (A) (B) (C) (D) (E)
47. (A) (B) (C) (D) (E)
48. (A) (B) (C) (D) (E)
49. (A) (B) (C) (D) (E)
50. (A) (B) (C) (D) (E)

51. (A) (B) (C) (D) (E)
52. (A) (B) (C) (D) (E)
53. (A) (B) (C) (D) (E)
54. (A) (B) (C) (D) (E)
55. (A) (B) (C) (D) (E)
56. (A) (B) (C) (D) (E)
57. (A) (B) (C) (D) (E)
58. (A) (B) (C) (D) (E)
59. (A) (B) (C) (D) (E)
60. (A) (B) (C) (D) (E)
61. (A) (B) (C) (D) (E)
62. (A) (B) (C) (D) (E)
63. (A) (B) (C) (D) (E)
64. (A) (B) (C) (D) (E)
65. (A) (B) (C) (D) (E)
66. (A) (B) (C) (D) (E)
67. (A) (B) (C) (D) (E)
68. (A) (B) (C) (D) (E)
69. (A) (B) (C) (D) (E)
70. (A) (B) (C) (D) (E)
71. (A) (B) (C) (D) (E)
72. (A) (B) (C) (D) (E)
73. (A) (B) (C) (D) (E)
74. (A) (B) (C) (D) (E)
75. (A) (B) (C) (D) (E)

76. (A) (B) (C) (D) (E)
77. (A) (B) (C) (D) (E)
78. (A) (B) (C) (D) (E)
79. (A) (B) (C) (D) (E)
80. (A) (B) (C) (D) (E)
81. (A) (B) (C) (D) (E)
82. (A) (B) (C) (D) (E)
83. (A) (B) (C) (D) (E)
84. (A) (B) (C) (D) (E)
85. (A) (B) (C) (D) (E)
86. (A) (B) (C) (D) (E)
87. (A) (B) (C) (D) (E)
88. (A) (B) (C) (D) (E)
89. (A) (B) (C) (D) (E)
90. (A) (B) (C) (D) (E)
91. (A) (B) (C) (D) (E)
92. (A) (B) (C) (D) (E)
93. (A) (B) (C) (D) (E)
94. (A) (B) (C) (D) (E)
95. (A) (B) (C) (D) (E)
96. (A) (B) (C) (D) (E)
97. (A) (B) (C) (D) (E)
98. (A) (B) (C) (D) (E)
99. (A) (B) (C) (D) (E)
100. (A) (B) (C) (D) (E)